THE ECONOMIC EVALUATION OF MENTAL HEALTH CARE

The Economic Evaluation of Mental Health Care

Edited by

MARTIN KNAPP

PSSRU
UNIVERSITY OF KENT
AT CANTERBURY

CEMH
CENTRE FOR THE ECONOMICS OF MENTAL HEALTH

arena

Published by
Arena
Ashgate Publishing Limited
Gower House
Croft Road
Aldershot
Hants GU11 3HR
England

Ashgate Publishing Company
Old Post Road
Brookfield
Vermont 05036
USA

British Library Cataloguing in Publication Data

Economic Evaluation of Mental Health Care
I. Knapp, Martin
362.20425

Library of Congress Catalog Card Number: 95-77013

ISBN 1 85742 211 2 (paperback)
ISBN 1 85742 207 4 (hardback)

Typeset by Jane Dennett at the PSSRU, University of Kent at Canterbury

Printed and bound in Great Britain by
Hartnolls Limited, Bodmin, Cornwall

Contents

	List of contributors	*vi*
	Preface	*vii*
1	The economic perspective: framework and principles *Martin Knapp*	1
2	Economic evaluations of mental health care: modes and methods *Shane Kavanagh and Alan Stewart*	27
3	Collecting and estimating costs *Jennifer Beecham*	61
4	Costs and outcomes: variations and comparisons *Martin Knapp*	83
5	Eight years of psychiatric reprovision: an economic evaluation *Angela Hallam, Martin Knapp, Jennifer Beecham and Andrew Fenyo*	103
6	Elderly people with dementia: costs, effectiveness and balance of care *Shane Kavanagh, Justine Schneider, Martin Knapp, Jennifer Beecham and Ann Netten*	125
7	Costing the care programme approach *Justine Schneider*	157
8	Comparative efficiency and equity in community-based care *Jennifer Beecham, Martin Knapp and Caroline Allen*	175
9	Reduced-list costings *Martin Knapp and Jennifer Beecham*	195
10	Decision analysis and mental health evaluations *Alan Stewart*	207
11	Have the 'lunatics taken over the asylums'? The rising cost of psychiatric services in England and Wales, 1860-1986 *James Raftery*	215
12	Mental health economic evaluations: unfinished business *Jennifer Beecham and Martin Knapp*	229
	Name index	243
	Subject index	247

List of Contributors

Caroline Allen, postgraduate student, University of Warwick. Formerly Research Officer, Personal Social Services Research Unit (PSSRU), and Junior Research Officer, University of the West Indies.

Jennifer Beecham, Research Fellow, PSSRU and Lecturer in Mental Health Economics, Centre for the Economics of Mental Health (CEMH), Institute of Psychiatry.

Andrew Fenyo, Senior Computing Officer, PSSRU.

Angela Hallam, Research Officer, PSSRU and Research Worker, CEMH.

Shane Kavanagh, Research Fellow, PSSRU.

Martin Knapp, Professor of the Economics of Social Care, PSSRU, and Professor of Health Economics and Director, CEMH.

Ann Netten, Research Fellow, PSSRU.

James Raftery, health economist with posts at district and regional levels.

Justine Schneider, Research Fellow, PSSRU, and Research Worker, CEMH.

Alan Stewart, Research Fellow, PSSRU.

Preface

The Personal Social Service Research Unit (PSSRU) undertakes research in all areas of community care, including multidisciplinary research on mental health services. One particular perspective which we bring to our research stems from economics, and more recently we have been able to develop this aspect of our work following the establishment of the Centre for the Economics of Mental Health (CEMH) at the Institute of Psychiatry. Many of the authors of chapters in this book are based part-time at CEMH, and all but James Raftery are currently or were recently based at PSSRU. Much of the research described in this book was funded by the Department of Health, although responsibility for what is written lies with the authors.

A number of people have helped in the process of the research or with the production of the book, yet do not feature as authors. Jenny Griffin, Elizabeth Parker and Glyn Lewis (Department of Health) oversaw and advised on the research. Maureen Weir typed and retyped most of the chapters and then corrected them many times over. This was always completed with speed and accuracy. Glenys Harrison, Sandra Semple and Audrey Walker also assisted in the preparation of some chapters. Jane Dennett subedited the whole book meticulously and generated the camera-ready copy, and helped the editorial process in more ways than is reasonable to expect, including chasing authors (especially the editor) and advising on content. Nick Brawn produced most of the excellent graphics which appear in the book. We are also especially grateful to the many service users and staff who have provided us with information in the course of our applied research, and to research collaborators who have constructed some of the projects which have generated data or helped us in other ways. Encouragement and advice — in different shapes and forms, but always constructive and welcome — have come from Julian Leff, Isaac Marks, David Melzer, Matt Muijen and Lou Opit.

Martin Knapp
Canterbury
April 1995

For Daniel and Emily

1 The Economic Perspective: Framework and Principles

*Martin Knapp**

1.1 Economic questions

The *Asylum Journal*, later the *Journal of Mental Science*, was first published in the 1850s. A lot of attention at that time was focused on how to secure the necessary finances for the provision of care for people with mental health problems. Early issues of the *Journal* contained few scientific articles of the kind found in academic journals today, but instead offered unique opportunities to disseminate practice developments and pose questions. In those early issues were a number of short articles, for example on the costs of mental health services, the pricing policies of private asylums, and comparisons between the public and private sectors. One extract, reproduced in Box 1.1, is fairly typical. It demonstrates a laudable balance between the pursuit of lower costs and the promotion of effectiveness through a caring environment.

Nearly a century and a half later, many years after the metamorphosis of the *Journal of Mental Science* into the *British Journal of Psychiatry*, there are rather fewer articles on the economic dimension. In 1993, for example, only eight articles out of a total of more than 200 could be said to include an economic perspective, and only two or three of them incorporated 'economic evaluations' in the way this term is generally understood by economists. These very modest numbers are not because the findings from economic studies are published elsewhere. There are, simply, few economic studies of mental health care. This is disappointing in view of the fact that one of the avowed aims of UK central government, the National Health Service (NHS), local authorities and other mental health providers and purchasers is to

Box 1.1
Reports of Lunatic Asylums, published during 1857 and 1859

The Report of the *Friends' Retreat at York* contains some interesting financial statements. This celebrated institution has lately been referred to in *The Times* newspaper, as an illustration of the good which can be effected by a well conducted private asylum. It is, however, to all intents and purposes, a public institution, coming under the legal category of Hospitals for the Insane, and, in this respect, it does not differ from the Coton Hill Asylum, the Warneford Asylum, and other public establishments of the same class. The inestimable benefit which its founders have conferred upon the insane by presenting in it the very first example of a public institution in which the insane were systematically treated on principles of humanity and intelligent forbearance, is in no slight degree enhanced by the example it presents of a public asylum for the middle classes, successfully conducted upon economical principles. It has, of late, been constantly repeated, that the most urgent want of the metropolis [London] is a self-supporting asylum, in which patients of the middle class may find treatment at an expense not exceeding one guinea per week. The Friends' Retreat presents an example of such an asylum. The actual expenditure during the year has been £5,920, of which £410 has been expended in repairs and alterations. Deducting this, the cost for care and maintenance of the 112 inmates has been, omitting fractions, 17s per week each. The sum includes everything except the rent of buildings and furniture. The management, as we can testify, is conducted on a thoroughly liberal scale, both of diet and appointment; as an example of which we may mention that carriage exercise is a regular part of the system. While the expenditure, irrespective of the building, has only been £5,510, the actual receipts from patients have been £6,556, and the receipts from all sources have been £6,992. It does not appear that this large amount of what may be called profits is any part of the plan of the founders, and indeed it is referred to as 'a result mainly consequent upon the proportion of the higher class of patients continuing to be large, and beyond the average of former years'. The inmates are classified in respect of payments as follows.

> Thirty-two who pay not more than 6s. per week; twenty-three more than 6s. but not exceeding 10s.; twenty-two more than 10s. but not exceeding 20s.; six more than 20s. but not exceeding 40s.; twenty-nine more than 40s. Of these 112 patients, twenty-one are unconnected with Friends by religious profession, and eleven others are not in membership with them. The number of patients who are members of the society is eighty.

Of course, all who pay less than 17s. per week are to that extent the recipients of a charity, which the Governors are to dispose from the successful financial remits of the enterprise of the founders.

Reproduced from the *Journal of Mental Science* (later the *British Journal of Psychiatry*) Vol. 5, No. 28, 1859.

promote cost-effectiveness in treatment, local management and system-wide allocations of resources.

Cost-effectiveness as an invocation is now certainly in vogue, if not altogether in favour. Some mental health professionals remain sceptical of the validity of health economics or the relevance of costs to clinical decision-making. Generally, however, the search for cost-effectiveness is being conducted at many levels of government, in most countries and health care systems. It has also been pursued from a number of perspectives, as will be illustrated later. These searches are sometimes known by other names — such as value-for-money scrutinies or efficiency drives — and are sometimes part of a wider initiative, such as medical audit or performance review. Although they may not share all the best features of an economic evaluation, these searches are often useful attempts to explore the resource consequences of policy or practice actions.

At the most general level, economic evaluations can address one or more of five types of question. Each question concerns the appropriateness of treatments or care modes in given circumstances. The term 'appropriate' could mean cost-effective, or efficacious, or equitable, depending on the evaluation criteria selected for the study or policy debate. The generic questions are:

- *What* treatment is most appropriate?
- *When* should it be provided?
- *Where* should it be provided?
- *To whom* should it be provided?
- *How* should it be provided?

One of the aims of this book is to illustrate how these questions are addressed in economic evaluations. We will also introduce the factors and trends which make economics relevant in the mental health field, set out the broad parameters and tools of economic evaluation, illustrate their application in some recently completed evaluations, and tease out some of the policy and practice implications of the methodologies and findings.

1.2 Anxieties and misunderstandings

A common view of economic evaluation is of a complex, controversial, unrealistic but nevertheless necessary component of policy or practice developments. It may be economists' jargon, or their love of algebraic explanations, or their seemingly unwavering adherence to implausible assumptions, or just their occasional need to be provocative which frightens non-economists. Or it may be that the frequent appearance of £ or $ symbols throughout a document is just too sordid for the financially squeamish, too diverting for the overworked care professional or manager, or maybe just too tedious. Or it may be that the regular recitation of cost per QALY (quality adjusted life year — see below) does not ring true to the professional, manager or researcher committed to the sensitive and multidimensional assessment of patient or user outcomes, or raises the kind of resource allocation question which those wedded to clinical freedom prefer not to have discussed outside the consulting room, and claim not to be relevant *within* it.

As we hope to show in this book, these fears and criticisms are largely groundless. Economic evaluations are not so very different from other evaluations of mental health care. Where they differ is in their tendency to examine a fuller range of causes and effects. The common theme of all evaluative research is to enquire if a particular service, treatment, drug or setting is worthwhile. The difference between economic and other evaluations is the meaning attached to the term 'worthwhile'. Economic evaluations add the resource dimension. However, they are not confined to costs — a common misunderstanding about economists working in health care — for economists are not glorified accountants.

Two other common misunderstandings or misinterpretations need to be cleared up. First, it must be emphasised that economic evaluation cannot replace the sound or informed judgements of decision-makers, whether politicians or managers at the systems level, or psychiatrists, psychologists, social workers, nurses or other professionals at the programme level. The primary aim of any evaluative research — and economic evaluation is no exception — should be to provide a sound and valid information base for policy and practice decisions. Some years ago, Burton Weisbrod (1979) made the important point that economic evaluations will never 'make decisions', but if they are vigorously pursued they will 'make decisions better informed'. The other misunderstanding is that economic evaluations are restricted to answering questions about cost-effectiveness or efficiency. This is not the case, for increasingly economists have sought to examine the *distributional* or equity implications of different treatment and other options.

1.3 Policy and practice contexts

The reforms introduced in the UK by the 1990 National Health Service and Community Care Act provide a context for understanding the relevance and application of economics in mental health service evaluations, although the needs for economics are considerably more pervasive and less context-bound. The 1990 reforms have generated or consolidated a number of demands for better cost information, a better understanding of cost-effectiveness, and the broader discussion of allocation criteria such as efficiency and equity.

The 1990 reforms comprise a number of strategic changes. They seek to alter the balance between institutional and community care, moving the emphasis away from long-term hospital provision in favour of treatment and support in community settings for people who probably do not need the intensity of 24-hour clinical supervision, and also moving the balance of provision away from nursing and residential care homes in favour of domiciliary-based support. More controversial, perhaps, has been the emphasis on market forces. The new 'internal markets' in health care separate purchasers and providers within the public sector NHS, and give fundholding general practices more freedom of manoeuvre and greater purchasing clout. The more 'external' or 'quasi-markets' in social care also separate purchasers and providers, the latter including a large number of private and voluntary sector organisations. The reforms stress the importance of decisions which are purchaser-dominated rather than provider-dominated: needs-led rather than supply-led. Care management and care programmes are becoming increasingly important elements in the new health and social care systems, more comprehensive and sensitive assessment procedures are being adopted, and users and carers are gradually acquiring greater influence and choice. There is also some realignment of responsibilities for decision-making and funding away from the NHS towards local government, although the process is not yet complete, and not without considerable complications. Greater provider pluralism is explicitly encouraged within the developing 'mixed economy' of mental health care.

These reforms are being introduced in pursuit of a number of familiar, broad policy aims. The White Paper setting out the government's intentions for health service reform, *Working for Patients* (Secretaries of State, 1989a), stressed two objectives:

> To give patients, wherever they live in the UK, better health care and greater choice of the services available; and greater satisfaction and rewards for those working in the NHS who successfully respond to local needs and preferences (para. 1.8).

The community care White Paper, *Caring for People* (Secretaries of State, 1989b), argued that the proposed policy changes would improve user choice, service innovation and quality. Both pre-legislation documents were unequivocal in their emphasis on cost-effectiveness. Not surprisingly, cost awareness now appears as an important national policy objective in the government's recommendations for mental health services. For example, the cost-effectiveness dimension appears as early as the fourth paragraph of the *Mental Illness Handbook*, a supplement to *The Health of the Nation* White Paper (Secretary of State for Health, 1992). A few paragraphs later, the *Handbook* argued:

> In a situation where 'need is limitless and resources finite', organisation of the available resources is critical to ensure that allocations are used as cost-effectively as possible in order to provide the maximum possible health benefits (Department of Health, 1993, p.13).

The demand for an economic perspective and for cost-effectiveness information should come as no surprise. Planning in a hierarchical, top-down, provider-led, single-agency manner — as was traditional in public administration — makes predictable, modest and uncomplicated demands on cost information systems. In the past, traditional line budgets were therefore often seen to be adequate in design and accessibility to satisfy most of the day-to-day operational needs of managers and the less frequent but more searching probity requirements of auditors. However, the 1990 Act required health and social care decision-making to become user-sensitive, bottom-up, needs-led and multiple-agency. Market-inspired allocations are now becoming more commonplace, introducing more financial incentives. System-wide implications are now more likely to be couched in terms of broader societal expenditures, rather than merely in terms of the drain on a single public sector agency's budget. In these new circumstances, policy-makers, planners, purchasers and providers need more and better cost and effectiveness information (Audit Commission, 1994).

Indeed, a growing number of agencies and professions are actively involved in mental health care delivery, funded from a growing diversity of sources. There is undoubtedly a need for new, broader and more refined data systems, as well as new attitudes regarding utilisation. Figure 1.1 summarises the mixed economy of mental health care, parametrised by the sources of demand (or types of purchase) and the sectors of provision. It is clear that many different services and funding arrangements come under the mental health banner, and that there are many types of 'transaction' linking them. The need for a strategic approach to resource utilisation and management is as pressing today as it has ever been.

1.4 The demand for health economics

There are probably five broad groups of demands for health economics (generally defined) which help to describe the issues which economic evaluations might address.

Accountability. Costs and other economic data are needed for the perennial performance reviews required for public probity, now often built around value-for-money audits and efficiency scrutinies. Clinical audit and quality assurance initiatives might also stimulate accountability demands for a health economics perspective. As with the other types of demand described here, it is the purposive combination of information from a variety of sources which will provide both the framework and the evidence needed for accountability.

Policy. As we have seen, among the specific changes which precipitate a need for a clear cost-effectiveness perspective in mental health care are developments in macro-planning and delegation of case coordination responsibilities. The community care plans drawn up by local and health authorities will have to be affordable, and their ramifications appreciated and accepted

Figure 1.1
The mixed economy of mental health care: service examples

Purchase, demand or funding	*Provision or supply of services*			
	Public sector	*Voluntary sector*	*Private sector*	*Informal sector*
Coerced collective demand	NHS psychiatric hospital	Day care under contract to a local authority	Publicly-funded placements in private nursing homes	Adult foster care
Uncoerced or voluntary collective demand	Voluntary organisation payments for public sector training programmes	Self-help group paying for expert advice from larger voluntary organisation	Purchases of goods and services by Mind or Alzheimer's Disease Society	Volunteers providing respite care organised through voluntary organisation
Corporate demand	Private residential home payments for LA registration and inspection	Corporate donations to charities	Counselling offered to company employees	Employer-funded stress days; redundancy payments for mental ill health
Uncompensated individual consumption	User charges for meals in LA day centre	Self-funding meal clubs run by voluntary organisation	Payment for private residential care by family or resident	Exchanges in kind between neighbours
Compensated individual consumption	LA hostel funded by social security entitlements	Income support payments to voluntary homes	Housing benefit and other user subsidies for private housing	Attendance allowance used to purchase informal care
Individual donation (for use by others)	Volunteers working in NHS psychiatric hospital	Donations to the National Schizophrenia Fellowship	Volunteers in private residential homes	Intra-family transfers of resources and care

by all relevant agencies. The perverse incentives inherent in the old system, which sometimes encouraged local and health authorities to shunt costs from their own budgets to someone else's (Audit Commission, 1986), should begin to disappear as better and more accessible cost-effectiveness evidence is gathered. The markets for health and social care generate new information needs for purchasers and providers: how to price services, how to compare costs across alternatives, how to make trade-offs between lower costs and greater effectiveness, how to respond to price or output changes by other providers or purchasing changes by other buyers, and so on. And, of course, at the highest policy level, all of the macro-, micro- and market developments need to be evaluated.

Practice. Care management and similar keyworker procedures — promoting the integrated, purposive, longer-term planning of interventions for individual service users — have their own cost information needs, particularly if budgetary responsibilities are devolved to fieldwork teams or individual professionals, and place some responsibility for cost-effective purchasing or care planning on the shoulders of local professionals. The introduction of *care programmes* to coordinate support for people with mental health problems is bringing new organisational costs, but may not have quite the same immediate information requirements as care management. Nevertheless, a care programme which is drawn up without awareness of the ability of professionals and agencies to supply services (and therefore awareness of the cost implications) is liable to run into difficulties (see Chapter 7).

Product development and distribution. In Australia, Quebec and Ontario, pharmaceutical companies must provide cost-effectiveness data before new products can be licensed (Drummond, 1992). The NHS has now been encouraged, though not yet mandated, to undertake economic evaluations of pharmaceutical products as part of the decision-making process about treatment (Department of Health Press Release, 19 May 1994; see Chapter 2). Increasingly, new products and procedures will be scrutinised not just for their efficacy, but also for their cost-effectiveness.

Research. As we can see, there are clearly many new demands for health economics to be added to the longer-standing demands for cost-effectiveness data and economics perspectives stemming, for example, from 'mere' intellectual curiosity. For instance, costs are the focus in the increasingly common and increasingly sophisticated 'burden of illness' calculations, although the results of these endeavours need to be employed carefully. Cost projections of a disease can be used to evaluate changes in the balance of care or treatment, but, in order to make allocative decisions, policy-makers require information about the interventions that realise the greatest health gain or the greatest improvement in quality of life, and at what marginal resource implications. More frequently, health economics research is being conducted in and by universities, research institutes, consultancy companies and others. Sometimes this endeavour produces only long-term or vague implications for accountability, policy, practice or product development, but generally the 'net worth' of health economics has been considerable.

Health economics has many potential points of entry to discussions of mental health care. Evidence from completed economic evaluations can assist the policy and practitioner worlds, inform accountability, underpin or regulate product development, licensing and distribution, and broaden academic and other research. Findings from mental health economics studies are beginning to accumulate, beginning to be influential, and beginning to be questioned in the healthy, lively manner of intellectual debate.

1.5 The challenge of scarcity

It is not the aim of health economics or economists to cut health spending or to pare down costs, but rather to improve both the efficiency with which health care and other resources are employed and the targeting of those resources on needs and demands. It might transpire that the pursuit of efficiency or equity requires cost or expenditure cuts in particular areas of clinical practice or community care, or reductions in access to care by some groups of people, but this should be because careful analysis has revealed that resources could be used better elsewhere.

Although the need for efficiency examinations might appear to be greater at a time when, say, the national economy is in some difficulty or when the annual round of public expenditure decisions produces a less generous settlement for the health service than had been anticipated, the relevance of health economics does *not* stem solely from the challenges of a recession-bound economy or government policy priorities. Public expenditure constraints in a country like the UK, which pays for almost all of its health care from general taxation, will obviously leave their mark, but economics has relevance whenever there is scarcity of resources relative to needs. This is virtually all the time, and all over the world.

Scarcity means that, relative to needs or demands, there are too few resources, for example in relation to drugs, therapy sessions, day treatment places or hospital beds. Demographic change exerts an important influence on scarcity, for example by pushing up the total level of need or the bombardment of demands through the ageing of the population, or by increasing the burden of payment for publicly-funded health care as either the size of the working population or the number of taxpayers diminishes. Another source of scarcity is the effect of raised standards of care or treatment: the requirement or recommendation that people with mental health problems should have more or better access to services, or better service quality. Closely allied to raised standards are the raised expectations of patients, relatives or carers about the quantity, quality and type of treatment which are offered.

Scarcity implies the need for choice, and a fundamental aim of economics — sometimes dubbed the 'science of scarcity' — is to offer information and analysis which can inform, analyse and ease such choices. The prevalence and problems of scarcity and the needs for economic evaluation can be illustrated by looking at three areas: schizophrenia, dementia, and psychiatric problems in childhood and adolescence.

Scarcity and dementia

The scarcity of resources and treatments relative to present and future needs and demands, and the consequent need for careful choices as to the allocation of resources, can be seen in relation to dementia. Chapter 6 describes the familiar prevalence pattern for dementia: a psychiatric problem whose incidence increases markedly with age and for which there is currently no cure and little likelihood of recovery. Predicted demographic changes for the UK imply that there will be an increase of about 600,000 people aged 75 or over by the year 2001, while there will be almost a million people aged 85 or over, a third higher than in 1991. Those people aged 85 or over will comprise some 13 per cent of all older people (OPCS, 1991). Elderly people with dementia, in the UK as elsewhere, need a considerable amount of support from the NHS, social services and other agencies. More than 60 per cent of people with moderate or severe dementia live in private households, most of them with a spouse or other relative, so that there is also the impact on informal carers to take into account (Gray and Fenn, 1993; Netten, 1993). The projected demographic changes thus present politicians and others with some major challenges.

Even though current levels of support are reckoned by many commentators to be inadequate, particularly the support for elderly people with dementia living outside specialist care settings, either alone or with relatives, the scale of provision is still enormous. As we will see in Chapter 6, the balance of provision for the estimated 320,000 elderly people with 'advanced cognitive impairment' in England in 1991 made considerable demands on the public purse, as well as on family members and other carers.

The ageing of the UK population over the next two decades will obviously add emphasis to the challenge of resource scarcity. Carers' organisations and elderly people are, with increasing regularity and with growing impact, voicing their expectations of greater availability of services of improved quality, while pharmaceutical companies, clinicians and researchers continue to search for pharmacological and other effective treatments for dementia. Standards of care may rise over the next few years as local authorities and health purchasers wave their new contractual sticks in generally threatening ways over the heads of providers, but these public bodies will also need to ensure that cost-effectiveness improves if good outcomes for users and their families are to be secured at an affordable price.

Scarcity and schizophrenia

Schizophrenia is another mental health condition which vividly illustrates the problems of scarcity and the challenges of resource allocation. A typical UK population of 500,000 people will include between 1,000 and 2,500 people with schizophrenia, although only between 33 and 50 per cent will be in contact with mental health services (Department of Health, 1993). There will be about 65 new cases each year (Goldacre et al., 1994). Most of these people will have more than one episode of the illness, and many will need long-term support or treatment. With the ageing of the population there may be a slight decrease in the number of people with schizophrenia needing care because of the early onset of the problem and its high relative mortality rates.

People with schizophrenia are much more likely to attempt suicide than members of the general population, and the mortality rate (all causes) is twice as high. As a consequence of the abnormalities of behaviour and speech exhibited by sufferers, schizophrenia is perhaps one of the most visible of mental health problems, especially in community settings. A small number of tragic or dangerous incidents involving schizophrenia sufferers — especially the killing of Jonathan Zito, and Ben Silcock's climb into the lion's enclosure at London Zoo — have added community anxiety to this visibility (Ritchie et al., 1994). These events have fuelled the current debate as to the adequacy of the service responses to schizophrenia from health, social services, housing and other agencies (Melzer et al., 1991; Conway et al., 1994; and see Chapter 8), and resource scarcity has become a major political issue for community mental health care. Hospital closures have been criticised for being precipitate, unplanned or underfunded, and it has been argued that there are not enough secure places or enough acute beds in the major cities. Care for people with schizophrenia thus raises a large number of resource issues (Kavanagh et al., 1995).

It is hoped by government that the introduction of supervision registers, supervised discharge orders, care programmes and care management will address these problems. Each seeks to improve standards, although each may push up the costs of care for some people, at least in the short term. In fact, as later chapters show, there is some UK evidence that care programmes, care management or similar arrangements might generate modest cost savings in the wider context (and see McCrone et al., 1994).

Raised expectations are particularly important for their potential impact on scarcity. Pharmaceutical companies are claiming big breakthroughs in the treatment of schizophrenia, which will, with the rapid spread of knowledge as to efficacy of new drugs, generate demands from schizophrenia sufferers and their families. The effect of new pharmacological developments on raised expectations can be clearly seen in relation to clozapine (Eichelman and Hartwig, 1990; Pelonero and Elliott, 1990; Healy, 1993). In the circumstances, it is understandable if patients and their families question clinical decisions to deny them access to these or other new drugs. The clinician has both a duty to the individual patient to prescribe the most efficacious treatment and a responsibility to the community of taxpayers to pursue efficiency in the broader provision of care. The tension between the two is not easily resolved.

The refocusing of government policy and the reconfiguration of health care aims have also contributed to, or at least highlighted, the scarcity of resources. Central to the UK health service reforms of 1990 was the creation of an internal market, separating purchasers (health authorities and fund-holding general practitioners) from providers (NHS trusts, directly-managed units and non-NHS facilities). Costs are now more transparent: they are being calculated for most health care procedures, and *real* money is changing hands. The need to use money wisely has always been there, of course, but the internal market and other changes greatly encourage the pursuit of value for money and effective targeting.

Problems in childhood and adolescence

Until recently, children who received psychiatric treatment rarely came to public attention through the media, unlike some of their adult counterparts. Growing concern about juvenile crime and a small number of high-profile cases — for example, the murder of James Bulger — may be changing public perceptions. Certainly there is concern that the level of psychiatric morbidity in children and young people is relatively high, and that many remain untreated (Williams, 1993). Evidence suggests that psychiatric disorder is common among children who frequently see their general practitioner with physical symptoms (Bowman and Garralda, 1993). At the same time, child and adolescent psychiatric services seem to be under threat in the face of cost constraints (Rutter, 1991). Resisting this trend, a case has been made for investing in mental health services for children, arguing that these not only produce immediate health gain, but also reduce long-term social and financial costs (Light and Bailey, 1993).

These issues raise a number of methodological and policy questions, for antisocial behaviour — which encompasses a broad range of activities such as aggressive acts, stealing, vandalism, cheating, lying and truancy — has implications which are not all directly related to health care. Failure to take these broader implications into account when considering how much of and what type of child psychiatry to purchase or provide could produce a worringly partial understanding of the impact of intervention in early childhood or adolescence, and may distort decision-making. Unlike most psychological characteristics, antisocial behaviour in childhood exhibits substantial continuity (Rutter, 1989). 'Conduct disorder' — antisocial behaviour that is clinically significant and clearly beyond the realm of 'normal' functioning (Kazadin, 1987) — has a low rate of remittance compared to other childhood disorders and often persists into adult life (Robins, 1966). A substantial proportion of children with conduct disorder go on to have psychiatric and other medical problems in adult life, but also a higher risk of poor social functioning, unemployment and broken marriages (Robins and Regier, 1991). Childhood depression is associated with higher rates of utilisation of health services in adulthood (Harrington et al., 1990). Antisocial behaviour by children is also a predictor of similar behaviour in their children (Rutter and Madge, 1976).

Economic evaluations of child and adolescent psychiatric problems are therefore needed but will face methodological and practical difficulties. For example, the costs and consequences of child psychiatry interventions fall not only to the health service but also to other sectors of society, and the financial burden will be unequally distributed across agencies. NHS purchasers are often faced with the choice between the high costs of early intervention to deal with antisocial behaviour and no treatment with an unknown risk of high longer-term social costs. Incentives in the UK and elsewhere are not well tuned to remedy the problem of costs and effects which are unequally distributed both over time and between agencies. Once again, economic evaluations can help by bringing the long-term social costs and effects into the same 'equation' as the short-term NHS treatment costs, providing a framework to reconcile the problems of differential timing and unequally distributed burdens and impacts.

Across the diagnoses

Choices *between* diagnoses or problem areas also pose challenges for local purchasers and systems-level decision-makers. How many mental health care resources should be allocated to the treatment and support of people with dementia and how much to schizophrenia? Should purchasers target more resources on affective disorders? Is there a mismatch between adult and child psychiatric provision? Should local authority social services departments spend more on mental health services and less on people with physical disability, or — if their base budgets are increased — which user group should benefit from more spending?

These are the kinds of question which conventional evaluative analyses cannot easily address, unless they can develop and employ instruments for the measurement of effects and costs which are equally valid for different diagnostic or user groups. The QALY — quality adjusted life year — has just this aim. It is intended that the QALY will be measured alongside other outcomes for a wide range of clinical procedures and health problems. Some economists have devoted considerable resources to the development of QALY measures and apply them in a growing number of contexts. In its relatively short life-span, the QALY has made a huge impact. However, the available measures for the QALY, though robustly developed and widely employed, have not yet been shown to perform sufficiently well in relation to people with mental health problems to provide any guidance to cross-diagnostic group or cross-user group comparisons and decisions (Chisholm et al., 1995).

We return to QALYs later in this chapter and in Chapter 2.

1.6 Efficiency and equity

Responding to scarcity does not just mean conducting cost-effectiveness analyses of alternative treatments, but also requires the examination of the patterns of employment, the forces of demand and supply, the roles of markets in resource and treatment allocation, and the incentives and disincentives to better practice. Good health economics textbooks illustrate this diversity of issues, activities and interests (McGuire et al., 1988; Donaldson and Gerard, 1993). However, it is not our intention in this book to attempt to provide a broad health economics education. We focus on the methods of economic evaluation and their application.

Our starting point is therefore a narrower allocation question. Faced with high levels of need in a context of scarcity, necessitating some tough resource allocation decisions, is it possible to make improvements to the nature, balance and quality of mental health treatment and care? And how do we judge whether improvements have been made?

In the early 1980s, the UK government's Financial Management Initiative (FMI) and the high-profile activities of the newly-established Audit Commission heralded the arrival in the public sector of what had become known in management-speak as the 'three Es': economy, efficiency and effectiveness. These are criteria for service or resource allocation. The three Es underpin the value-for-money drives, performance reviews, medical audits and the like of the last ten years. There is, of course, also a need to include a fourth E — equity (or distributive justice) — which often seemed to be overlooked in the early years of the Thatcher premiership. Other possible criteria would be autonomy, liberty and diversity.

The first criterion, economy, is the saving of resources. It is frugality. The pursuit of economy obviously requires detailed and accurate cost information, but — in its strictest sense — pays no heed to the impact of lower spending upon people with mental health problems, their families, or the wider society. Clearly, therefore, this first criterion is relevant — indeed, probably necessary — but not sufficient.

Effectiveness is equally insufficient on its own for most allocation decisions. Strictly speaking, the pursuit or promotion of effectiveness pays no particular regard to costs. Improving effectiveness means enhancing patient health and quality of life or moving a providing or purchasing agency closer to its chosen operational objectives (for example, increasing the numbers of patients served, drugs dispensed or referrals processed). But many of the most important facets of effectiveness are especially hard to gauge, even though psychologists and other researchers in the mental health field have developed large batteries of impressive instruments to scale and score most behavioural problems, symptoms, self-care capacities and subjective perceptions.

Efficiency, a third criterion for allocation or rationing, combines the resource and effectiveness sides: for example, pulling together treatment inputs and user outcomes. The pursuit of efficiency could mean reducing the cost of producing a stated level of outcome or effectiveness, or improving the level of effectiveness or the volume and quality of outcomes achieved from fixed budgets. Efficiency is a controversial term and concept but, properly understood and properly located within a comprehensive, multiple-objective policy framework, it ought to be beyond criticism as a rationing criterion. As has already been argued, efficiency does not have to mean 'cutback', for efficiency can often be best promoted by spending more, not less. There are different types of efficiency with various implications at the programme and system levels, each of them combining information on the resources used with insights or data on outcomes or effectiveness (see, for example, Knapp and Beecham, 1993, 1995).

The fourth criterion — equity (not the same as equality) — is easily overlooked when acute scarcity and the urgent need for constrained choice or rationing produce a headlong rush for what might look like better 'value for money'. Allocating budgets, services or drugs so as to achieve a more equitable, fair or just distribution is an aim of most health care systems, although it can be difficult to frame a discussion in such a way as to engage the general public in debates about equity. The distinction can be made between horizontal and vertical equity, the former being the equal treatment of equals (individuals with the same 'needs' should receive an equivalent amount of care or treatment), and the latter being the unequal treatment of unequals (the differential allocation of treatments or outcomes to individuals with different needs). Targeting services on needs is the most common example of the pursuit of greater equity, and it is therefore also legitimate to question the efficiency with which equity is pursued — the so-called target efficiency (Bebbington and Davies, 1983).

In broad terms, the concepts of efficiency and equity are straightforward, although there are many alternative definitions and concepts for practical applications. (Donaldson and Gerrard, 1993, offer a useful discussion.) Common parlance might use the word efficiency as a euphemism for cheap, but it should really be reserved for a criterion which looks at both achievements and resources, outcomes and costs, ends and means. It would also be wrong to equate equity with equality, for what is generally sought is a fair and acceptable way to distribute resources or services *unequally*. The empirical research described in later chapters of this book illustrates how these criteria can be operationalised.

1.7 Economic evaluation — an overview

The production of welfare

It is helpful for the discussion of these four allocation criteria, and imperative for the interpretation of any empirical measures, to locate them within an appropriate conceptual framework (see Figure 1.2). A useful and entirely general framework for the job is the *production of welfare* approach, although it has to date only been developed in detail in relation to social care services, especially for elderly people (Davies and Knapp, 1981, 1988; Knapp, 1984; Davies et al., 1990). The framework distinguishes the key elements in the provision of services, particularly:

Figure 1.2
The production of welfare

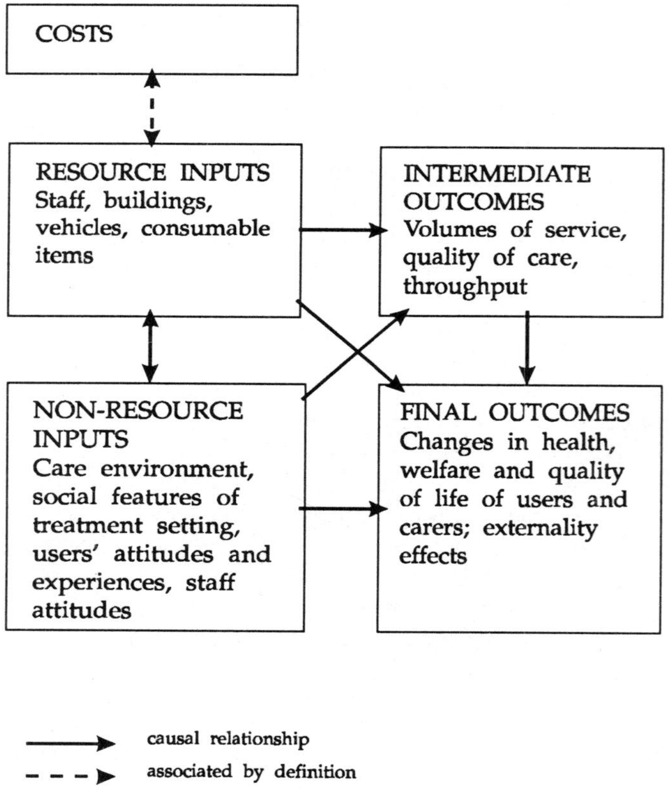

- the *resource inputs* to mental health care, mainly staff, capital and consumables;
- the *costs* of those resource inputs expressed in monetary terms;
- the so-called *non-resource inputs* to the care or treatment process, these being the influences on the achievement of outcomes which do not have an identifiable price or are not currently marketed (such as the social milieu of a treatment setting, staff attitudes and patient histories);
- the *intermediate outcomes,* which are the volumes of service output and/or the quality of care, perhaps weighted in some way for user characteristics, produced from combinations of the resource and non-resource inputs; and
- the *final outcomes,* which are changes over time in the health, welfare and quality of life of users and their carers.

The final outcomes of a mental health intervention will depend upon the nature of the treatment, the resources employed, the social environment of care, and so on.

It is then possible, for instance, to define effectiveness as the achievement of goals expressed in terms of any or all of the component elements of the production of welfare framework. Efficiency and equity can also be defined and measured in terms of component elements within the framework (singly or in combination). A point to be emphasised is that it is usually a complex combination of factors which determines the level of effectiveness, efficiency or equity. Thus, the allocation of mental health services on the strength of information on just one or two elements risks a misleadingly partial view of the treatment process and its implications, and thus also risks recommending or implementing inappropriate allocations of scarce resources.

The production of welfare approach — which encapsulates the economist's perspective on the organisation and allocation of services and user-level achievements — is thus a summary of the complex linkages between services and achievements and the resource and non-resource inputs that make them possible. It is a framework on which to hang an evaluation. The various influences on outcome — the inputs — are highly inter-correlated but this should not be a cause for conceptual concern or empirical difficulty. The production relations approach is capable of disentangling these inter-correlations and, indeed, using them to good effect.

There is nothing peculiar or particular about the production of welfare approach to evaluation, nor the economist's approach to resource allocation in general from which it is derived. The approach is simply an ordered collection of likely and proven causal connections between the factors within the control of decision-makers, staff and carers (and perhaps also of users), and the achievements made possible, either at a service level or in terms of improvements in the wellbeing of individual members of society.

The approach can contribute to the understanding of mental health care practice and policy in a number of ways. First, it offers a theoretical framework within which to locate many of the current views on the organisation and delivery of services. Because it suggests clear hypotheses about the links between different resource availabilities, personnel activities, user preferences and identifiable changes in circumstances and characteristics, the framework is testable. If it is carefully constructed and responsively restructured, the framework can embody the results of empirical research. There are, for example, many assumed and statistically corroborated causal relationships between aspects of care, carers and users. While the approach cannot contain all the perspectives put forward, it provides a coherent conceptual framework in which to locate and examine inter-relationships. What is more, the approach suggests which relationships should be examined and how these may be interpreted. The production of welfare approach provides a repertoire of eminently usable empirical tools — theoretically valid constructs with extensive supportive statistical techniques — with which to address practice and policy questions. The book should provide cogent illustrations of the power of the approach.

Outcomes

The two primary dimensions of economic evaluation are cost and outcomes. Health care evaluations usually define outcomes as changes over time in the health and the broader welfare of service users and their families. Outcome dimensions commonly include clinical measures of symptomatology, psychopathology, quality of life, user satisfaction, family carer impact, social networks and self-care abilities. There are, of course, well-developed instruments for measuring wellbeing along each of these and other dimensions.

As noted above, some health economists have taken a different tack, looking to measure outcomes using 'utility' indices which combine individual preferences on quality of life and data on enhanced life duration to produce measures such as quality adjusted life years. The QALY has been seen as a useful generic measure of health status that can be combined with cost data to produce, for example, estimates for the marginal cost per QALY for different treatment modalities (Maynard, 1993). The logical corollary is to advise that resources are allocated to interventions or diagnostic groups which achieve a given number of QALYs at lower marginal cost. However, as Shane Kavanagh and Alan Stewart argue in Chapter 2, the QALY is generally currently too simplistic and reductionist *on its own* for other purposes. Ethical objections have also been raised, for example because the QALY might be held to discriminate against groups such as elderly people (Rosser, 1990), although the ethical case can be exaggerated.

Obviously, the limitations of today's specific QALY measures do not mean that quality of life considerations must be excluded from mental health evaluations, or that QALYs might not eventually be an integral part of evaluation instrumentation, or that the search for unidimensional utility measures is fruitless. Selai and Rosser review the main QALY measures and their relevance for mental health evaluations. They conclude that quality of life 'measures are invaluable in psychiatry for identifying need, evaluating therapies, monitoring change, and assisting in decisions about the allocation of scarce resources' (Selai and Rosser, 1993, p.70), but that there is as yet no simple or appropriate measure for mental health service uses.

Costs

There are four broad types of cost. The *direct costs* are the health services provided to people with mental health problems, the largest cost item often being inpatient hospital care, with others including community nursing and medications. *Indirect costs* are the necessary complements to direct expenditure from local authorities and other agencies. The *hidden costs,* as their label suggests, are not immediately identifiable but are nevertheless measurable. Examples are family and volunteer support and other informal care. Finally, there are probably some *immeasurable costs,* necessary elements of a package of care which are difficult or perhaps impossible to express in monetary terms, such as premature mortality, family anxiety or the impact of informal care on relatives. In fact, some economists have attached costs to some of these elements, but the methods and figures remain contentious (McGuire et al., 1988; Netten, 1993).

Each of these costs should, where possible, be measured as long-run marginal opportunity costs (Knapp, 1993). This helps to ensure that a long-term perspective on resource implications is employed, that only those effects on resources attributable to the programme or service user are counted, and that costs are reckoned as opportunities forgone, not just money expended. In Chapter 3, Jennifer Beecham shows how these principles can be converted into estimates of unit costs for the most commonly-used mental health care services.

Modes of evaluation

Economic evaluations combine outcome and costs data, most commonly in cost-effectiveness, cost-benefit and cost-utility analyses (CEA, CBA and CUA, respectively). There are also simple cost or cost minimisation evaluations. Each mode of evaluation sets out to measure costs comprehensively in accordance with the principles just outlined. The main differences between them relate to outcome measurement (see Chapter 2). Simple cost evaluations do not measure outcomes at all, and are therefore of limited usefulness. CEAs compare the costs of different policies in achieving an identical outcome, such as a uniform reduction in hospital re-admission rates or different degrees of success, such as cost per re-admission avoided. A multivariate CEA admits more than one outcome and seeks to examine the different cost-outcome links *statistically* (see Chapter 4). A CBA values all outcomes in monetary terms. This is useful in that it allows the policy-maker to compare treatment costs with benefits using the same measure of value, but has the disadvantage of sometimes squeezing multifarious, complex effects into a monetary strait-jacket. The simple comparison of costs incurred with costs saved is *not* a CBA. It may be a worthwhile exercise, but it neglects to look at the impacts of services or treatments on patients — it is a simple cost comparison. A CUA compares cost with a global measure of outcome such as the QALY, allowing treatments to be compared in terms of cost per QALY.

1.8 Principles of evaluation

Economists have produced a few 'good practice' guides to the conduct of economic evaluations. One of the earliest and best within the health economics genre is Drummond's (1980) book on economic appraisal, subsequently extended with accounts of more recent evaluative tools and a broader span of evidence (Drummond et al., 1987). There has been no equivalent in the mental health field. However, four basic principles for *costs* research have been suggested (Knapp and Beecham, 1990), and these also lie at the core of economic evaluation. They can be used to structure the arguments and evidence in this book.

The first principle is *comprehensiveness*: costs and outcomes should generally be measured broadly, covering all relevant services and other financial implications, and all possible or likely impacts on users, carers and the broader society. There are circumstances when exceptions can be made, as discussed below. The second principle is to recognise that there will be cost and outcome *variations* between service users, facilities and areas of the country, and to recommend their examination for policy, practice and other insights. Third, *like-with-like comparisons* should be attempted: the influences of extraneous factors should be removed or qualifications made to ensure that comparable samples of users or facilities are studied in comparable contexts. Finally, the fourth principle urges the integration of cost information with information on user and other *outcomes*. These four basic principles of economic evaluation are really no different in intent from the principles of clinical or other evaluations. Although blind adherence would be inadvisable, the wider adoption of these principles should aid the policy and practice processes, as we can now illustrate.

Comprehensiveness

The well-conducted economic evaluation will measure costs and outcomes comprehensively, or will employ partial measures advisedly. Davies and Drummond's (1993) evaluation of clozapine for treatment-resistant schizophrenia needed to include the costs of the regular blood tests to guard against agranulocytosis, as well as the costs of outpatient attendances, GP consultations, and so on. The evaluations of services in South London by the PRiSM team at the Institute of Psychiatry are using instruments to measure needs, diagnoses, related clinical characteristics as well as the comprehensive costs of treatment and support. The evaluation of community reprovision in North London for long-stay psychiatric hospital residents embodies comprehensive measures of costs and outcomes (see Chapter 5). Other things being equal, the greater and the more diverse a patient's or user's needs, the broader the range of services likely to be utilised and the greater the number of outcome dimensions which an evaluation will need to include in order to gauge impact.

The influence of user choice and the extension of the mixed economy of health and social care may broaden the range of services available in a locality, and simultaneously increase the variety of services used by individuals (see Figure 1.1 on page 7). An evaluation which addresses the resource dimension might therefore be called upon to cost a large number of services. In some circumstances it may not be necessary to cost every component of a care 'package', for example when an evaluative trial is sufficiently narrow and when randomisation can guarantee the equivalence of some service utilisation (Burns et al., 1993), although such occasions will probably be rare. In the interests of research economy and efficiency, there might also be occasions when it is sufficient to look at a *reduced list* of just the most expensive services to gain a general indication or an informed second-best estimate of costs (Chapter 9). However, comprehensiveness should never be abandoned lightly: such action could produce dangerously partial research.

Exploring variations

Reliance on a reduced list will probably not be sensible if the research aims to illuminate inter-individual differences, which — as argued in Chapter 4 — is desirable in the context of the health and community care arrangements being developed in the UK during the 1990s. Exploring inter-individual variations is also relevant with almost any clinical or other treatment intervention. Why, for example, are costs or outcomes different for one user when compared to another? What factors push up costs or effects? Without closer examination of variations, evaluations can give only incomplete guidance to the mental health care provider looking for a way to target available treatment resources on assessed needs in order to improve service or system efficiency or equity. Could there, as Bosanquet and Zajdler (1993, p.30) ask, 'be less distance between the average standard of treatment and the best available?' Is it possible within a broad organisational arrangement (such as community care) or a standard medication response (such as prescription of neuroleptics or SSRIs) to identify and 'explain' different service utilisation patterns or individual patient outcomes?

Like-with-like comparisons

Economic evaluations should aim to make comparisons between treatments or policies on a careful like-with-like basis. This is why it is so important to design certain types of economic evaluation around or linked to randomised controlled trials. Alternatively, like-with-like comparisons can be sought by employing matched designs or statistical standardisation analyses in an attempt to control for extraneous factors. Some of the economic evaluations described in Chapter 4 built upon or are integral parts of randomised design studies, but the reprovision research reported in Chapter 5 did not follow this approach and instead relied on matching (for comparisons between hospital and community care) and statistical controls (for comparisons between the various community care settings). These issues are explored further in Chapter 2, with a look at meta-analyses and decision trees in Chapter 10.

Cost-outcome linkages

Accountants the world over produce and analyse good-quality costs data, and clinical evaluators collect and interpret outcome information. Less commonly undertaken, but revealing, are examinations of the links between costs and outcomes. Setting comparisons of costs alongside comparisons of outcomes should generally be insightful, but there is also a pressing need to analyse more thoroughly the links between the two. Do better outcomes follow from higher levels of spending, once other factors have been held constant? What is the marginal cost of a given improvement in user health or welfare? The links between costs and *needs* should also be examined. What, for example, are the user characteristics and needs which push up or reduce costs? The associations between costs, needs and outcomes are explored in a number of the chapters of this book, in particular those on community reprovision and variations and comparisons (Chapters 4 and 5), and underpin the balance of care discussions in Chapter 6.

1.9 Conclusions

The efficiency imperative is making itself felt at the policy and practice levels, and the adequacy of targeting (equity) is being called into question in relation to a number of mental health problems. These two allocation criteria are regularly addressed by economists in their evaluations of public policies, new products and other practice initiatives. However, there have to date been few economic evaluations in the mental health area, and the impact of economic research has been substantially less than might have been expected. The substantial libraries of British and international literature on the outcomes of mental health interventions compare with a half-empty filing cabinet of completed economic evaluations. Sometimes when there is an 'economic component' it is little more than glorified accountancy: a cursory description of some of the costs of a service with no real attempt fully to integrate costs with other data. The empirical studies described in this book go beyond the mere description of costs, also examining user needs and outcomes. However, they can only be *illustrations* of how economic evaluations might inform decisions about mental health care strategies and individual interventions. A huge amount of work remains to be done.

Economics is as much craft as science, more a way of organising thought than of mechanically allocating resources. It cannot replace the judgements of decision-makers, but it ought to be able to supplement and inform them.

Note

* This chapter builds in part on arguments presented in Knapp (1994, 1995).

References

Audit Commission (1986) *Making a Reality of Community Care*, HMSO, London.

Audit Commission (1994) *Finding a Place: A Review of Mental Health Services for Adults*, HMSO, London.

Bebbington, A.C. and Davies, B.P. (1983) Equity and efficiency in the allocation of the personal social services, *Journal of Social Policy*, 12, 309-30.

Bosanquet, N. and Zajdler, A. (1993) Psychopharmacology and the ethics of resource allocation, *British Journal of Psychiatry*, 162, 29-32.

Bowman, F.M. and Garralda, M.E. (1993) Psychiatric morbidity among children who are frequent attenders in general practice, *British Journal of General Practice*, 43, 6-9.

Burns, T., Raftery, J., Beadsmoore, A., McGuigan, S. and Dickson, M. (1993) A controlled trial of home-based acute psychiatric services. II: Treatment patterns and costs, *British Journal of Psychiatry*, 163, 55-61.

Chisholm, D., Healey, A. and Knapp, M.R.J. (1995) QALYs and mental health care, Working Paper 26, Centre for the Economics of Mental Health, Institute of Psychiatry, London.

Conway, A.S., Melzer, D. and Hale, A.S. (1994) The outcome of targeting community mental health services: evidence from the West Lambeth schizophrenia cohort, *British Medical Journal*, 308, 627-30.

Davies, B.P. and Knapp, M.R.J. (1981) *Old People's Homes and the Production of Welfare*, Routledge, London.

Davies, B.P. and Knapp, M.R.J. (eds) (1988) *British Journal of Social Work*, 18, Supplement.

Davies, B.P., Bebbington, A.C. and Charnley, H. with Baines, B., Ferlie, E.B., Hughes, M. and Twigg, J. (1990) *Resources, Needs and Outcomes in Community-Based Care*, Avebury, Aldershot.

Davies, L.M. and Drummond, M.F. (1993) Assessment of costs and benefits of drug therapy for treatment-resistant schizophrenia in the United Kingdom, *British Journal of Psychiatry*, 162, 38-42.

Department of Health (1993) *Health of the Nation: Mental Illness Handbook*, HMSO, London.

Donaldson, C. and Gerard, K. (1993) *Economics of Health Care Financing*, Macmillan, Basingstoke.

Drummond, M.F. (1980) *Principles of Economic Appraisal in Health Care*, Oxford University Press, Oxford.

Drummond, M.F. (1992) Cost-effectiveness guidelines for reimbursement of pharmaceuticals: is economic evaluation ready for its enhanced status?, *Health Economics*, 1, 85-92.

Drummond, M.F., Stoddart, G.L. and Torrance, G.W. (1987) *Methods for the Economic Evaluation of Health Care Programmes*, Oxford Medical Publications, Oxford.

Eichelman, B. and Hartwig, A. (1990) Ethical issues in selecting patients for treatment with clozapine: a commentary, *Hospital and Community Psychiatry*, 41, 880-82.

Goldacre, M., Shiwash, R. and Yeates, D. (1994) Estimating incidence and prevalence of treated psychiatric disorders from routine statistics: the example of schizophrenia, *Journal of Epidemiology and Community Health*, 48, 3, 318-22.

Gray, A. and Fenn, P. (1993) Alzheimer's disease: the burden of the illness in England, *Health Trends*, 25, 1, 31-7.

Harrington, R., Fudge, H., Rutter, M., Pickles, A. and Hill, J. (1990) Adult outcomes of childhood and adolescent depression. I: Psychiatric status, *Archives of General Psychiatry*, 47, 465-73.

Healy, D. (1993) Psychopharmacology and the ethics of resource allocation, *British Journal of Psychiatry*, 162, 23-9.

Kavanagh, S., Opit, L., Knapp, M.R.J. and Beecham, J.K. (1995) Schizophrenia: shifting the balance of care, *Social Psychiatry and Psychiatric Epidemiology*, forthcoming.

Kazadin, A.E. (1987) Treatment of anti-social behaviour in children: current status and future directions, *Psychological Bulletin*, 102, 187-203.

Knapp, M.R.J. (1984) *The Economics of Social Care*, Macmillan, London.

Knapp, M.R.J. (1993) Principles of applied cost research, in A. Netten and J. Beecham (eds) *Costing Community Care: Theory and Practice*, Ashgate, Aldershot.

Knapp, M.R.J. (1994) The health economics of schizophrenia treatment, *The Clinician*, 12, 1, 39-52.

Knapp, M.R.J. (1995) Community mental health services: towards an understanding of cost-effectiveness, in P. Tyrer and F. Creed (eds) *Community Psychiatry in Action*, Cambridge University Press, Cambridge.

Knapp, M.R.J. and Beecham, J.K. (1990) Costing mental health services, *Psychological Medicine*, 20, 893-908.

Knapp, M.R.J. and Beecham, J.K. (1993) Health economics and psychiatry: the pursuit of efficiency, in D. Bhugra and J. Leff (eds) *Principles of Social Psychiatry*, Blackwell Scientific Publications, Oxford.

Knapp, M.R.J. and Beecham, J.K. (1995) Programme-level and systems-level health economics considerations, in G. Thornicroft and H.C. Knudson (eds) *Mental Health Service Evaluation*, Cambridge University Press, Cambridge.

Light, D. and Bailey, V. (1993) Pound foolish, *Health Service Journal*, 11 February, 16-18.

Maynard, A. (1993) Cost management: the economist's viewpoint, *British Journal of Psychiatry*, 163, Supplement 20, 7-13.

McCrone, P., Beecham, J.K. and Knapp, M.R.J. (1994) Community psychiatric nurse teams: cost-effectiveness of intensive support versus generic care, *British Journal of Psychiatry*, 165, 218-21.

McGuire, A., Henderson, J. and Mooney, G. (1988) *The Economics of Health Care*, Routledge, London.

Melzer, D., Hale, A.S., Malik, S.J., Hogman, G.A. and Wood, S. (1991) Community care for patients with schizophrenia one year after hospital discharge, *British Medical Journal*, 303, 1023-6.

Netten, A. (1993) Costing informal care, in A. Netten and J. Beecham (eds) *Costing Community Care: Theory and Practice*, Ashgate, Aldershot.

Office of Population Censuses and Surveys (OPCS) (1991) *National Population Projections Number 17*, (1989-based), HMSO, London.

Pelonero, A.L. and Elliott, R.L. (1990) Ethical and clinical considerations in selecting patients who will receive clozapine, *Hospital and Community Psychiatry*, 41, 878-80.

Ritchie, J., Dick, D. and Lingham, R. (1994) *The Report of the Inquiry into the Care and Treatment of Christopher Clunis*, HMSO, London.

Robins, L.N. (1966) *Deviant Children Grown Up: A Sociological and Psychiatric Study of Sociopathic Personality*, Williams and Wilkins, Baltimore. (Reprinted and published by Robert E. Kreiger Publishing Co., New York, 1974.)

Robins, L.N. and Regier, D.A. (eds) (1991) *Psychiatric Disorders in America: The Epidemiologic Catchment Area Study*, The Free Press, New York.

Rosser, R. (1990) From health indicators to Quality Adjusted Life Years: technical and ethical issues, in A. Hopkins and D. Costain (eds) *Measuring the Outcomes of Medical Care*, Royal College of Physicians Press, London.

Rutter, M. (1989) Pathways from childhood to adult life, *Journal of Child Psychology and Psychiatry*, 30, 23-51.

Rutter, M. (1991) Services for children with emotional disorders: needs, accomplishments and future developments, *Young Minds Newsletter*, 9, 1-5.

Rutter, M. and Madge, N. (1976) *Cycles of Disadvantage: A Review of Research*, Heinemann, London.

Secretaries of State (1989a) *Working for Patients*, Cm 555, HMSO, London.

Secretaries of State (1989b) *Caring for People: Community Care in the Next Decade and Beyond*, Cm 849, HMSO, London.

Secretary of State for Health (1992) *The Health of the Nation*, Cm 1523, HMSO.

Selai, C. and Rosser, R. (1993) The role of quality of life measurement in psychiatry, *Current Medical Literature — Psychiatry*, 4, 67-71.

Weisbrod, B.A. (1979) A guide to benefit cost analysis as seen through a controlled experiment in treating the mentally ill, Discussion Paper 559-79, Institute for Research on Poverty, University of Wisconsin, Madison.

Williams, R. (1993) Psychiatric morbidity in children and adolescents: a suitable cause for concern, *British Journal of General Practice*, 43, 3-4.

Wistow, G., Knapp, M.R.J., Hardy, B. and Allen, C. (1994) *Social Care in a Mixed Economy*, Open University Press, Buckingham.

2 *Economic Evaluations of Mental Health Care: Modes and Methods*

Shane Kavanagh and Alan Stewart

2.1 Introduction

Health care is one of the few services that is at least partly funded by the public sector in most industrialised countries. Service delivery decisions are thus guided not just by market forces but also by social criteria (Maynard and Hutton, 1992). Economic data and analyses are playing an increasingly large role in the decision-making processes of those who commission and deliver care. For example, in Australia and Ontario pharmaceutical companies are required to subject new medicines to economic as well as clinical analyses before their products can attain reimbursement by government. Such analyses are not yet mandatory in the United Kingdom, but their potential importance has been recognised by the Department of Health. A set of guidelines has been issued (Department of Health, 1994) — drawn up in collaboration with the pharmaceutical industry — to ensure good practice in the economic evaluation of new medicines. In mental health care the growing importance of economic evaluation has not been confined to new pharmaceutical products (Davies and Drummond, 1993; Jönsson and Bebbington, 1993), but has also played a part in the debate surrounding de-institutionalisation (Korman and Glennerster, 1990; Knapp et al., 1992, 1993; Donnelly et al., 1994) and the organisation of hospital and community services more generally (Weisbrod et al., 1980; Goldberg, 1991; Burns et al., 1993; Knapp et al., 1994; McCrone et al., 1994; Jackson et al., 1995).

This chapter explores and illustrates the methodological issues relating to the economic evaluation of health and social care interventions. The Department of Health guidelines — although targeted at the evaluation of pharmaceuticals — provide a useful template for identifying issues (Box 2.1).

2.2 General evaluative issues

The first four DH guidelines in Box 2.1 relate to epidemiological and clinical evaluation standards for health care evaluation rather than economic methods. This is entirely appropriate as the application of even the most powerful economic and statistical techniques is worthless if the underlying design of a study is flawed due to inadequate planning or implementation. This problem has been described as 'building castles on sand' (Maynard and Bloor, 1994).

The first of the guidelines appears quite basic in that it states that the study should 'clearly set out the question that is being addressed'. For example, to state that a study compares hospital to community care is rather vague. These terms cover a variety of different types of hospital and community services and disparate groups of patients. It is therefore good practice to state clearly on whom the treatment is targeted, and their relevant demographic characteristics, diagnoses and previous psychiatric histories.

Choosing a comparator intervention

The main focus of any service evaluation is to demonstrate whether there are outcomes — gains in welfare or quality of life — attributable to the service or treatment under scrutiny. It is therefore necessary to have a comparator so that the changes in welfare or quality of life can be compared to those that would have been achieved in the absence of the treatment or with an alternative treatment. The UK guidelines — unlike those in either Australia (Commonwealth of Australia, 1990) or Ontario (Ontario Ministry of Health, 1991) — are not explicit about which comparator should be employed, but state that 'the conceptual and practical reasons for choosing the comparator should be set out and justified'. The open-ended nature of this statement reflects the difficulty of choosing an appropriate comparator and the dangers of being excessively prescriptive in general guidelines.

Many clinical trials of medicines employ a placebo as the comparator. While this is adequate in determining the efficacy and likely side-effects of treatment, it fails to provide sufficient information for decision-makers faced with real world choices. There are a number of potentially more useful alternatives than placebo, such as the most commonly used form of alternative treatment or the cheapest alternative treatment. Other issues arise, such as the dose levels at which medications are prescribed, which have an important impact on efficacy. For example, prescribing of tricyclic antidepressants at subtherapeutic levels is well documented (Johnson, 1981; Thompson and Thompson, 1989; Forder et al., 1994). In choosing a comparator, the analyst

Box 2.1

Guidelines for the economic evaluation of pharmaceuticals

1. The question being addressed by the study, including the demographic characteristics of the target population group, should be identified and be set out at the start of the report of the study.
2. The conceptual and practical reasons for choosing the comparator should be set out and justified in the report of the study.
3. The treatment paths of the options being compared should be identified, fully described, placed in the context of overall treatment, and reported. Decision analytic techniques can be helpful in this regard.
4. In choosing the method of data capture and analysis, the use of one of, or a combination of, prospective or retrospective randomised clinical trials, meta-analysis, observational data and modelling should be considered. The reasons for choice of method and, where relevant, for choice of trials should be reported.
5. The perspective of the study should ideally be societal, identifying the impact on all parts of society, including patients, the NHS, other providers of care, and the wider economy. However, costs and outcomes should be reported in a disaggregated way so that the recipients of costs and outcomes can be identified. Attention should be drawn to any significant distributional implications. Indirect costs should normally be included in a societal perspective although care should be taken to avoid any double-counting and results should be reported including and excluding these costs.
6. The study should use a recognised technique. These include cost-minimisation analysis (CMA), cost-effectiveness analysis (CEA), cost-utility analysis (CUA), and cost-benefit analysis (CBA). Any one of these could be appropriate according to the purpose of the study. The report of the study should include justification of the technique chosen.
7. Assessment of the question should include determining and reporting what additional benefit is being provided at what extra cost using incremental analysis of costs and outcomes.
8. Outcome measures should be identified and the basis for their selection reported. Where CUA is used, proven generic measures of quality of life are preferred.
9. All relevant costs should be identified, collected and reported. Physical units of resource use should be collected and reported separately from information about the costs of the resources. Costs should reflect full opportunity cost, including the cost of capital and administrative and support costs where relevant. Average cost data is often acceptable as a proxy for long-run marginal cost.
10. Discounting should be undertaken on two different bases:
    – all costs and outcomes discounted at the prevailing rate recommended by the Treasury, currently 6 per cent per annum;
    – all costs and monetary outcomes discounted at the Treasury rate, currently 6 per cent, but non-monetary outcomes not discounted.
    Both sets of results should be reported. The physical units and values of costs and outcomes prior to discounting should also be reported.
11. Sensitivity analysis should be conducted and reported. The sensitivity of results to all uncertainty in the study should be explored. This should involve the use of confidence intervals and/or ranges for key parameters, as appropriate. The ranges and choice of parameters to vary should be justified.
12. Comparisons with results from other studies should be handled with care. Particular attention should be paid to differences in methodology (such as the treatment of indirect costs) or differences in circumstances (such as different population groups).

Source: Department of Health (1994).

is faced with a choice between an ideal situation where dose levels are appropriate and a more likely situation where subtherapeutic prescribing is common. At an even more fundamental level, the question becomes one of whether non-pharmaceutical alternatives or supplements such as counselling or cognitive therapy should be compared with medications (Drummond, 1992). A potential conflict of interest therefore exists between the decision-maker, who would like to be presented with a full range of care options, and those commissioning or conducting the research, who often have a vested interest in marketing a new pharmaceutical product or encouraging a pioneering new treatment to be adopted. Freemantle and Maynard (1994) and the response by Jönsson (1994) provide a particularly lively debate of these issues with particular reference to antidepressants.

Structure and process

In order to ascertain the replicability of the results of any health care evaluation, it is necessary to identify the well-known elements of 'structure' and 'process' (Donabedian, 1980) analogous to resource inputs and intermediate outcomes in the production of welfare framework (see Chapter 1). This clarifies not only what staff, equipment and medicines are used, but also how they are combined in the process of care. Häfner and an der Haden (1991) provide a useful review of these concepts with respect to psychiatry. The guidelines therefore require that 'the treatment paths of the options being compared should be identified, fully described, placed in the context of overall treatment, and reported'.

Determining effectiveness

Economic evaluation requires data on the clinical effectiveness of the interventions being compared. A variety of methods for data capture and analysis exists and the guidelines are — perhaps suitably — open-ended in their recommendations for methods to employ, stating that 'the use of one of, or a combination of, prospective or retrospective randomised clinical trials, meta-analysis, observational data and modelling should be considered'. We now consider each of these options.

Economic evaluation and RCTs. In mental health, as in all areas of modern medicine, the bedrock of clinical research has been the randomised controlled trial (RCT). The use of random allocation permits chance to determine the assignment of subjects to interventions. Properly designed and implemented RCTs have the advantage of eliminating selection bias and therefore create groups that are comparable with respect to factors that may influence outcomes (Mausner and Kramer, 1985; Pocock, 1991). A variety of strategies can be adopted for randomising subjects between interventions. Burns et al. (1993) compared the costs and effects of standard hospital-based care with home-based psychiatric services, and used randomisation to allocate subjects between interventions. In contrast, Jackson et al. (1995) compared care provided by a specialist community mental health team to standard care, and allocated subjects to interventions by randomly allocating the entire primary care practice to which they belonged. Two options exist for the economic evaluation of RCTs. Data from a trial that is already completed can be utilised or economic data can be collected prospectively alongside the clinical data. Both approaches have advantages and disadvantages.

An economic evaluation using data from an RCT that has already been completed, or indeed from a meta-analysis of previously conducted RCTs, faces the difficulty that data such as utilisation of services (particularly for services not directly related to the specific treatment intervention), time lost from work and time spent caring for a relative are rarely collected as part of the trial protocol. The economist is then faced with either trying to collect these data retrospectively and/or making a large number of assumptions. Alternatively, an economic study may be included within the trial protocol with the collection of economic data being performed alongside the process of collecting and measuring information on health care interventions and effects. The prospective approach depends on there being a suitable clinical study available, with investigators willing to cooperate with an economic evaluation. This is not always the case, and even if suitable clinical studies can be found, there is often a long time lag before results can be generated and analysed.

Both prospective and retrospective economic evaluations of RCTs come to acquire the same strengths and weaknesses as the clinical studies on which they are based. A particular problem with RCTs is that they examine a constrained set of treatment options and responses that may not be typical of routine care. Trials are usually based in atypical settings, such as an academic teaching hospital, where the cost structures as well as treatment regimes differ from those found in standard care settings. RCTs are often criticised for failing to allow an adequate period of follow-up to determine longer-term outcomes, and this problem is no less applicable when the economic impact of interventions is considered. The unusual service utilisation profile generated by the trial protocol may affect both the outcomes attained and also the costs of care, with the potential consequence that the results of the study may not be realisable in standard care (Drummond, 1992). Despite these problems, RCTs provide a useful basis for economic evaluations.

Economic evaluation and quasi-experimental studies. RCTs cannot be conducted for every care intervention. Investigators face the dilemma that it is impossible to get approval for an RCT unless there is insufficient evidence to suggest that either of the treatment interventions is more effective. If sufficient evidence were available, then it would be unethical to provide care which was viewed as sub-optimal. Further factors such as the need for informed consent from subjects and the desirability of blinding (of subjects, care professionals and investigators from the treatment being given) can also make RCTs difficult to implement. Where RCTs are not feasible, then the use of quasi-experimental studies may be appropriate. A number of alternatives exist. One method is to employ historical controls where a cohort of subjects receiving one form of care is compared to a subsequent cohort who receive a more innovative intervention. Natural experiments are also possible where similar areas adopt different care interventions for similar groups of subjects. An example of this type of study is the retrospective design employed in the evaluation of care provided in a district general hospital compared to a psychiatric hospital (Goldberg and Jones, 1980; Jones et al., 1980). Two demographically similar catchment areas were identified, and subjects experiencing their first admission for schizophrenia from one catchment area received care in the district general hospital while similar subjects in the other area received care in the psychiatric hospital.

However, the problem with these study designs is that other factors influencing prognoses and outcomes may confound the results. In some instances the policy decision about the provision of care may precede the evaluation, and the choice of study designs available to the investigator is constrained. A good example is the case of de-institutionalisation. The studies of hospital discharge for former long-stay patients in Northern Ireland (Donnelly et al., 1994), in an English demonstration programme (Knapp et al., 1992) and in North London (see Chapter 5) were faced with such a constraint. The comparison between hospital and community care is difficult due to the lack of a control group. However, comparisons could be made before and after hospital discharge, by careful matching with people who did not (initially) move from hospital. In addition, multivariate analyses were employed to control for the myriad of factors influencing wellbeing, and provided useful evidence on the impact of different community settings on users. These methods are considered in more detail in Chapter 4.

Modelling effectiveness. Decision analysis is advocated as a means for clarifying the process of care. This technique breaks 'complex problems down into manageable component parts and analyses those parts in detail' (Thornton et al., 1992; see Chapter 10). A decision tree presents a simple flow diagram representing the effects of decisions in terms of the probabilities of consequent events. Decisions and events are displayed in the order of occurrence. Where events are subject to chance, a range of probability values can be employed to predict the likely impact of decisions on future events.

Prospective studies (both RCTs and quasi-experimental designs) often require time to plan, implement, collect and analyse data. In the short term, decision-makers are often faced with pressure to choose between available interventions before the results from prospective studies are available. Under these circumstances, economic evaluation can use modelling techniques to assess the possible impact on both costs and outcomes. An example of such an approach is the comparison of clozapine with standard neuroleptic therapy for people with schizophrenia (Davies and Drummond, 1993). The authors constructed a model using decision analytic techniques, and previously published work was used to estimate efficacy, care packages received and costs. By incorporating these factors into a decision tree, the authors were able to estimate costs, efficacy and life years gained for patients treated with clozapine. Another study comparing the cost-effectiveness of dothiepin to sertraline in the treatment of depression employed delphic panels to supplement existing clinical data, and again used decision analytic methods (Hatziandreu et al., 1994). While such results do not have the same status as an economic evaluation of actual clinical practice, they can indicate where more detailed investigation is required and where cost variations have a potentially significant impact on the costs of treatment.

2.3 Whose perspective?

The purchasing and provision decisions of a range of public and other agencies — not just the health service but also social services, housing, education and criminal justice — have important impacts on the wellbeing of people with mental health problems and on the costs borne by other agencies, families and society at large. The DH guidelines recognise these problems and state that 'the perspective of the study should ideally be societal, identifying the impact on all parts of society, including patients, the NHS, other providers of care and the wider economy' (see Box 2.1).

For example, inadequate primary care may lead to an emergency inpatient admission with high costs for both family and hospital. A shortage of appropriately trained educational psychologists may generate inappropriate referrals to child psychiatric services, or heavier burdens of responsibility for child welfare services. Alternatively, good care by one provider may produce savings for other providers and families. Similarly, in terms of outcomes the effects of care on any individual may have a reflexive impact on their family. On the one hand, the amelioration of a parent's psychiatric symptoms may improve the wellbeing of other family members. However, a good outcome for one individual may be achieved at the expense of reduced wellbeing for another (Opit, 1988). Substituting inpatient hospital care with community-based services may improve a patient's quality of life but increase the family burden (Grad and Sainsbury, 1963). Conversely, respite care can reduce carer stress, though possibly at the cost of poorer outcomes for the mentally ill person.

By disaggregating costs and outcomes, it becomes easier to identify perverse incentives, such as cost shifting (Kavanagh and Knapp, 1995a,b) or potential budgetary shortfalls that may prevent the implementation of a potentially successful intervention. The distributional implications of care between agencies, budgets and families are important, but there has been a lively debate among economists about how equity should be defined (see Pereira, 1992 for a review). Some economists have argued that access to care should be given greatest consideration (Mooney, 1994), while others argue that health itself is the desired maximand (Culyer and Wagstaff, 1993). One perspective on equity — developed in the context of social care — is to consider the 'target efficiency' of services (Bebbington and Davies, 1983, 1993) — the efficiency with which people are recruited and retained as service users. If people are assigned to need groups in order of priority (by service providers) on the basis of whether they have a welfare shortfall that could be (partly) removed, then:

- horizontal target efficiency is the proportion of those in priority need who receive the service; and
- vertical target efficiency is the proportion of recipients of a service who satisfy the criteria of priority need.

The concept of target efficiency is couched in terms of need. Need is itself a difficult concept but is often considered in terms of ability to benefit (Williams, 1978). Someone whose welfare shortfall would not be reduced by receiving a service can therefore be considered not to need it. Welfare shortfall is a broad concept. In the context of social care it is generally considered in terms of compensation for disability, for example through providing support to someone who has difficulties with the activities of daily living (Knapp, 1984). In health care it tends to be considered as the ability of an intervention either: to prevent the onset of disease, to alter the prognoses of a disease or to reduce the symptoms of a disease that has already developed.

2.4 Measuring costs

The guidelines recommend that

> all relevant costs should be identified, collected and reported. Costs should reflect full opportunity cost, including the cost of capital and administrative and support costs where relevant. Average cost data is often acceptable as a proxy for long-run marginal cost.

Opportunity cost is an important economic concept, which often varies significantly from accounting cost. It is a measure not merely of actual amounts of money spent but of the resource implications of opportunities forgone, that is the true private or social value of a resource as measured by its best alternative use. This may be a market price, but not every resource or service is marketed, hence some opportunity costs are social values, for example time from unpaid volunteers and informal carers. Long-run marginal costs refer to the situation where the mix of inputs and use of resources can be varied from that which currently exists. And the marginal cost is the addition to total cost that will follow from the inclusion of one more client or the provision of one more unit of output. A fuller account of the theoretical and practical issues relating to costs is given in Chapter 3.

An additional requirement in the DH guidelines is that 'physical units of resource use should be collected and reported separately from information about the costs of the resources'. This is particularly useful in that alternative cost assumptions can be applied that are applicable in other settings where the costs structure is different. Service utilisation profiles can illustrate where small numbers of people contribute disproportionately to the costs within treatment groups. The usefulness of examining cost data closely is clearly demonstrated by Häfner and an der Haden (1991), who compared the costs of inpatient care to care by community services for people with schizophrenia. While community care was on average much less costly than hospital care, the authors showed that this was not true for all patients. A small number of patients using community services incurred costs greater than the average hospital inpatient cost. The authors argue that further discharge of psychiatric hospital inpatients would cause a greater proportion of people using community services to incur costs in excess of the cost of a hospital inpatient place thus increasing the average cost of community care. (See Chapter 5 for equivalent evidence for the UK.)

When a wider societal perspective is employed, costs and outcomes which are difficult to define and measure must be considered. These include: reduced productivity at work, the psychic costs to relatives of caring for someone with mental health problems and the psychic costs to members of the community through the risk of violence in the community which, although objectively rather small, can generate disproportionate fear and anxiety. There are many problems of definition, measurement and valuation, and caution is needed to avoid double-counting. For example, the impact on everyday activities could be included as both a cost in terms of inability to carry out gainful employment but also as an outcome in terms of reduced quality of life. The DH guidelines therefore state that it is useful to report results 'including and excluding these costs'.

2.5 Modes of economic evaluation

There are a variety of techniques for conducting economic evaluations. The most common are cost-minimisation analysis (CMA), cost-effectiveness analysis (CEA), cost-utility analysis (CUA), and cost-benefit analysis (CBA). (These terms are not always consistently applied by the economics profession or others, so careful reading is required to ensure that a study is what it purports to be.) There is much debate among health economists as to the validity of the different techniques and the DH guidelines are therefore not prescriptive about which method should be employed, stating that 'any one of these could be appropriate according to the purpose of the study' provided sufficient justification is furnished. Each of the modes of evaluation sets out to measure costs comprehensively, paying due regard to marginal costs, opportunities forgone, long-run versus short-run adjustments, and so on (see Chapters 1 and 3). Differences between the modes of evaluation relate primarily to their treatment and measurement of outcomes.

Cost-effectiveness analysis

Cost-effectiveness analysis compares the costs of different treatment interventions in achieving an identical outcome or the costs of different degrees of success in achieving a given outcome. Where two interventions achieve an identical level of success with respect to a desired outcome, such as a uniform reduction in the re-admission rate, then the evaluation compares which intervention achieves this at lowest cost. This particular form of cost-effectiveness evaluation is often known as cost-minimisation analysis and is predicated on the availability of clinical evidence of sufficient quality which shows no significant difference in terms of the desired outcome. It is not just a simplistic comparison of cost.

However, the interventions may achieve a varying degree of success. If a particular intervention is both more successful in achieving the desired outcome — such as reducing the inpatient re-admission rate — and also less costly than the alternative intervention, then it is said to dominate in terms of both costs and outcomes and is clearly the cost-effective option. Unfortunately, the results of studies are not always so clear cut. An intervention can often be more successful in achieving the desired outcomes but at a higher cost compared to the alternative intervention. In such cases the comparison becomes one of costs per unit of success (such as re-admission avoided) or unit of success for a given cost (number of re-admissions avoided per £10,000 spent). A decision rule is then employed to select between the alternative interventions where 'the criterion for cost-effectiveness is the ratio of the net increase in health care costs to the net effectiveness' (Weinstein and Stason, 1977, p.718). Consider the following example where two forms of community psychiatric services are compared. Service B is more successful in reducing re-admissions compared to A: 60 re-admissions avoided compared to 50. However, the costs are also greater: £15,000 rather than £10,000. Using the decision rule posited by Weinstein and Stason (1977), service A is the more cost-effective because the ratio of costs to desired outcomes is lower — £200 (10000/50) rather than £250 (15000/60) — or in simple terms the cost per re-admission avoided is lower.

The example above discussed the costs of care interventions in reducing re-admissions. While re-admissions are often considered to be synonymous with relapse and recidivism, their usefulness as a proxy measure of improved mental health is contaminated by factors independent of the quality of care such as: the availability of hospital beds and/or the availability of alternative services (Häfner and an der Haden, 1991). Strictly speaking, re-admissions indicate health service activity or process rather than outcome. Economic evaluations therefore try to focus on actual user outcomes as the desired maximand for services rather than the level of activity. But performing such a CEA and producing figures for each comparator does not actually make a decision between the options. The economist is merely presenting decision-makers with information to enhance the eventual decision.

Cost-effectiveness analysis requires a comparison of measures of clinical or social outcome, in addition to assessment of costs. Cost-effectiveness studies often include measures of outcome and dependency commonly employed in epidemiological and evaluative studies, such as the Present State Examination (Wing et al., 1974) and the Brief Psychiatric Rating Scale (Overall and Gorham, 1962). The following examples demonstrate the use of such measures for two forms of care intervention: community psychiatric nursing and the drug treatment of schizophrenia.

Examples of cost-effectiveness analysis. An example of a well-executed cost-effectiveness evaluation is the study by Mangen et al. (1983), who compared psychiatric care based on community psychiatric nurses and standard care by psychiatrists in outpatient clinics. Services were targeted at patients suffering from chronic neurotic disorder (a small proportion had a primary diagnosis of personality disorder or affective psychosis). A prospective RCT design was employed, although the sample sizes were relatively small. Service utilisation for a wide range of public sector agencies was recorded and costed. Patient outcomes were measured on a variety of dimensions (Paykel et al., 1982): symptoms using the Clinical Interview for Depression (Paykel et al., 1970) and the Three Area Depression scale (Raskin et al., 1970), social role performance using the Social Adjustment Scale (Weissman and Paykel, 1974), family burden using a modified schedule from Grad and Sainsbury (1968), and consumer satisfaction (Catalan et al., 1980). Outcomes were similar for the two groups with the exception of consumer satisfaction which favoured the CPN service. A narrow examination of the costs to psychiatric services showed that the CPN service was significantly less costly (£148 per patient per year, at 1977 prices) compared to the outpatient services (£165). The CPN group was therefore dominant in terms of both costs and outcomes.

The study is useful in that it highlights some of the methodological issues raised earlier in the chapter. First, the differential impact of services on resource use often accrues in the longer term. The assessment at six months showed a significantly higher cost in the CPN group compared to the outpatient group, while the costs over the first twelve months showed little difference between the groups. It was only when the costs were compared over an eighteen month period that the cost advantage to the CPN group became apparent.

Second, the study highlights the importance of costs to parts of the health and social services other than psychiatric services. The broad public sector costs for health and social care services in the CPN group were higher (£1,117) compared to the outpatient group (£720). Local authority social services accounted for most of the difference, with the worrying implication that cost-shifting had occurred. However, disaggregation of the costs and service utilisation data demonstrated that the cost difference was largely driven by two individuals in the CPN group who had children in care. Closer investigation led the research team to conclude that the situation was unattributable to the level or type of psychiatric care. However, this analysis clearly illustrates the importance of disaggregating costs and service utilisation data.

The evaluation by Mangen et al. (1983) and Paykel et al. (1982) was clearly influential in the rapid expansion of CPN services in the UK during the 1980s (White, 1990). However, as the service has developed, concern has grown that CPNs are working in isolation and are therefore unable to provide well-coordinated care to their patients (Wooff et al., 1988). A recent study compared the cost-effectiveness of two different service configurations of CPN-based care for people with long-term mental health problems (McCrone et al., 1994; Muijen et al., 1994). The study is useful in that, like the Mangen et al. (1983) study, it identifies the costs to different service providers and illustrates the changing profile of costs over time both for total and component costs (see Chapter 4).

Two further cost-effectiveness studies examined the treatment of schizophrenia using clozapine, compared to treatment with neuroleptics medication such as chlorpromazine and haloperidol. Revicki et al. (1990) conducted a retrospective cohort analysis of patients in the United States: one group received care with clozapine while the other group received care using neuroleptics. Patients in the former group were recruited from patients receiving 'humanitarian' treatment with clozapine before it was made commercially available. Members of the comparator group were recruited from two sources: hospital inpatients and from an epidemiological study of tardive dyskinesia. Service utilisation data were collected from medical records. Outcome data were available — using the Brief Psychiatric Rating Scale and the Clinical Global Impression scale — for the clozapine group and those in the epidemiological study, but were not available for hospital inpatients. Assessment of the treatment costs for the two years following treatment showed that care with neuroleptics was marginally less costly than clozapine, although no statistical tests were reported. The treatment costs for both groups declined between the year prior to treatment and two years post-treatment, and the authors state that use of clozapine can reduce overall treatment costs over time. The ratings on the Brief Psychiatric Rating Scale favoured the neuroleptic group when treatment commenced, but the difference was reduced during the course of treatment. The study examines a particularly pertinent question, but deficits in the design — acknowledged by the authors — make the results provisional. These deficits are failure to conduct complementary analysis on the basis of intention to treat (those who discontinued treatment with clozapine were excluded); missing outcome data for a subsample of the neuroleptic group; and selection bias and the presence of other confounding factors.

Davies and Drummond (1993) built on the work of Revicki et al. (1990) to estimate the costs and outcomes for care using clozapine compared to neuroleptics in the UK. Data from the Revicki et al. (1990) study were supplemented with data from the literature and assessments by a delphic panel of psychiatrists and employed in a decision analytic design. The results suggested that clozapine led to an additional 5.7 years of life with either no disability or mild disability. Cost predictions from the model also suggested that clozapine was less costly. An extensive sensitivity analysis was performed which tended to support the initial findings. However, the authors themselves acknowledge the provisional nature of the results due to data limitations and the number of assumptions required to model care. These include deficits in the design of the Revicki et al. study, the assumptions of the delphic panel and the use of values for key variables from the literature.

Both studies provide useful information with respect to a newly available treatment in the absence of data from a prospective study. However, Davies and Drummond (1993) conclude that the results require validation from a properly implemented prospective study.

Discussion. Formal cost-effectiveness analysis requires a single measure of outcome, but as the examples demonstrate there is rarely a single common measure by which treatments can be compared. Service interventions affect many aspects of a person's wellbeing, and also affect their expected length of life. In the examples discussed above, this issue was not a problem because the results were reasonably clear cut. Mangen et al. (1983) demonstrated cost-effectiveness for CPN service because the intervention was dominant with respect to both costs and outcomes. Although a range of outcome measures were employed, the CPN service was at least as good, and in the case of consumer satisfaction was better. Similarly, Davies and Drummond (1993) found that treatment with clozapine dominated neuroleptic therapy in terms of both outcomes and costs. Although the Muijen et al. (1994) and McCrone et al. (1994) study employed a range of outcome measures, no difference was found between treatment groups, and costs were lower (at least in the short term).

A more difficult situation arises where different dimensions of outcome move in different directions, making it difficult to complete a simple cost-effectiveness analysis. Extending the methodology to admit multivariate analyses so as to ensure that outcomes are 'statistically identical' is certainly feasible, and this issue is dealt with in some detail in Chapter 4. An alternative approach is to collapse these different dimensions of wellbeing into a single measure, such as the quality adjusted life year (QALY).

Cost-utility analysis

Cost-utility analysis is a particular form of cost-effectiveness analysis where the QALY is employed as the unit of effectiveness. Ratings for quality of life can be derived using a variety of techniques. Nord (1992) identifies five methods that have been used to elicit preferences for health states from individuals:

A Ratings scales ask individuals to place states on a graphical scale from 0 to 100 with one end representing the most preferred health state and the other end the least preferred health state.
B Magnitude estimation asks direct questions about the relative value of time spent in one state compared to another.
C Standard gambles ask individuals to choose between the certainty of living in a health state versus a chance of regaining full health at a probability p and dying at a probability 1-p.
D Time trade-offs elicit how much time an individual would exchange living in one health state versus being perfectly healthy.
E Person trade-offs ask individuals to choose between curing a certain number of individuals in one disability class versus another number in a different class.

The purpose in each case is to derive a quality adjustment factor for a particular health state relative to death (rated as zero) and perfect health (rated as 1). The survival duration is then multiplied by the quality adjustment factor to derive the number of QALYs produced by the programme. If a health state is rated as 0.5, then a treatment which produces ten years of survival in this state is deemed to be equivalent to a similar programme that produces five years in perfect health. The basis for this adjustment comes from the theory of expected utility (von Neumann and Morgenstern, 1947). However, only one of the techniques — the standard gamble — is actually based within this theory (Torrance, 1986). Nord (1992) and Loomes and McKenzie (1989) question whether an individual whose preference for a health state is rated as 0.5 is actually indifferent between living ten years in this state as opposed to five years in perfect health. Both authors call for empirical testing to see if the results are compatible.

The techniques for calculating QALYs are not all similar. Methods C, D and E employ equivalence techniques where people are faced with two choices for the state of the world. Methods A and B are more abstract and people are asked to place numerical values to clinical conditions. It is unsurprising that the different techniques produce different ratings by the same people for the same health state: the results of studies are sensitive to the technique employed (Buxton et al., 1987; Nord, 1992).

Examples of cost-utility analysis. Cost-utility analysis is rarely employed in mental health care. A recent bibliography of economic evaluations (Backhouse et al., 1992) identified only one CUA out of a total of 60 publications relating to mental health.

Two studies that examine the effects of maintenance therapy for depression both employ cost-utility analysis. Kamlet et al. (1993) used modelling techniques to compare the effectiveness of inter-personal therapy (a form of psychotherapy) with imipramine, both singly or in combination, for similar cohorts of women aged 40. Data from the Pittsburgh study of depression (Frank et al., 1989) were used to estimate the probability of recurrence and the length of time between episodes. Data on expected length of life, likely suicide rate, the cost of treatment and the utility values of differing states of health were estimated using data from the relevant literature. Results showed that imipramine is more cost-effective than inter-personal therapy. However, the authors themselves state that the data limitations and the assumptions employed make this paper more interesting for its methodology than for its results. Hatziandreu et al. (1994) compared maintenance treatment for depression using sertraline with episodic treatment using dothiepin. Two delphic panels — one composed of five general practitioners and the other of five psychiatrists — were employed to provide the likelihood of further episodes of depression and the likely time between episodes. Standard gamble techniques were employed to ascertain how the panels rated various health states. Modelling techniques similar to those employed by Kamlet et al. (1993) show that the lifetime cost per additional QALY gained using maintenance treatment with sertraline is £2,172 for women aged 35.

Both studies illustrate the factors likely to influence the cost-effectiveness of particular treatments. However, the disadvantages are that the models employed are often excessively reductionist, build lifetime models on the basis of current treatment practices, and lack the data that only prospective studies can provide.

A further two studies examine the cost per QALY gained for differing treatment programmes for caring for elderly people with dementia. Wimo et al. (1994) evaluated two forms of community care for elderly people with dementia in Sweden. One group received the standard range of care services, while the experimental group additionally received specialist day care. Randomisation was not possible, so the reference group was drawn from people on the waiting list for day care and matched with respect to demographic characteristics and dependency within a prospective quasi-experimental design. The change in quality of life ratings between entry to the study and one year later were not statistically different between the two groups. However the costs of care were significantly lower in the group receiving day care due to the reduction in the use of institutional care. The study suggests that day care may be more cost-effective, but the possibility of selection bias or confounding cannot be precluded.

Health and social care interventions often have an impact on the families of mentally ill people, particularly where a carer is providing care and support (Fadden et al., 1987; Twigg, 1992; Kuipers, 1993). The position of informal carers has received increased political attention in recent years, and research in this area is growing. Drummond et al. (1991) examined the effects of a service that particularly targets care towards caregivers of elderly people with dementia. An RCT design was employed, and subjects were randomised between standard care services — based largely on conventional community nursing care — and a caregiver support programme. Time trade-off techniques were employed to elicit the caregiver rating of their quality of life using the Caregiver Quality of Life Instrument (CQLI; Mohide et al., 1988). The trial showed a 20 per cent differential between the control and experimental groups in terms of the CQLI. The incremental cost per 'QALY' was $20,000. However, the sample size was insufficiently large to demonstrate a statistically significant difference.

Discussion. Wilkinson et al. (1992) examined the costs of care and derived QALY measures for people in contact with specialist psychiatrist services in Buckinghamshire. They acknowledge that their study is not a true CUA because of the absence of a proper comparator. However, the study usefully identifies the attenuated clinical sensibility of the Rosser index (Rosser and Kind, 1978) with respect to mental health. This is in keeping with the work of Donaldson et al. (1988) who demonstrated that QALYs based on the Rosser index lack sensitivity in picking up changes in quality of life for elderly people (some of whom had dementia) compared to specific scales such as the Crichton Royal Behaviour Rating Scale (Wilkin et al., 1979). Wimo et al. (1994) also report that, although the QALY measure employed in their study showed no statistically significant change between groups, other more specific instruments were able to pick up statistically significant differences.

A person's valuation of a particular health state is unlikely to be independent of the length of time spent in that state. People may provide lower ratings for an adverse health state if they are likely to spend considerable time in that state compared to their ratings if they are faced with a similar state for a brief period. The QALY methodology is based on the separability of the valuation of a health state and the time spent in that state. An alternative approach is to employ healthy year equivalents (HYEs) — again based on expected utility theory — where the expected length of time in the health state is actually integrated into the individual's preferences (Mehrez and Gafni, 1989). Another approach has evaluated healthy active life expectancy (HALE): this concentrates on years of healthy life gained from reduction or elimination of particular health conditions causing disability (Bebbington, 1991, 1992).

Future developments in quality of life measurement. There has been a huge increase in the development and use of non-condition-specific indices and questionnaires for measuring health status. Some general measures include: Short Form 36 (SF36; Brazier et al., 1992), WHOQOL (Sartorius, 1993), and disability adjusted life year (DALY; Murray, 1993; World Bank, 1993).

Quality of life measures specific to psychiatry are also being developed. These include the Lancashire Quality of Life Instrument (Oliver, 1991) and the IHQL-P, a psychiatry-specific version of the Index of Health Related Quality of Life currently being developed by Rachel Rosser, one of the pioneers of quality of life measurement in the UK.

Cost-benefit analysis

The title 'cost-benefit analysis' is often mistakenly applied to all categories of economic evaluation, but it is actually a specific category of analysis, rooted firmly in principles of welfare economics and facilitating the comparison of programmes with a varying range of inputs and outcomes. It is more commonly used in areas other than health care, for example in the evaluation of transport projects.

The strength of CBA is in evaluations where the outcomes of alternative programmes are not identical and cannot be expressed using the same physical measure, or where it is just not practical to measure outcomes in terms of a single effect. There may be multiple effects or they may vary between the different alternatives. Therefore a common denominator is required to facilitate comparison, and in the analyst's search for a common measure of value this is usually money. This requires the translation of physical effects, such as disability days avoided or life years gained, into monetary values. In some circumstances, depending on the nature of the effects, this may be appropriate and it will be feasible to perform this type of conversion. A critical factor in a cost-benefit study is that there must be comprehensive costing of all relevant items, taking in all costs that accrue because of the intervention and all benefits that flow from the intervention. Some of the costs and benefits that should be included are shown in Box 2.2.

The valuation of costs and benefits can follow a number of different methods. Drummond et al. (1987) describe some of the most commonly used valuations:

- ***Market valuation*** — taking actual market prices where they exist, such as for most consumables, or deriving a value by using the price of a similar commodity (informal carer's time could be valued by reference to the wages of domestic help).
- ***Willingness-to-pay estimates*** — these can be assessed either directly by asking people what they would pay to acquire goods or services, a process known as contingent valuation (McGuire et al., 1988), or indirectly by observing their behaviour, such as the trade-offs they make between expenditure and travel time savings, an approach described as implicit valuation.
- ***Policy-makers' views*** — these can be explicitly stated or can be implicit and observed from actions, for example the value of a life could be imputed by the amount of resources devoted to a road scheme designed to reduce the number of fatal traffic accidents.

Box 2.2
Cost benefit: two sides of the equation

Costs	**Benefits**
Capital used	Capital released
equipment and buildings	equipment and buildings
Revenue used	Revenue released
salaries	salaries
extra consumables required	fewer consumables used
Higher workload for staff	Lighter workload for staff
Costs to individuals	Benefits to individuals
dissatisfaction with poor service	satisfaction with good service
time lost	time saved
inconvenience	convenience
personal expenses incurred	personal expenses saved
Less healthy patients	Healthier patients
less relief of clinical problem	better treatment of clinical problem
lower level of care	higher level of care
Decreased productivity	Increased productivity

A fuller description of the relevant costs and benefits can be found in McGuire et al. (1988)

- ***Practitioners' views or professional opinions*** — as above, these may be explicitly stated, or they can be imputed from other areas: Drummond et al. (1987) suggest that the value of an injury could be imputed from relevant court awards of compensation.

It is the evaluation of both costs and benefits in the same unit that is distinctive to CBA. The results of this can be expressed as a simple monetary sum or difference (possibly negative) representing the net benefit or loss of one programme, for comparison with alternatives.

Calculating a monetary sum requires comparison of benefits and costs across the period of interest to decision-makers, that is the whole lifetime of a project or intervention. The general framework for such an evaluation can be expressed as the following equation:

$$V_j = B_j - C_j$$

where:
V_j = Value of project j
B_j = Benefits expected from project j
C_j = Costs expected from project j

If the value of V_j is greater than zero, then CBA rules would say that the project evaluated is worth proceeding with.

This approach theoretically gives guidance on the absolute benefits of an intervention, that is the value of the resources used as compared to the value of the resources that might be saved or created. Within this analysis there is a clear assumption that there is always a 'do nothing alternative' with zero costs and benefits, against which any new intervention is always being implicitly compared. This is a slightly unreal assumption, as there are very few instances where absolutely no intervention would in fact occur.

Cost-benefit ratios are often misleadingly referred to — or indeed employed as — the criterion for comparing alternative projects. This is not simply a misnomer but can actually alter the conclusions reached about the relative merits of competing care interventions. Consider the following example where there are two projects P and Q. Project P incurs costs of £5,000 and produces benefits valued at £7,500; project Q, on the other hand, incurs costs of £2000 and produces benefits of £4,000. If the difference between costs and benefits is employed as the decision-making criterion, then project P will be selected (net benefit of £2,500 compared to £2,000 for project Q). However, if a cost-benefit ratio is employed as the appropriate criterion, then project Q would be chosen because the ratio is greater than the ratio for P (for Q £4,000/2,000 = 2, for P £7,500/ £5,000 = 1.5). The problem with the use of ratio criterion is that its validity rests on two assumptions that rarely hold: first, that programmes for care are divisible — you can have as much or as little of the programmes as you choose; and second, that these are constant returns for scale — the relationship between inputs (costs) and the quantity of output (benefits) remains constant regardless of the size of the programme (Mishan, 1975). Furthermore, the use of the ratio rule is arbitrary, the value of the ratio can be affected by whether a particular component — such as reduced quality of life — is included as a negative benefit or as a cost — through lower productivity. The cost-benefit difference rule is more satisfactory (providing of course that double-counting can be avoided).

A recurring problem in CBA is how to impute a value to human life or illness, an important element in many analyses using this technique. One common method has been described as the human capital approach: human life is valued as the present value of the discounted stream of future expected earnings. This approach has been heavily criticised: it appears to imply that life after retirement age has no value, hence health care for persons over 65 years old can never be justified. There are other distributional and equity implications that it may have for the allocation of health care resources: for example, the implication that higher-income persons should receive higher priority than others. For these and other reasons, the human capital approach has not been widely popular in the evaluation of health care programmes.

Examples of cost-benefit analyses. Weisbrod (1983) conducted a cost-benefit evaluation of the well-known evaluation of assertive community treatment (ACT) compared to traditional hospital-based care pioneered by Stein and Test (1980). The paper identified a series of factors that represented costs and benefits: there were both direct and indirect treatment costs and also such items as 'law enforcement costs' (police, jails, courts, etc.), maintenance costs and family burden costs attributable to lost earnings due to the patient; the monetary benefits came in the form of earnings from increased participation in the workforce. Assessing these figures for the experimental and control groups showed net figures (benefits – costs) of –\$5,729 and –\$6,128 (1973 prices) respectively, representing a saving of \$399 from switching to the community-based programme. The Weisbrod study provides a good example of a well-executed cost-benefit analysis. However, the narrow definition and measurement of benefits which concentrated mainly on increased earnings — with the problems inherent in the human capital approach outlined above — make the results somewhat provisional.

Shifting psychiatric care from hospital to community settings is a long-standing policy aim in the UK. Hyde et al. (1987) compared care in a hostel ward for new long-stay patients with care in conventional wards in a district general hospital (DGH) in Manchester, in a study described as a 'modified' CBA.

Comparison of the revenue and capital costs showed a clear advantage in the cost per inpatient day in the hostel ward compared to the ward in the DGH. Further analyses of the costs to various public agencies for the two years after entry to the study — when patients could move into less supported settings or back to hospital — showed that the costs for the group assigned to hostel ward care were lower, although no statistical tests were reported. Indirect costs such as the burden on carers or the effects of (un)employment were not included because they were believed to be similar in the two groups. The benefits of the study were measured with respect to patients' skills, functioning and absence of symptoms using a number of instruments (Wing et al., 1974; Folstein et al., 1975; Krawiecka et al., 1977; Jablensky et al., 1980; Wykes, 1982). However, these benefits were not translated into money terms and the study could better be described as a cost-effectiveness study, with the hostel ward dominating in terms of both costs and outcomes. However, the authors acknowledge the small sample sizes limited both the validity and the generalisability of the results.

An earlier study — also from Manchester — compared clinical and social outcomes for two groups of patients in the four years after a first admission for schizophrenia using a quasi-experimental design (described earlier) (Jones et al., 1980). One group received treatment in a district general hospital and the other in an area mental hospital (AMH). Data on a wide range of costs and benefits were collected. Interestingly — and unlike many other studies in this area — the study incorporated the effects on other family members of their relative's state of health and the impact of care services. Outcome data were collected using a variety of clinical instruments.

However, the definition and measurement of benefits — and to a lesser extent costs — for the actual calculation of costs-benefit difference were narrow and focused almost exclusively on the valuation of time spent in (un)employment. (The problems with this approach have been outlined earlier.) Furthermore, the use of transfer payments within the cost-benefit framework is problematic (Mishan, 1975; Knapp, 1984). Analysis of the narrow costs to public sector service providers — excluding transfers of money by other government departments — and the outcome data appear to support the authors' finding that the 'DGH(T) unit is economically superior to the AMH' (Jones et al., 1980, p.493).

Another example of this type of approach is the evaluation of nurse therapy in primary care settings for the treatment of neuroses (Ginsberg et al., 1984). The authors assessed the costs and benefits of an innovative approach to treatment using nurse therapists to provide behavioural psychotherapy, compared to an implicit 'do nothing' alternative of continuation of standard care from GPs. Data on a range of costs and outcomes were collected. The analysis showed a decline in costs in the treatment group over the first year of treatment, while costs in the control group rose over the same period. The study provides a useful description of the service use by patients and identifies the disproportionate contribution to costs of a small number of individuals using relatively costly hospital care. However, as in the other studies reviewed, the main benefits included in the cost-benefit difference are those resulting from (un)employment. In addition, insufficient attention is paid to the costs within the period of treatment rather than the change in costs, and the use of cost-benefit ratios as the decision criterion invokes the problems described earlier.

It will be clear from the studies that the measurement of certain less tangible costs and benefits, and the calculation of a monetary valuation, is not unproblematic. Perhaps, for this reason, this type of analysis is rarely performed for specific health care interventions: such evaluations are more likely to adopt other evaluative frameworks, such as cost-effectiveness analysis.

2.6 Incremental or marginal analysis

The DH guidelines recommend that evaluations should determine and report what additional benefit is being provided at what extra cost using incremental analysis of costs and outcomes. These factors are important when considering specific interventions and also wider health care programmes. With any evaluation, the result of a cost-effectiveness analysis will often change when different levels of service provision are costed and analysed. At the margins of provision, decisions on health care are often focused on the level of extra funding for specific options or which of a range of options should receive additional funding. Such incremental analysis can be applied to all of the evaluation techniques described in this chapter.

In a paper discussed earlier (Hatziandreu et al., 1994), incremental analysis is applied to a CUA to determine benefits from switching from episodic treatment of depression using a TCA to maintenance treatment using an

SSRI. The authors calculated the incremental cost per QALY gained from this change as the ratio of the change in lifetime costs over the incremental gain in QALYs. The lifetime costs were £3,407 with SSRIs and £1,648 with TCAs (1991 price levels), and the QALYs gained were, respectively, 14.94 and 14.13. The ratio of the differences is thus:

$$\frac{£3{,}407 - £1{,}648}{14.94 - 14.13} = £2{,}172\ per\,QALY\ gained$$

Switching between the treatment options results in a gain in outcome measure (QALYs), but the cost per patient treated is greater, hence the decision to be made is whether the cost of the incremental gains is acceptable.

The application of such incremental approaches to alternative programmes is described as marginal analysis. It is increasingly being adopted for programme budgeting, where providers are establishing where and to what extent to shift funds between budgets for different programmes. This is dealing with issues at the core of welfare economics, one of the intellectual roots of health economics. By making incremental or decremental changes at the margins of programmes, the objective is to arrive at a position where the ratio of incremental (or marginal) benefits to incremental (or marginal) costs is equal for all programmes under review, a position that may be seen as the most efficient allocation of resources between alternative programmes.

Making these comparisons requires a common measure that can be applied to all interventions, and has led to innovations such as QALY league tables, where health care interventions are ranked in terms of the cost per QALY gained (see Hatziandreu et al., 1994, for an example of a QALY league table). The use of league tables raises the issue of comparability. For example, studies may use different costing ideologies or perspectives, and QALYs may be measured using different techniques, with different ratings obtained for the same health status (Nord, 1992). Furthermore, the incremental changes — in the cost per QALY — may be measured across different interventions. This emphasises the warning in the DH guidelines about comparing results from different studies. Another point made by Gerard and Mooney is that 'QALY league tables do not deal with total programmes' and that they have nothing to offer on the relative efficiency of total programmes. They merely analyse 'what happens if the resources available to the [interventions] in the table are changed on the margin' (1992, p.19). Birch and Gafni (1994) fundamentally question the use of such criteria for resource allocation. However, despite such problems, they do represent an advance on other attempts at prioritisation such as purely epidemiologically-based needs assessment (Donaldson and Mooney, 1991). The area of marginal analysis can also be accommodated within the analytic techniques of the cost function and the production function (see Chapter 4).

2.7 Present and future values

In drawing up its guidelines, the DH also suggests that discounting is employed for future costs and benefits. This reflects the fact that care interventions can affect both present and future outcomes for service users and their carers and thus present and future resource requirements. Commissioners of care often have to trade-off future costs and outcomes against current costs and outcomes of care. Economic analyses therefore have to incorporate these trade-offs within the evaluative framework.

Theoretical basis for discounting. The basis for discounting costs and outcomes is that individuals place different values on similar costs and outcomes in the present than they would for similar costs and outcomes in the future, described as time preference. Generally speaking, individuals prefer income (or rather good outcomes) in the present and prefer to incur costs in the future. For example, an individual would not be indifferent between having £100 now and £100 in one year's time. The individual may require £110 to forgo having £100 in the present, which is known as pure time preference. The person's rate of time preference can therefore be observed to be 10 per cent. A number of additional factors also influence people's decisions relating to preference over time (McGuire et al., 1988; Sheldon, 1992). Myopia in relation to future events (Pigou, 1946) will encourage the irrational discounting of the future too heavily in favour of the present. Uncertainty about future events may also play a part; for example, people may be unsure about whether they will actually be alive in the future. Alternatively, they may also expect real incomes to rise with the passage of time, and therefore additional income may have a marginally lower impact on their standard of living in the future than in the present. An individual will also require additional income in the future compared to the present because £100 forgone today can be invested in capital and may be worth more than £100 in the future.

The state therefore has to set a discount rate for public sector projects to reflect the preferences of its citizens in relation to future costs and benefits. In an idealised economy the interest rate would approximate to this social time preference rate, but market imperfections and distortions cause the two to diverge. The state may also wish to take account of other factors such as excluding the effects of individuals' myopia and to include concerns with distributional issues (see Mishan, 1975; Sugden and Williams, 1978). The distributional issues may be important, as individuals' personal rates of time preference may diverge from the discount rate that they would like to see employed in collective decisions (Sen, 1967). This may reflect concerns for others' wellbeing (Culyer, 1971), or even concern for the wellbeing of future generations (Marglin, 1963).

A dual approach to discounting is recommended by the DH guidelines: first, that all costs and outcomes should be discounted at the Treasury rate

(6 per cent); and, second, that non-monetary outcomes are not discounted. The recommendation reflects the ongoing debate among health economists about individuals' time preference with respect to health as opposed to their preferences with respect to income. Some economists claim that people's preferences for health in the future are greater because when people get older their health is poorer relative to when they were younger. Thus the impact of a health improvement may be greater. Disentangling preferences for health at different stages in life from preference for health over time is another area of debate; however, such issues are beyond the scope of this chapter (see Cairns, 1991, 1992; Olsen, 1992, 1993; Parsonage and Neuberger, 1992; Sheldon, 1992; Murray, 1993).

Examples of the effects of discounting in practice. Figure 2.1 illustrates the effects in practice of employing discounting. Consider two programmes of care where the analysis uses QALYs as a measure of people's relative well-being. Intervention 1 produces more immediate effects in terms of the number of QALYs attained in the early period of treatment, but its effects in the longer term are limited. Intervention 2, on the other hand, produces fewer QALYs in the early period of treatment — perhaps as people adjust to a particular form of therapy which has short-term side-effects — but has a relatively greater impact on health as measured by QALYs in the longer term. Over the entire period — without discounting — intervention 2 produces a greater number of QALYs. That is, the difference in favour of intervention 1 in the early period — equal to area A in Figure 2.1a — is less than the additional number of QALYs produced by intervention 2 in the longer term — area B in Figure 2.1a. However, if discounting is applied (see Figure 2.1b), then the relative impact of intervention 2 in the longer term is reduced. Area D is much smaller than area B. The additional discounted QALYs produced by intervention 1 in the early period — area C — is greater than the additional discounted QALYs produced by intervention 2 in the later period — area D. The rate employed in discounting obviously affects the results: the use of higher rates will favour interventions which produce more immediate gains in health.

Discounting can be most easily applied to cost-benefit analysis where discounting is applied to both costs and benefits; alternatively, the difference between costs and benefits for each year can be discounted. If we update the equation on page 44 to include discounting of the streams of costs and benefits, then the cost-benefit calculation takes the form:

$$V_j = \sum_{t=1}^{T} \frac{B_{jt} - C_{jt}}{(1+r)^t}$$

where:

Figure 2.1
The impact of discounting on health outcomes

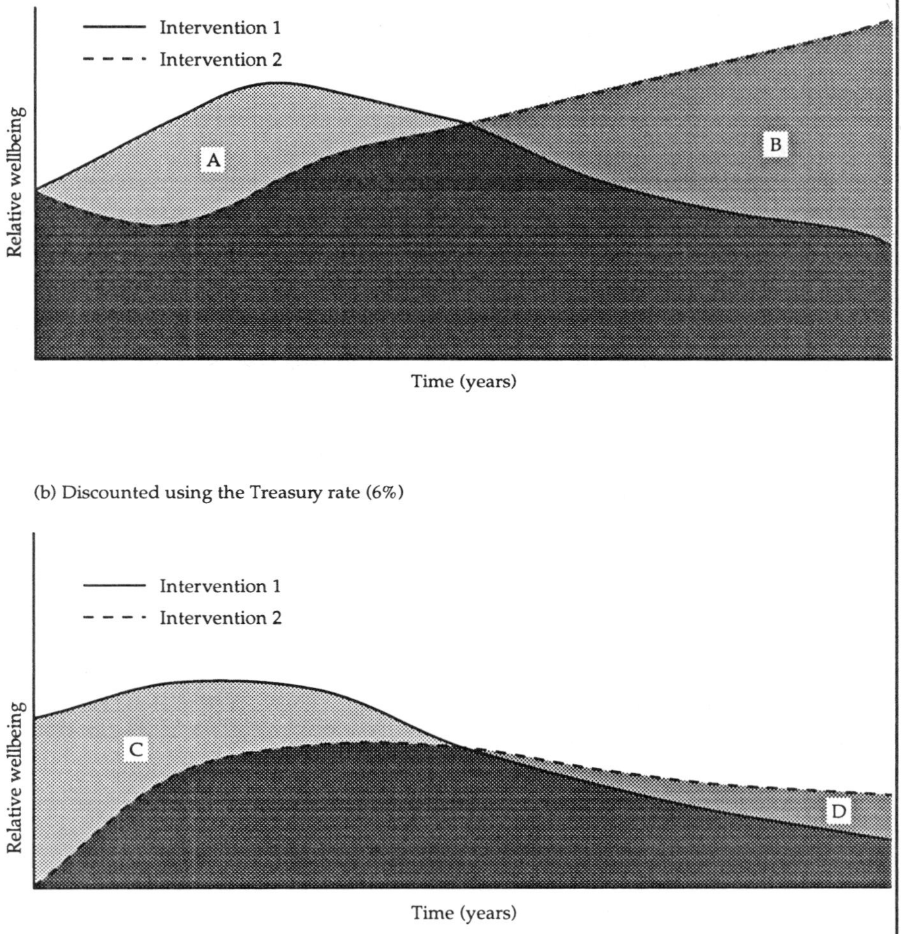

V_j = Value of project j
B_{jt} = Benefits expected from project j in year t
C_{jt} = Costs expected for project j in year t
T = Planning horizon (expected lifetime of project/intervention)
r = Discount rate.

Discounting in cost-utility analyses is more difficult. The appropriateness of discounting QALYs is contentious given that elements such as uncertainty are already included in measurement techniques such as the standard gamble (Nord, 1992; Sheldon, 1992). However, the discounting of outcomes within cost-effectiveness analysis is particularly problematic. For example, the analyst must decide whether it is valid to discount scores on particular psychiatric symptoms scales or if a measure of outcome such as suicides avoided can be discounted.

2.8 Dealing with uncertainty

The technique of sensitivity analysis is advocated to ensure that the 'sensitivity of results to uncertainty in the study is explored'. The analyst must identify areas where data may not be robust or reliable or where specific assumptions on costs and treatment programmes may not be valid in different care settings. The values used in the original analysis (the 'base case') can then be varied in a structured manner to identify the effect on the results obtained.

A number of available techniques can be applied, depending on the problems being assessed and the data available (Briggs et al., 1994, provide a useful review). The most basic form is stepped sensitivity analysis, where the values of specific parameters are adjusted by defined steps in magnitude, with results being recalculated for each change. This may even be multi-dimensional, with more than one parameter being adjusted and results being obtained for variations in input figures. Monte Carlo analysis is a more sophisticated technique where, instead of a series of fixed values for each parameter, the analyst defines a distribution curve which can be varied. A series of random selections are then made from these distributions and used to recalculate results, generating a distribution curve for the results of the analysis. A further potentially useful technique is threshold analysis. Specific parameters are varied in value until a point is identified where the cost-outcome advantage between the two interventions becomes neutral. For example, the cost of cognitive therapy sessions could be varied until there was no difference in cost-effectiveness ratio between cognitive therapy and treatment using antidepressants. In this way, the circumstances can be identified whereby the advantages of a particular intervention over a comparator are no longer present.

Differences in costing or accounting procedures can often significantly affect the conclusions of a study. McGuire (1991) illustrates the importance of sensitivity analysis by examining the assumptions used for estimating the capital cost of public psychiatric facilities in the study of community- versus hospital-based care by Weisbrod (1983) described earlier. Weisbrod used an assumption of 8 per cent for the estimated value of the land and buildings adjusted for depreciation. The finding of the study was that the innovative community programme produced a net benefit of US $399 (1973 prices) compared to traditional treatment. However, McGuire illustrates that if Weisbrod had followed the typical public sector accounting practices of the time and assumed a zero cost for capital, then the net benefit of $399 would have been altered to a net cost of $542. Under these circumstances McGuire questions whether the ACT model would have appeared so attractive to policy-makers. This form of sensitivity analysis is sometimes referred to as 'scenario analysis'. It explores the implications of different 'states of the world', each of which implies different values for the parameters used for the evaluation.

The McGuire study illustrates some important points about the technique of sensitivity analysis. The set of values used ranged from a zero cost of capital, reflecting typical public sector accounting practices, through to 8 per cent per annum, allowing for depreciation and forgone interest on the capital values. These values all reflected some form of current practice and hence represent plausible extremes for the analysis. And in testing the impact of the costs of capital, McGuire identified that the value of this factor was critical to the outcome of the economic evaluation. This picks out one of the important roles of sensitivity analysis, which is to highlight which elements of resource use or of treatment outcomes contribute to the evaluation's results and hence where changes are required if different results are to be achieved.

2.9 Summary

The final item in the Department of Health guidelines advises that care should be exercised in making comparisons between results from different studies, which may use different methodologies and which may be evaluating very different states of the world.

Variations in methodology between studies can be crucially important, given the range of evaluation techniques covered in this chapter: using a different technique may give different answers to the same question with the same data. And differences in the population groups are also very important in mental health evaluations. Alternative studies may use the same economic methodology, but if there are differences in the level of dependency of the client populations being evaluated, then there is likely to be a significant difference in the costs and the results from the economic studies (see Chapter 4).

Even where studies appear to use the same methods, there may be problems with cross-comparisons. For example, so-called QALY league tables have been compiled, ranking health care interventions by the cost per QALY gained. One such table is used by Hatziandreu et al. (1994) in their study of antidepressants as an illustration of why maintenance therapy is a good use of resources. Even the authors admit that not all the studies listed in their table are fully comparable: there are variations in the discount rates used and the range of costs included.

This chapter has given an overview of some of the techniques and concepts used in economic evaluations, both of health care in general and of mental health care in particular. More detailed discussion of all the techniques described can be found elsewhere (e.g. Drummond et al., 1987; Knapp, 1984).

The increasing use made of these techniques reflects a current set of pressures on health care budgets and on health care providers. In the UK, as in other Western economies, governments are anxious to control the seemingly inexorable rise in health services expenditure and so are increasingly drawn to seek the most productive uses for limited resources. Many of the recent changes to the organisation of the NHS and social services have provided more opportunities and greater flexibility in pursuit of these objectives. Health care providers are increasingly able to shift spending between different budgets, seeking the location for spending where it will achieve the greatest outcomes. Where purchasers have access to alternative technologies or modes of care, the techniques of economic evaluation can be used to give comparative assessments in an overt and objective manner, before making final resource allocation decisions.

References

Backhouse, M.E., Backhouse, R.J. and Edey, S.A. (1992) Economic evaluation bibliography, *Health Economics*, 1, Supplement.

Bebbington, A.C. (1991) The expectation of life without disability in England and Wales 1976-88, *Population Trends*, 66, 26-9.

Bebbington, A.C. (1992) Expectations of life without disability measured from the OPCS disability surveys, *Studies on Medical and Population Subjects*, 54, 23-32.

Bebbington, A.C. and Davies, B.P. (1983) Equity and efficiency in the allocation of the personal social services, *Journal of Social Policy*, 12, 309-30.

Bebbington, A.C. and Davies, B.P. (1993) Efficient targeting of community care: the case of the home help service, *Journal of Social Policy*, 22, 373-91.

Birch, S. and Gafni, A. (1994) Cost-effectiveness ratios: in a league of their own, *Health Policy*, 28, 133-41.

Brazier, J.G., Harper, R., Jones, N.M.B., O'Cathain, A., Thomas, K.J., Usherwood, T., and Westlake, L. (1992) Validating the SF-36 health survey questionnaire: new outcome measure for primary care, *British Medical Journal*, 305, 160-64.

Briggs, A., Sculpher, M. and Buxton, M. (1994) Uncertainty in the economic evaluation of health care technologies: the role of sensitivity analysis, *Health Economics*, 3, 95-104.

Burns, T., Raftery, J., Beadsmoore, A., McGuigan, S. and Dickson, M. (1993) A controlled trial of home-based acute psychiatric services. II: Treatment patterns and costs, *British Journal of Psychiatry*, 163, 55-61.

Buxton, M., Ashby, J. and O'Hanlon, M. (1987) Alternative methods of valuing health states, Mimeo, Health Economics Research Group, Brunel University.

Cairns, J. (1991) Health, wealth and time preference, Discussion Paper 07/91, Health Economics Research Unit, University of Aberdeen.

Cairns, J. (1992) Discounting and health benefits: another perspective, *Health Economics*, 1, 76-80.

Catalan, J., Marsack, P., Hawton, K.E., Whitwell, D., Fagg, J. and Bancroft, J.H.J. (1980) Comparison of doctors and nurses in the assessment of deliberate self poisoning patients, in R.D.T. Farmer and S. Hirsch (eds) *Suicide and Parasuicide*, Croom Helm, London.

Commonwealth of Australia (1990) *Guidelines for the Pharmaceutical Industry on Preparation of Submissions to the Pharmaceutical Benefits Advisory Committee: Including Submissions Involving Economic Analyses*, Department of Health, Housing and Community Services, Woden, ACT.

Culyer, A.J. (1971) The nature of the commodity 'health care' and its efficient allocation, *Oxford Economic Papers*, 23, 189-211.

Culyer, A.J. and Wagstaff, A. (1993) Equity and equality in health and health care, *Journal of Health Economics*, 12, 4, 431-57.

Davies, L.M. and Drummond, M.F. (1993) Assessment of costs and benefits of drug therapy for treatment-resistant schizophrenia in the United Kingdom, *British Journal of Psychiatry*, 162, 38-42.

Department of Health (1994) Press release 94/251.

Donabedian, A. (1980) *The Definition of Quality and Approaches to its Assessment*, Health Administration Press, Ann Arbor, Michigan.

Donaldson, C. and Mooney, G. (1991) Needs assessment, priority setting and contracts for health care: an economic view, *British Medical Journal*, 303, 1529-30.

Donaldson, C., Atkinson, A., Bond, J. and Wright, K.G. (1988) Should QALYs be programme specific?, *Journal of Health Economics*, 7, 239-57.

Donnelly, M., McGilloway, S., Mays, N., Perry, S., Knapp, M.R.J., Kavanagh, S., Beecham, J.K., Fenyo, A.J. and Astin, J. (1994) *Opening New Doors: An Evaluation of Community Care for People Discharged from Psychiatric and Mental Handicap Hospitals*, HMSO, London.

Drummond, M.F. (1992) Cost-effectiveness guidelines for reimbursement of pharmaceuticals: is economic evaluation ready for its enhanced status?, *Health Economics*, 1, 85-92.

Drummond, M.F., Stoddart, G.L. and Torrance, G.W. (1987) *Methods for the Economic Evaluation of Health Care Programmes*, Oxford University Press, Oxford.

Drummond, M.F., Mohide, E.A., Tew, M., Streiner, D.L., Pringle, D.M. and Gilbert, R.J. (1991) Economic evaluation of a support program for caregivers of demented elderly, *International Journal of Technology Assessment in Health Care*, 7, 2, 209-19.

Fadden, G.B., Bebbington, P.E. and Kuipers, L. (1987) The burden of care: the impact of functional psychiatric illness on the patients family, *British Journal of Psychiatry*, 150, 285-92.

Folstein, M.F., Folstein, S.E. and McHugh, P.R. (1975) Mini-mental state: a practical method for grading the cognitive state of patients for the clinician, *Journal of Psychiatric Research*, 12, 189-198.

Forder, J., Kavanagh, S. and Fenyo, A.J. (1994) A comparison of sertraline versus tricyclic antidepressants in primary care. I. Efficacy and effectiveness. II. Service use and costs, Discussion Paper 1070/2, Personal Social Services Research Unit, University of Kent at Canterbury.

Frank, E., Kupfer, D.J. and Perel, J.M. (1989) Early recurrence in unipolar depression, *Archives of General Psychiatry*, 46, 397-400.

Freemantle, N. and Maynard, A. (1994) Something rotten in the state of clinical and economic evaluations?, *Health Economics*, 3, 63-7.

Gerard, K. and Mooney, G. (1992) QALY league tables: three points for concern — goal difference counts, Discussion Paper 04/92, Health Economics Research Unit, University of Aberdeen.

Ginsberg, G., Marks, I. and Waters, H. (1984) Cost-benefit analysis of a controlled trial of nurse therapy for neuroses in primary care, *Psychological Medicine*, 14, 683-90.

Goldberg, D.P. (1991) Cost-effectiveness studies in the treatment of schizophrenia: a review, *Schizophrenia Bulletin*, 17, 453-9.

Goldberg, D.P. and Jones, R. (1980) The costs and benefits of psychiatric care, in L. Robins, P. Clayton and J.K. Wing (eds) *The Social Consequences of Psychiatric Disorder*, Brunner/Mazel, New York.

Grad, J. and Sainsbury, P. (1963) Mental illness and the family, *Lancet*, I, 544-7.

Grad, J. and Sainsbury, P. (1968) The effects that patients have on their families in a community care and a control psychiatric service: a two year follow up, *British Journal of Psychiatry*, 114, 265-78.

Häfner, H. and an der Haden, W. (1991) Evaluating effectiveness and cost of community care for schizophrenic patients, *Schizophrenia Bulletin*, 17, 441-52.

Hatziandreu, E.J., Brown, R.E., Revicki, D.A., Turner, R., Martindale, J.J., Levine, S. and Siegel, J.E. (1994) Cost-utility of maintenance treatment of recurrent depression with sertraline versus episodic treatment with dothiepin, *Pharmacoeconomics*, 5, 3, 249-64.

Hyde, C., Bridges, K., Goldberg, D.P., Lowson, K., Sterling, C. and Faragher, B. (1987) The evaluation of a hostel ward: a controlled study using modified cost-benefit analysis, *British Journal of Psychiatry*, 151, 805-12.

Jablensky, A., Schwarz, P. and Tomas, T. (1980) WHO collaborative study on impairments and disabilities associated with schizophrenic disorder, *Acta Psychiatrica Scandanavica*, supplement 285, 152-9.

Jackson, G., Gater, R., Goldberg, D.P., Jennett, N., Lowson, K., Saraf, T. and Warner, R. (1995) The care of patients with chronic schizophrenia: a comparison between two services, *Psychological Medicine*, forthcoming.

Johnson, D.A.W. (1981) Depression: treatment compliance in general practice, *Acta Psychiatrica Scandanavica*, 63, supplement 290, 447-53.

Jones, R., Goldberg, D.P. and Hughes, H. (1980) A comparison of two different services treating schizophrenia: a cost-benefit approach, *Psychological Medicine*, 10, 493-505.

Jönsson, B. (1994) Economic evaluation and clinical uncertainty: response to Freemantle and Maynard, *Health Economics*, 3, 305-7.

Jönsson, B. and Bebbington, P.E. (1993) What price depression? The cost of depression and the cost-effectiveness of pharmacological treatment, *British Journal of Psychiatry*, 164, 665-73.

Kamlet, M., Wade, M., Kupfer, D. and Frank, E. (1993) Cost-utility analysis of maintenance treatment for recurrent depression: a theoretical framework and numerical illustration, in R. Frank and W.G. Manning (eds) *Economics and Mental Health*, Johns Hopkins University Press, Baltimore, Maryland.

Kavanagh, S. and Knapp, M.R.J. (1995a) At the crossroads of health care policy, health economics and family policy: whose interest to provide a family-orientated service?, in M. Göpfert and J. Webster (eds) *Disturbed Mentally Ill Parents and Their Children*, Cambridge University Press, Cambridge.

Kavanagh, S. and Knapp, M.R.J. (1995b) Rationing, market rationales and rationality? The mixed economy of mental health care in England, *Health Affairs*, forthcoming.

Knapp, M.R.J. (1984) *The Economics of Social Care*, Macmillan, London.

Knapp, M.R.J., Cambridge., P., Thomason, C., Beecham, J.K., Allen, C. and Darton, R.A. (1992) *Care in the Community: Challenge and Demonstration*, Ashgate, Aldershot.

Knapp, M.R.J., Beecham, J.K., Hallam, A. and Fenyo, A.J. (1993) The costs of community care for former long-stay psychiatric hospital patients, *Health and Social Care in the Community*, 1, 193-201.

Knapp, M.R.J., Beecham, J.K., Koutsogeorgopoulou, V., Hallam, A., Fenyo, A.J., Marks, I., Connolly, J., Audini, B. and Muijen, M. (1994) Service use and costs of home-based care versus hospital-based care for people with serious mental illness, *British Journal of Psychiatry*, 165, 195-203.

Korman, N. and Glennerster, H. (1990) *Closing a Hospital: A Political and Economic Study*, Open University Press, Milton Keynes.

Krawiecka, M., Goldberg, D. and Vaughan, M. (1977) A standardised psychiatric assessment scale for rating chronic psychotic patients, *Acta Psychiatrica Scandanavica*, 55, 299-308.

Kuipers, L. (1993) Family burden of care: the impact of functional psychiatric illness on the patients family, *Social Psychiatry and Psychiatric Epidemiology*, 28, 207-10.

Loomes, G. and McKenzie, L. (1989) The use of QALYs in health care decision making, *Social Science and Medicine*, 28, 299-308.

McCrone, P., Beecham, J.K. and Knapp, M.R.J. (1994) Community psychiatric nurse teams: cost effectiveness of intensive support versus generic care, *British Journal of Psychiatry*, 165, 218-21.

McGuire, A., Henderson, J. and Mooney, G. (1988) *The Economics of Health Care*, Routledge, London.

McGuire, T.G. (1991) Measuring the economic costs of schizophrenia, *Schizophrenia Bulletin*, 17, 375-88.

Mangen, S.P., Paykel, E.S., Griffith, J.H., Burchall, A. and Mancini, P. (1983) Cost-effectiveness of community psychiatric nurse or out-patient psychiatric care of neurotic patients, *Psychological Medicine*, 13, 407-16.

Marglin, S. (1963) The opportunity costs of public investment, *Quarterly Journal of Economics*, 77, 95-111.

Mausner, J.S. and Kramer, S. (1985) *Epidemiology: An Introductory Text*, 2nd edition, W.B. Saunders Company, Philadelphia, Pennsylvania.

Maynard, A. and Bloor, K. (1994) Building castles on sand, paper presented to the Workshop on the Costs of Schizophrenia, Venice.

Maynard, A. and Hutton, J. (1992) Health care reform: the search for the Holy Grail, *Health Economics*, 1, 1, 1-4.

Mehrez, A. and Gafni, A. (1989) Quality-adjusted life-years, utility theory and healthy-year equivalents, *Medical Decision Making*, 9, 142-9.

Mishan, E.J. (1975) *Cost-Benefit Analysis*, 2nd edition, George Allen and Unwin, London.

Mohide, E.A., Torrance, G.W., Streiner, D.L., Pringle, D.M. and Gilbert, R. (1988) Measuring the well-being of family care-givers using the time trade-off technique, *Journal of Clinical Epidemiology*, 41, 5, 475-80.

Mooney, G. (1992) *Key Issues in Health Economics*, Harvester/Wheatsheaf, London.

Muijen, M., Cooney, M., Strathdee, G., Bell, R. and Hudson, A. (1994) Community psychiatric nurse teams: intensive support versus generic care, *British Journal of Psychiatry*, 165, 211-17.

Murray, C. (1993) Quantifying the burden of disease: the technical basis for disability adjusted life years, Health Transition working paper series no. 93.03, Harvard Center for Population and Development Studies, Harvard School of Public Health, Cambridge, Massachusetts.

Nord, E. (1992) Methods for quality adjustment of life years, *Social Science and Medicine*, 34, 559-69.

Oliver, J.P.J. (1991) The social care directive: development of a quality of life profile for use in community services for the mentally ill, *Social Work and Social Science Review*, 3, 1, 5-45.

Olsen, J.A. (1992) On what basis should health be discounted?, *Journal of Health Economics*, 12, 39-53.

Olsen, J.A. (1993) Time preferences for health gains: an empirical investigation, *Health Economics*, 2, 257-65.

Ontario Ministry of Health (1991) *Guidelines for Preparation of Economic Analysis to be Included in Submission to Drug Programs Branch for Listing in the Ontario Drug Benefit Formulary/Comparative Drug Index*, Ministry of Health, Toronto.

Opit, L.J. (1988) The measurement of health service outcomes, in W.W. Holland, R. Detels and G. Knox (eds) *Oxford Textbook of Public Health, Volume 3, Applications in Public Health*, 2nd edition, Oxford Medical Publications, Oxford.

Overall, J.E. and Gorham, D.R. (1962) The Brief Psychiatric Rating Scale, *Psychological Reports*, 10, 799-812.

Parsonage, M. and Neuberger, H. (1992) Discounting and QALYs, *Health Economics*, 1, 71-9.

Paykel, E.S., Klerman, G.L. and Prusoff, B.A. (1970) Treatment setting and clinical depression, *Archives of General Psychiatry*, 22, 11-21.

Paykel, E.S., Mangen, S.P., Griffith, H.J. and Burns, T.P. (1982) Community psychiatric nursing for neurotic patients: a controlled trial, *British Journal of Psychiatry*, 140, 573-81.

Pereira, J. (1992) What does equity in health mean?, *Journal of Social Policy*, 22, 19-48.

Pigou, A.C. (1946) *Economics of Welfare*, 4th edition, Macmillan, London.

Pocock, S.J. (1991) *Clinical Trials: A Practical Approach*, Wiley, Chichester.

Raskin, A., Reatig, N. and McKeon, J. (1970) Differential response to chlorpromazine, imipramine and placebo: a study of sub groups of hospitalized depressed patients, *Archives of General Psychiatry*, 23, 164-73.

Revicki, D.A., Luce, B.R., Brown, R.E. and Adler, M.A. (1990) Cost-effectiveness of clozapine for treatment resistant schizophrenics, *Hospital and Community Psychiatry*, 41, 850-54.

Rosser, R. and Kind, P. (1978) A scale of valuations of states of illness: is there a social consensus?, *International Journal of Epidemiology*, 7, 4, 347-58.

Sartorius, N. (1993) A WHO method for the assessment of health related quality of life, in S.R. Walker and R.M. Rosser (eds) *Quality of Life Assessment: Key Issues in the 1990s*, Kluwer Academic Publishers, London.

Sen, A. (1967) Isolation, assurance and the social rate of discount, *Quarterly Journal of Economics*, LXXXI, 112-24.

Sheldon, T. (1992) Discounting in health care decision making: time for a change? *Journal of Public Health Medicine*, 14, 250-56.

Stein, L.I. and Test, M.A. (1980) Alternative to mental hospital treatment. I: Conceptual model, treatment program, and clinical evaluation, *Archives of General Psychiatry*, 37, 392-7.

Sugden, R. and Williams, A. (1978) *The Principles of Practical Cost-Benefit Analysis*, Oxford University Press, Oxford.

Thompson, C. and Thompson, C.M. (1989) The prescription of antidepressants in general practice. I: A critical review, *Human Psychopharmacology*, 4, 91-102.

Thornton, J.G., Lilford, R.J. and Johnson, N. (1992) Decision analysis in medicine, *British Medical Journal*, 304, 1099-1103.

Torrance, G.W. (1986) Measurement of health state utilities for economic appraisal: a review, *Journal of Health Economics*, 5, 1-30.

Twigg, J. (1992) *Carers: Research and Practice*, HMSO, London.

von Neumann, J. and Morgenstern, O. (1947) *Theory of Games and Economic Behaviour*, Princeton University Press, Princeton, New Jersey.

Weinstein, M.C. and Stason, W.B. (1977) Foundations of the cost-effectiveness analysis for health and medical practices, *New England Journal of Medicine*, 296, 716-21.

Weisbrod, B.A. (1983) A guide to benefit-cost analysis, as seen through a controlled experiment in treating the mentally ill, *Journal of Health Politics, Policy and Law*, 808-45.

Weisbrod, B.A., Test, M.A. and Stein, L.I. (1980) Alternative to mental hospital treatment. II: Economic benefit-cost analysis, *Archives of General Psychiatry*, 37, 400-405.

Weissman, M.M. and Paykel, E.S. (1974) *The Depressed Woman: A Study of Social Relations*, University of Chicago Press, Chicago, Illinois.

White, E. (1990) Surveying CPNs, *Nursing Times*, 86, 62-6.

Wilkin, D., Mashiah, T. and Jolley, D.J. (1979) Changes in behavioural characteristics of elderly populations of local authority homes and long-stay hospital wards, *British Medical Journal*, 276, 1274-6.

Wilkinson, G., Williams, B., Krekorian, H., McLees, S. and Falloon, I. (1992) QALYs in mental health: a case study, *Psychological Medicine*, 22, 725-31.

Williams, A. (1978) 'Need': an economic exegesis, in A.J. Culyer and K.G. Wright (eds) *Economic Aspects of Health Services*, Martin Robertson, London.

Wimo, A., Mattsson, B., Krakau, I., Eriksson, T. and Nelvig, A. (1994) Cost-effectiveness analysis of day care for patients with dementia disorders, *Health Economics*, 3, 6, 395-404.

Wing, J.K., Cooper, J.E. and Sartorius, N. (1974) *The Description and Classification of Psychiatric Symptoms*, Cambridge University Press, London.

Wooff, K., Goldberg, D.P. and Fryer, T. (1988) The practice of community psychiatric nursing and mental health social work in Salford, *British Journal of Psychiatry*, 153, 30-37.

World Bank (1993) *World Development Report: Investing in Health*, Oxford University Press, Oxford.

Wykes, T. (1982) A hostel-ward for 'new' long-stay patients: an evaluation study of 'a ward in a house', in Wing. J.K. (ed.) *Long-Term Community Care Experience in a London Borough, Psychological Medicine*, Monograph Supplement 2, 55-97.

3 Collecting and Estimating Costs

*Jennifer Beecham**

3.1 Introduction

This chapter has two aims: to describe the instrumentation developed for collecting service utilisation data and to calculate comprehensive costs. The process of costing can be broken down into three connected tasks: the collection of service receipt or utilisation data by individual clients or patients over a consistently defined period; the costing or pricing of each of the services used; and the combination of these two sets of information in order to cost full care packages. Each of these tasks is described below. For simplicity the methodology has been described by reference to a single research project — the economic evaluation of psychiatric reprovision services in North London — although the flexibility of the approach and instrument should be stressed.

3.2 Collecting service utilisation data

In order to calculate the costs of community care a new instrument, the Client Service Receipt Interview (CSRI) was developed. The CSRI built on previous research, particularly on child care and young offender services (see Knapp and Robertson, 1989, for partial reviews), and incorporated relevant parts of previously developed instruments in the mental health field, particularly the Economic Questionnaire of Weisbrod et al. (1980). The instrument needed to be tailor-made to fit the research context. An early requirement was easy adaptability, for the CSRI was also to be employed in the evaluation of the Department of Health's Care in the Community demonstration programme of 1984/88 under which more than 800 people left hospital. Twenty-eight projects were funded to develop community alternatives to long-stay hospital care for adults with needs associated with old age, mental health problems, learning disabilities or physical disabilities (Renshaw et al., 1988; Knapp et al., 1992; Cambridge et al., 1994).

The CSRI was piloted in the summer of 1986 in the Maidstone service for people with learning difficulties. Under this Care in the Community demonstration project, a wide range of services had been developed, affording the chance to test the instrument under different conditions. A second round of instrument refinement was based on use of the CSRI in another three Care in the Community projects. Since its introduction the CSRI has been used in more than 40 evaluation studies (see, for example, Marks et al., 1988; Melzer et al., 1991; McCrone et al., 1994; Donnelly et al., 1994; and later chapters of this book).

In this chapter the description of the CSRI refers to its development for the North London study of people with a history of long-stay hospital residence moving to the community under a planned and well-funded reprovision programme (Leff, 1993). This research is undertaken in collaboration with the Team for the Assessment of Psychiatric Services and some results are reported in Chapter 5. Clients entering the study were likely to have a key carer or case manager, or would be living in a group home where a diary would be kept of residents' activities (especially contacts with health, social care and related services, and with peripatetic professionals). The questionnaire was therefore originally designed for administration by an interviewer from the research team to a principal carer, often a member of staff at the residential unit. On occasions it was impossible to identify a carer, for example when a client was living in an independent flat, and the questionnaire was then successfully completed in an interview with the client. It has also been completed by staff without an interview, although it is not specifically intended for use in that way. Although in some research projects the key questions of the CSRI have been incorporated into other schedules, experience has confirmed that a trained interviewer is needed to tease out accurate and comprehensive information.

This version of the questionnaire is ten pages long and takes about 40 minutes to complete. The questions are largely structured, some with a multiple choice answer format but, given the complexity of community care arrangements, it is not surprising that a few semi-structured questions are also asked. The questionnaire design includes blank spaces to write additional comments or interpret the occasionally confused responses of the interviewee. A series of 'prompt cards' supplements the CSRI. These cards contain indicative lists of accommodation types, different services and social security benefits.

The CSRI collects retrospective information on service utilisation, service-related issues and income. The retrospective period (prior to the date of the interview) is a compromise between the accuracy that comes from not asking respondents to cast their minds back too far and the comprehensiveness which can only come by allowing sufficient time to elapse for some occasional but potentially expensive services to be used. To solve this dilemma, questions on service utilisation are divided into two parts, one covering the previous month — in the North London study this is the twelfth month after discharge from hospital — and the other asking about less regularly received services (such as dentists or GP appointments) over the past twelve months. These durations are not fixed, and can be varied to fit particular uses. In one study a single retrospective period of three months was used (see Chapter 8). Repeated use of the CSRI in a longitudinal design allows one to ask only about the period between interviews, and data collected at all interviews can be recorded on the same schedule. The interviewer can also use data from the previous interview to prompt or guide questions. This was the approach used in the Daily Living Programme (see Chapter 4).

Background and client information. The first section of the CSRI records client code number, gender, marital status and date of birth. For the North London project, questions on past admissions and discharges from hospital, participation in special programmes, registration with GP and medication were included. The opening section also records the date and place of interview and identifies both the interviewee and the interviewer.

Accommodation. Accommodation is usually a major component in both provision and costs of community care. The section thus covers:

- address, partly for the purposes of identifying facility type and budget, and partly because location influences cost and some adjustment may be needed (London is more expensive than the rest of the country, for example);
- tenure of accommodation (council or private rent, residential home, owner occupied);
- a simple description of the size of the unit (the number of different types of rooms and the number of other residents);
- the amount paid by the client or household in rent or other payments; and
- receipt of housing benefit.

Where several clients live in the same unit, some of these questions need be completed only once and can be separated from the other parts of the questionnaire. This approach was used in the evaluations of residential facilities and services provided by Domus and SENSE-in-the-Midlands (Beecham et al., 1992, 1993).

Most clients leaving long-stay hospital care live in specialised facilities such as residential or nursing homes, hostels or group homes. The interviewee is asked for their classification of the facility, although later this may need to be altered, as we use a standardised categorisation based on other information on tenure, staffing arrangements and managing agency. Other clients who have not moved from long-stay hospital care are more likely to live in domestic accommodation, perhaps with other members of their families. The CSRI has been adapted to fit these circumstances by extending the accommodation section to ask about the composition of the household and whether the clients themselves have any care responsibilities. More attention is also paid to how household expenses are covered. These clients are likely to move from one address to another, and the CSRI records such changes of address, including hospital re-admissions. Instability of accommodation obviously complicates the cost calculation, and it can have dire consequences for clients' abilities to work, entitlements to social security or indeed mental health itself.

Employment and income. Research has shown that concerns about money can have an adverse effect on some mental health conditions (Brugha et al., 1985; Granzini et al., 1990). Many people in this client group have low incomes, due in part to the heavy reliance on social security benefits (never renowned for their generosity) and also to problems associated with underclaiming of benefits, low wages if work is found, and unstable work patterns. Information on *employment history, earnings and other personal resources* provides an important data source. Questions on employment are not usually relevant to clients with a history of long-term hospital residence, and it is more important to clarify receipt of social security benefits. Although in strict economic terms these benefits should be considered as transfer payments, not representing an aggregate cost to society, they are good proxies for living expenses as many clients rely on these benefits as their only source of income. In the North London study, few people had any other sources of income and only very rarely had they been able to accumulate any savings. Data on *changes* in benefit status over the past year are also collected. In some of the accommodation units managed by voluntary organisations or by private individuals, carers receive benefits on behalf of the clients. Details of these and of clients' regular outgoings, such as fines, debts or local taxes, are collected in this section.

Former long-stay hospital residents rarely find (open) employment, but employment and its loss are important facets of both service effectiveness and cost. For some applications, therefore, more questions are needed in the CSRI on employment history and current employment activities. The costs of lost employment resulting from mental ill health or inpatient treatment will fall to clients (lower income) and to society (lost production), the actual values to be attached depending on a variety of labour market and individual circumstances (Jenkins, 1985; Thompson and Pudney, 1990; Kavanagh et al., 1993).

Service receipt. This section is at the core of the CSRI, and can take up most of the interview time. Community care is delivered and received in a 'fragmented' system, with many agencies providing a variety of services. There is certainly no standard package of psychiatric care, and so there will be a great deal of variation between clients' packages of care. At this point the questionnaire identifies receipt of services which are not funded within the accommodation budget: either health or social care services available to everybody or specialist mental health services. Information is collected on services which the client leaves the accommodation to attend, such as day centre activities, hospital-based services or appointments at the GP surgery. Some professional support or services are provided for the client at home: for example, home help, community psychiatric nurse or field social worker visits. These service utilisation fields are both divided into two parts; the first allows collection of information pertaining to the twelfth month since discharge from hospital (representing some form of 'steady state', for to record service use since the first day after discharge will pick up the high transition costs which were not the focus of this particular study) and, second, to allow adjustment of this picture to account for regularly but infrequently used services such as outpatient appointments.

For each service outside the place of residence, information is collected on: type of service, such as day care or outpatient appointment; name of providing establishment, for example the name of a day centre or hospital attended; providing agency, such as MIND or the named health authority; professionals involved, such as psychiatrist; frequency of attendance or contact per week; duration of attendance, such as one day or one hour; mode of clients' travel to and from the service; time spent travelling; and any charges made for the service. For domiciliary services the interviewer asks for a similar range of information, but this field includes a question on the total number of clients sharing the service. This is important when a professional visits an establishment to see several clients for a group session (as with occupational therapy) or will see them sequentially (as with GP visits) and the allocation of cost to individuals must take the scope of the visit into account.

Three questions complete this section. One asks about use of personal aids (for example, zimmer frame) or adaptations to property (such as a wheelchair ramp). Although more relevant for other client groups, these are used quite frequently by older people with mental health problems. The next question asks for details of time spent by the *principal paid carer* both on direct care activities (face-to-face contact) and indirect care activities (telephone calls, record-keeping, contacting other agencies to arrange services and the like). Within residential units, little variation in principal carer input has been found between residents. The final question in this section asks whether there has been above-average administrative or managerial involvement with the client. In general, virtually no input from administrative personnel has been found once the client has been living in the community for a year unless a serious threat has been posed to other residents or the wider community.

Informal support. The importance of clients' informal care networks has been highlighted in recent policy documents such as the White Paper on community care (Secretaries of State, 1989), and the CSRI includes questions on the input of informal carers in terms of time spent (frequency and duration of visit) and tasks undertaken (personal care, shopping, domestic tasks and social visits). The availability of informal care for people leaving long-stay psychiatric hospitals appears to be limited (see Chapter 5) although where a number of study members are known to be living with other family members, more weight is given to this dimension in the interview.

Satisfaction with services. Two aspects of satisfaction with services are covered in the interview, and gaps in service availability are identified. Neither is needed for cost calculation, but both offer useful insights. Because the interview refers to a single client, the same GP or day care facility may be considered appropriate or satisfactory for one client but not for another. Service availability is assessed very broadly on a four-point scale: usually sufficient, sometimes insufficient, usually inadequate, or service not required. Quality of contact is similarly measured: usually helpful, sometimes unhelpful, generally unhelpful, or not applicable (where the service is not used). Although this approach is not as detailed as that developed by others (Larsen et al., 1979; Attkisson and Zwick, 1985), it provides a broad picture, sufficient for this evaluation. The final question on the CSRI schedule on gaps in service availability fulfils two functions. It draws the interview to an end by providing a discussion point for the interviewee and, when completed, it obviously provides information on 'service gaps' in the client's total care package, thus supplementing the data on satisfaction. Where service gaps were identified, inadequacy and inappropriateness of day care activities and lack of personal resources were frequently noted. Aggregation of these responses can point to gaps in service provision within a particular district or locale.

3.3 Costing health and social care services

Principles, reality and the model

The second major task in measuring the costs of mental health services is the costing or pricing of the various services used by clients. Ideally, a unit cost is produced which accurately measures what it is supposed to measure, and is correct by the criteria of the theoretical baseline on which it is built. It is usually possible to adhere to principles suggested by theory, but for pragmatic reasons it is often more difficult to achieve accuracy. The aim, however, is for a valid representation of cost, which is at the same time reliable in the sense that the measure used yields the same result whenever it is applied to similar data (Kirk and Miller, 1986, p.19). The following principles, derived from economic theory, provide guidelines for the costing exercise and later sections point to short-cuts which do not contravene these principles. Service costs should be *inclusive* of all service elements, take into account *cost differences*, should be calculated as the *long-run marginal cost* of an *appropriate service unit* and should have taken into account issues of *time*.

For cost evaluations the calculation of costs should encompass the resource implications of all elements of a service even though some service planners may primarily be interested in the cost to their own agencies. Thus the amount of social services finance routed to a voluntary sector day care unit shows the cost of that service to the social services department but does not necessarily give the total (or comprehensive) service cost. Health authority funding, central government grants or private fundraising may also play a part. The calculation of unit costs for services should also take account of cost differences caused by input factors, such as the variation in land and property values throughout the country. Services in London are considerably more expensive than elsewhere in England (Bebbington with Kelly, 1993) and additional salary points may be offered to encourage people to work in particular areas. Client characteristics, service outcomes and changes in client welfare also exert an influence on costs. These are discussed in later chapters (in particular, see Chapters 4 and 6).

Economic theory advocates basing cost measures on *long-run marginal opportunity costs*. In practice, long-run means moving beyond the immediate development of community care which could probably be achieved by using present services more intensively. Since national policy intentions are to substitute community services for most long-term hospital beds, it would hardly be credible to measure only short-run cost implications. Marginal cost reflects the addition to total cost attributable to the inclusion of one more client; opportunity costs reflect the resource implications of opportunities forgone rather than amounts spent. The opportunity cost measures the true private or social value of a resource or service, based on its value in the best alternative use. In a perfectly informed and frictionless market economy, this 'best alternative use value' would be identical to the price paid in the market. Not everything is marketed, not every market works smoothly, and information is rarely complete, with the result that observed prices and opportunity costs diverge. Thus the recorded depreciation payments on capital equipment or buildings will not usually reflect the opportunity costs of using these durable resources, nor will the (zero) payments to volunteers and informal carers usually indicate their social value.

Use of long-run marginal costs allows examination of the difference which the option under study (community-based mental health services) will make to the available resources. Short-run marginal costs are inappropriate for most costing tasks as they only include revenue costs and do not take account of the full costs of *creating* new services. However, knowledge about the present time is more certain than knowledge of the future, so the convention is to use short-run *average* costs which include both revenue and capital elements as an approximation for long-run marginal costs. This is based on the widely-held assumption that, in the long run, relative prices will remain stable although absolute price levels may change (see also Jones et al., 1980; Mangen et al., 1983; Davies and Challis, 1986; Wright, 1987).

Once calculated, long-run marginal costs should be disaggregated to an appropriate unit of measurement to get as close to client-level data as possible. Clients use services in discrete units; for example, hospital service use is counted by the number of inpatient days or outpatient attendances. More complex analyses allow more detailed levels of disaggregation, such as ward-level hospital costs (Haycox and Wright, 1984; Knapp et al., 1990) or the disaggregation of residential care costs, in recognition of residents' dependency levels (Darton and Knapp, 1984; and see Chapter 4).

The final guiding principle for costing concerns timeliness. The year chosen to calculate the costs data should be as up-to-date as possible to enhance the validity and utility of the results. Ideally, service costs information should apply to the time period in which the policy is to be implemented or the service used. Too much delay between policy and the presentation of costs data may mean that intervening variables, such as inflation, render costs data less valid. If different service costs rise by equal (proportionate) amounts, the problem of out-of-date information is less serious, especially if purchasing budgets rise equally. However, costs may change in relation to each other. The annual inflation rate for health services in 1990/91 was 7.4 per cent and was slightly higher (8.8 per cent) for personal social services. But for the period 1986-1989 the health service annual inflation rate was the higher. Decisions based on inaccurate information about relative costs are invalid and are likely to lead to inefficiency.

These principles and the economist's concept of opportunity costs underlie the methodology for costing services and should guide the search for practical solutions to costing problems. Reality presents two main obstacles to achieving an ideal costing: the scarcity of research resources, including researcher time, with which to undertake costing; and the lack or inaccessibility of data. The desire for quick results, presented concisely, to be provided within a limited budget counteracts efforts to achieve perfection. Compromises may be necessary, but these should be made on the basis of the principles set out above.

In translating cost principles into practice, three points can be made. First, the degree of effort expended in picking up cost differences should depend on an estimate of the size of those differences. Employment costs for a health service worker of a certain profession on a certain grade will not vary throughout the country (except where regional weighting applies). However, building costs are likely to vary considerably with local land and property prices. Linked to this point, the degree of effort expended in pursuing costs data should be roughly proportional to the benefit of the data in terms of meeting the objectives of the evaluation or other exercise. Thus, where a service is likely to make up a large proportion of the total cost of care packages, more effort should be made to achieve accuracy.

Second, the level of detail required for the collection of cost information depends crucially on the objectives of the study. A study that describes the costs of services provided by one day activity unit (see, for example, Bebbington, 1993) requires a very different level of disaggregation to that required for services used by clients in the North London evaluation. Similarly, if an exercise is focused on national policies then detailed information on regional variations may be unnecessary.

Third, the methodologies described below will identify some hidden costs. For example, the full description of a social services day care centre will reveal some service elements (costs) that are 'hidden' if only the facility accounts are considered, such as sessional staff funded by the health authority. Similarly, calculation of the long-run marginal costs recognises the cost implications of buildings which do not always appear in revenue accounts. In practice, therefore, costs are only hidden in relation to the starting point of the costing process and are, theoretically, indirect costs.

A four-stage building-block approach to costing services is described below (see Figure 3.1) which also allows classification of services into two categories which determine the choice of costing methodology.

Figure 3.1
Service costing model

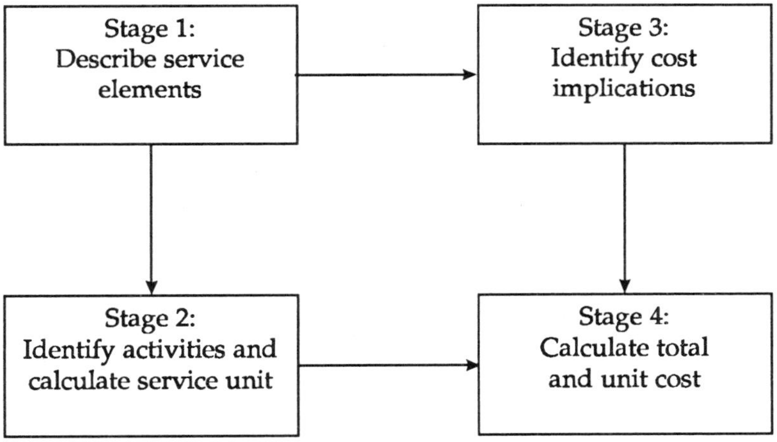

Stage one: identify and describe the elements of the service. Before costing can begin, a detailed description of the service is required. This should include all elements of the service, including those provided by other agencies and those which appear to have no cost relevance. Dimensions might include the building used, the number, grade and hours of staff in different professions and roles, provision of other elements such as food and travel, and the number of clients or the size of the caseload.

This description allows services to be divided into two categories for which different costing methodologies are appropriate: *facility-based services* where groups of clients visit a building in which the service is provided, for example, residential or hospital-based services and day care; and *peripatetic services* which are usually delivered by a single member of staff to individual clients or groups of clients. Clients may be seen either at an office or clinic, but staff also have the flexibility to travel to see clients in their own homes or at other locations. Examples of peripatetic services are social work and community nursing.

Stage two: calculate a constant and relevant service unit to which a cost can be attached. Routinely-prepared expenditure accounts usually span one year and there may be times when it is most useful to present costs information annually. It is often easier, however, to understand the cost consequences of policy and practice if data are presented in smaller units. Moreover, clients rarely use the whole of a service for a year; they use services in smaller units, perhaps seeing a social worker for twenty minutes a month, or attending day facilities for three days each week. For a social worker, therefore, it is useful to calculate the cost per minute (so that this unit can be multiplied by the number of minutes used by each client per week) or per appointment. In contrast, there can be very few purposes for which it would be useful to represent the costs of day care per minute, so a cost per session may be more appropriate.

The choice of a unit of measurement for each service and the method by which it is calculated is an integral part of the costing exercise. The unit should be relevant to the service, relevant to the objectives of the exercise and take into account the nature of the available data. It should also remain constant for each type of service, although elements of the costs may be calculated separately. Thus, a home help visit may be costed as the number of minutes, but the travel costs may be more easily expressed as a cost per visit.

Stage three: identify and collect data on the cost implications of all service elements. For each service element there are different cost implications. A building in which a service is located is usually intended to last considerably longer than one year: it represents a long-term investment of resources. On the other hand, the running costs associated with use of that building are recurrent expenditures, usually presented annually. Provider agencies can be approached for building valuations and facility expenditure accounts which provide the basis for costing. Staff time presents different problems. The cost of employing a member of staff includes their salary, as well as additional costs such as the employer's national insurance contributions. Travel may be a staff-related cost but could also be provided for clients. At this stage *hidden costs* can also be identified, such as costs to the clients of using a service (a charge or personal expenditure) or direct management costs.

Obtaining access to this information is not always easy, and data specific to some items may not be readily available. Information that allows an estimate will be required to set alongside the description of the service. Price indices are also important when data are obtained for a different year to that used to calculate service costs. Earnings indices for public administration, education, health and personal social services (Department of Employment, Department of Health), the retail price index (Central Statistical Office), a variety of local authority statistics (Chartered Institute of Public Finance Accountants) and the Housing and Construction Statistics (Department of the Environment) have also been used in the construction of a unit cost list.

Stage four: calculate the unit cost for the service. The service description and the collection of cost information allow the total cost of the service to be calculated. This final stage is more complex and is explained in detail in the following sections. The aim is to calculate a relevant cost for each service which reflects the long-run marginal (opportunity) cost of an appropriate unit, calculated by dividing the total cost of the service by the unit of measurement.

Costing facility-based services

Box 3.1 identifies the main groups of service elements which comprise a facility-based service and the data requirements that allow a cost to be attached to each element. The text below discusses in some detail the cost calculations for buildings and other *capital expenditure* and continues by examining *revenue cost* implications using routinely-produced annual accounts.

Box 3.1
Costing facility-based services

Service elements	Information required
Building: location and size Equipment, furniture and fittings	Valuation of capital
Building-related expenses: power, rates, maintenance	Expenditure accounts
Full staff complement: professions and grades	Salary-related costs and expenditure accounts
Other service-related expenses: food, stationery, transport	Expenditure accounts
Ex-budget services: other agency-funded resources, direct management, client-borne costs	Salary-related costs and expenditure accounts

Capital costs. Many community services are based in a building which is visited by clients. To estimate the long-run marginal (opportunity) costs of these services, the cost implications of the buildings (capital resources) must be included in the total costs. Furthermore, it is useful if they are calculated in a way that is commensurate with revenue costs, allowing the total costs to be presented as one figure. The convention for calculating the opportunity costs of capital is to assume that the best alterative use would be to invest the resources to earn interest over the lifespan of the building, commonly estimated at 60 years. (Shorter periods, such as five or ten years, can be used for other items such as equipment which reflects their shorter life expectancy.) Thus the value of the resources includes interest which could have been earned had the money not been tied up in buildings. The opportunity cost of capital, therefore, is often calculated as the constant stream of cash payments, or *annuity*, which will deplete the lump sum over the lifetime of the capital (Bromwich, 1976). Annuitisation necessitates the choice of an appropriate value for the resources 'tied up', estimated with regard to the likely future use of the building. Most mental health services are expanding to meet demand and it is appropriate to value buildings at 'new-build' replacement costs. Data available from the NHS capital charging system may facilitate these calculations, but the valuations should be treated with caution (Mayston, 1990). However, many long-stay psychiatric hospitals are due to close and a more appropriate value may be the resale value of the property, adjusted to reflect its future use.

The second component to calculate capital costs is the appropriate rate of interest or rate of return and one that is applicable in the market where the resources would be invested should be selected. For example, in calculating the costs of public services, the real (inflation-adjusted) rate of return on public sector investments is appropriate, currently estimated by the Treasury at 6 per cent (HM Treasury, 1989). Standard interest rate tables show the annuity generated by (the replacement costs of a building estimated at) £1 million is £61,876. This represents the annual opportunity cost of the capital investment in that building.

There are, of course, cases where this approach cannot be used. For example, when costing private sector residential or nursing homes, valuations for buildings and other capital-intensive items are rarely available and convention suggests that the fee or charge (for shelter and care) is set at a level that covers both revenue and capital costs. Given the public policy focus of many mental health cost evaluations and the likely proximity of the fee (as a market price) to the real cost, using the fee to reflect the cost is an acceptable compromise. Similarly, when costing privately-rented accommodation, it is often inappropriate to ask residents or landlords for the value of a property, and convention suggests that the rent (fee for shelter) covers the cost implications of the original capital investment.

Domestic accommodation sits a little uneasily in the category of facility-based services for, although a building is provided, the services relate to that specific facility. Public sector-rented properties, for example, provide shelter for many clients of care services, but disaggregated data on the cost implications of these properties are not available. The cost calculations, therefore, need to be built up from a variety of sources, including the resident's level of living expenses (see below) and information on the value of different-sized properties (available from the local authority valuation officer). In addition, statistics compiled by the Chartered Institute of Public Finance and Accountancy (CIPFA) suggest that the local authorities' housing departments also bear costs of supervision and management of properties, repairs and maintenance, debt management and some miscellaneous expenditure. These data allow the cost of subsidies to be calculated per household. Similar data for housing association-owned properties are available from the Housing Corporation.

Revenue costs. Routinely-produced annual income and expenditure accounts provide the starting point for calculating the revenue costs of facility-based services provided by the public and voluntary sectors. To these accounting costs are added those borne by other agencies — a form of hidden costs. In residential care an example would be forgone local taxes (such as rates and council tax). These are 'forgone' because residents are rarely eligible, so the local authority must bear the cost of not receiving them. It may be necessary to remove items from the revenue accounts. For example, rent paid for the property or expenditure on structural alterations is removed as the cost implications of capital investment have already been costed (double-counting is as great a sin as incomplete costings). However, expenditure on recurring maintenance is a revenue cost. In a residential facility, staff attached to outreach or day care services for non-residents are not resource inputs to the residential service but the costs of another service that is based in the same building. These joint costs are often difficult to allocate but expenditure on these services should be dealt with separately.

Residential services and day activity facilities exhibit tremendous inter-facility variation in objectives, services provided, client characteristics and so forth. Facilities should therefore be costed separately. In costing day care, the description of the service is particularly important as the labels (for example, day care, social club or drop-in centre) rarely describe the service. Some facilities cater for a particular client group, others are open to everyone; some are based in a special building, others are provided in village halls or community centres; the service may be available each day of the week or for just one or two sessions; staff/client ratios vary with the function each facility performs and the clients served. Each of these is a potential *cost-raising factor* so the choice of an appropriate unit of time measurement is crucial. Special attention should be paid to the level of resources which do not come from the main provider agency, such as sessional workers or income generated from fundraising, otherwise total costs are easily underestimated.

Hospitals also show wide variation in purpose and scale, and warrant facility-based costing exercises (Knapp and Beecham, 1990). They may range in size from more than 650 beds to perhaps 50, providing services in acute or long-term care and any combination of in-, out-, day patient and accident and emergency services. Information from individual hospital expenditure accounts is ideal as this allows costs to be more accurately allocated to each of the service units; per day for in- and day patient services and per attendance for outpatient and accident and emergency services. These data are not always available and so other estimates must be made. Unfortunately, since 1987/88 hospital expenditure data have been aggregated at regional level by specialty categories, for example, psychiatric care or surgical specialties. These costs are misleading as they include only direct patient treatment services and exclude support services such as maintenance, estate management, fuel and catering. Furthermore, specialty costs cross *types* of hospital, amalgamating costs from psychiatric hospitals and wards in general hospitals. The Körner Report also recommended altering some of the workload definitions: day patients are now rarely identified separately and may either be regarded as outpatients or inpatients. In 1989/90, the cost per patient day of patients using a bed in the psychiatric specialty was reported as £45.28, and £35.20 for an outpatient attendance (from the FR12A forms submitted by district health authorities to the Department of Health). A brief study of hospitals in five regional health authorities suggests that patient treatment services account for only 71.5 per cent of the total revenue costs so these figures should be adjusted to include an estimate for general services. To the adjusted revenue figure should be added costs borne by other agencies, such as social work provided by local authorities or clients' living expenses, and the resource implications of capital as described above.

Client living expenses. It is particularly important to take into account the client-borne costs of services when comparing different modes of care that include residential services. The calculations are complex as there is a great deal of variation in the extent to which living expenses are met from the accommodation budget. In residential homes the fee paid includes provision of food, furnishings, domestic and social care as well as shelter. The resident retains only a small allowance ('pocket money') for personal expenditure. In other specialised accommodation and care settings (hostels, for example), personal expenditure may have to cover food or other living expenses. In non-specialised or domestic settings (private households), the amount of money available to the client after paying for shelter is larger, but the client will often have to pay other household expenses, such as for heat, light and leisure. These variations have been reduced by the introduction of new financing arrangements under the 1990 National Health Service and Community Care Act. Even so, to ignore the client-borne costs of living expenses would underestimate the total costs of care and, in comparative evaluations, the level of underestimation will vary for each setting.

The calculations become even more complex where the client lives with family or friends. The precise amounts of expenditure or income may be unclear as the allocation of income within the household is unknown. The most practical assumption to make is that total household income is divided evenly between household members. *Family Expenditure Survey* data can be used where more accurate client-based data are not available, but this may overestimate expenditure where a client's income comes mainly from social security benefits. In these cases benefit levels for the relevant year should be used as a proxy for personal consumption costs.

Following the above procedures the total revenue costs per annum can be added to the annuitised capital cost of the facility to obtain the total long-run marginal cost per annum. The choice of a unit to which costs are attached depends on the function of the facility. Thus, for short-term or relief care a resident-day may be appropriate, but for long-term residential care a resident-week may be more useful. Both should be calculated by taking into account the number of residents at the facility's long-term level of provision, multiplied by the number of weeks per year the facility is open. (There are actually 52.18 weeks per year.) This is the divisor with which the *unit cost* is calculated.

Accurate recognition of the cost implications of these facility-based services cannot be overestimated as these services are costly to provide. For example, in 1989/90 adult residential services still absorbed nearly 30 per cent of the personal social services gross current expenditure (Department of Health, 1991). In addition, the type of accommodation (and therefore the cost) affects the other range of services a client might receive. Thus, residents of a nursing home would be unlikely to receive home help visits as domestic services are usually provided within the residential service. People living in private households rarely receive waking night cover from professional staff, but may use several other peripatetic services.

Costing peripatetic staff

As with facility-based services, the focus of the evaluation guides pragmatic decisions on the level of detail required to cost peripatetic staff. The methodology set out below illustrates the building-block approach with national data and can be used for a range of staff groups, such as field social workers, community nurses, chiropodists and home helps. The costs are calculated cumulatively using the elements identified at stage one (see Box 3.2).

Salary-related costs. The decision to use national-level data on *pay scales* can short-cut a number of research tasks without losing too much detail. Many staff groups have nationally-applicable pay and conditions and it is often difficult to identify precise pay scale points for different staff members. If the costing exercise is focused on one local authority, the following methodology can still be used, but local working conditions should be substituted for the national-level data.

Most categories of employees are paid on a variety of scales, each with

Box 3.2
Costing peripatetic services

Service elements	Information required
Staff: profession, grade, hours	Salary-related costs (salary scales, regional weighting, NI and superannuation rates, travel and subsistence payments)
Office/clinic: location, size	Valuation of capital
Building-related expenses: power, rates, maintenance	Expenditure accounts
Service-related expenses: supervision and clerical support	Salary-related costs and expenditure accounts

incremental points. The appropriate salary level is calculated using either the likely grade for staff providing care to the client group under study or the numbers of staff in each grade. In the latter case, the average pay in each grade is multiplied by the number of whole-time equivalent staff in that grade. Dividing the total pay by the total number of whole-time equivalent staff gives a weighted average pay. The appropriate *regional weighting* is added and then the percentage rate for employer's *national insurance* and *superannuation contributions* for each professional group.

Although staff do not always travel to provide care for clients, the payment of *travel and subsistence expenses* is a cost to the service provider. The approach taken in the North London study was to spread the cost of travel evenly throughout the cost of the service and add the travel time to contact time. An alternative approach, requiring much more detail on staff activities, is to calculate the cost of travel per visit separately, perhaps the relevant bus fares, and add this to the cost of each visit.

Overheads. The immediate overheads are the support provided by clerical and supervisory staff (calculated as salary-related costs) and the resource implications of the office or clinic base. The capital cost implications can be calculated using the methodology described for facility-based services where an appropriate size of office space is attributed to each staff member and multiplied by the average value of office space for that year. Running costs for the building, such as fuel, can be apportioned from the revenue accounts.

The focus of the evaluation again dictates what other overheads should be included in the cost calculations. For example, should the costs of the finance department, the social services director or community care planning groups be included? What are the cost implications of the purchaser/provider split in health services? There obviously must be a practical limit to any service costing exercise. These administrative sections may have an important support function for, say, a social worker, but the cost of this support will be only a small proportion of the cost of providing a social work visit. Unless this disaggregation task has already been adequately undertaken, the benefit of such a time-consuming allocation of resources is too small for most evaluations. Moreover, with a public policy focus, the assumption is that, in the long run, the input from these sections into individual services is unlikely to change as a result of an expansion of the service.

There are two exceptions to this approach: first, where there is a specific input into a particular client's care package, perhaps where an assistant director chairs a meeting or authorises an unusual course of action; and second, where a middle-management arrangement has been set up to oversee a particular service. A new post might have been created (costed as peripatetic services) or a resource centre developed (costed as a facility-based service) which provides centrally-based services. It is often difficult to apportion these costs in any other way than allocating them equally across service users.

A top-down approach

For some services it is more difficult to build up an average cost per minute or per consultation using the above procedures because of the complexity of payment for these professionals. General practitioner services (provided by family health services authorities) usefully illustrate this point as their income (as non-fundholders) largely depends on the amount and type of work done. There are different fees for different types of service, such as the removal of stitches or for the provision of contraceptive services, and higher capitation fees for patients aged over 65. There are different fixed payments depending on seniority, or whether the GP is on study leave. GPs are also directly reimbursed for some practice expenses including some staff, premises, improvements to premises, drugs and dispensing, and the level of reimbursement varies with the nature and location of the practice. A pragmatic solution to this complex problem is to take the total cost of general medical practitioner services for the appropriate year and to divide the cost by the number of practitioners.

Similarly, data on the time implications of general practitioner activities are not easy to collect so global estimates of the likely length of appointments were examined. Using data in the Butler and Calnan study (1987) on GP workloads, Allen (1988) calculated that GPs spend 9.3 minutes on the care of a patient seen in surgery, and 27.1 minutes for a home visit, including time spent on administration, reading, writing, training and travel where appropriate. These figures compare well with the other estimates (Department of Health and Social Security, 1987). Using the cost (calculated per minute) and these activity data, a unit cost per surgery or domiciliary appointment is calculated.

3.4 Costing full care packages

The Client Service Receipt Interview is a means to an end rather than an end in itself: the interview collects the data that enable packages of care to be identified. This information must be manipulated and joined with information on the costs of those services. This data preparation stage allows service receipt to be allocated at a constant unit over a defined period of time. The unit of calculation for service receipt should be the same as that used for the calculation of service costs. The period of time is often defined by the research: for the North London community reprovision study the follow-up period was one year after discharge from hospital. Data are now collected for five years after discharge. Follow-up periods of between three and 36 months have been defined in other research projects.

These data manipulation tasks employ a particular methodology. To facilitate the process, the Service Entry and Numeration form (SEAN) has been developed which enables the components of a client's package of care to be listed, alongside the amount of that service received. It is most usefully presented as receipt per week for each individual. The third and final task is also completed on the SEAN form, to combine each client's average weekly use of services with the unit costs for each service so as to calculate total care cost. A computerised version of the SEAN form reduces much of the routine work where large samples are involved, but it requires careful modification to ensure detailed information is not lost.

In the North East Thames Regional Health Authority evaluation in North London, client-level service receipt data were collected with the aim of calculating how much care each client received from each service or professional in a week, although adjusted for less frequently-used services. For facility-based services, this service receipt calculation can be complex. Although clients may use the services in discrete units (per week for accommodation services, per day for hospital care, or per session for day care activities), they do not always use them at a constant rate. Thus, a client may move to three or four different accommodation types within the year or may have been re-admitted to hospital for one or more short stays. The cost consequences of such patterns of service receipt must be incorporated into the average weekly service receipt picture. Thus, for example, four outpatient appointments per year equals 0.077 appointments per week. Each client in the study is likely to exhibit a different service profile and particular care must be taken to ensure the pattern of use of these costly elements is calculated correctly.

The most appropriate unit to which the costs of peripatetic staff can be attached is one minute. This allows building-related costs to be calculated over a whole year, as most premises function throughout the year, and salary-related costs to be divided by the official length of the working year for each professional. The working year can be based on contracted hours, thus allowing for holidays and statutory days leave, or may also include an estimation for sick leave and other absences. The most basic unit cost, therefore, is a cost per minute which can be multiplied up in recognition of service receipt data or the objectives of the exercise. For example, where a client sees a social worker once during a thirteen week period for 30 minutes, the social worker's contact time per week is calculated as 30 minutes divided by 13 (weeks) or 2.31 minutes. If a domiciliary visit is made, travel time might take an extra 20 minutes. The length of time spent on providing care would then be 50 minutes, or 3.85 minutes per week. If several clients were seen on one visit, the time spent providing care is divided by the number of clients seen.

If cost per minute is not appropriate for the work undertaken, then a relevant unit can be calculated from activity data. For example, if the only information available is on face-to-face contact, this may underestimate the total cost of providing social work support. Other dimensions of workload activity may be: time spent on non-direct client-based activities such as case conferences, writing reports or advocacy; time spent travelling to appointments; time spent attending meetings; and time spent on general administration. Dunnel and Dobbs (1983) provide useful data on the time implications of nurse's activities as well as methods of travel and office allocations, but there is little activity information for local authority staff or most mental health services staff.

3.5 Summary

The activities undertaken within the process of costing care packages are threefold: the collection of service related data; costing of services used; and the combination of these data at the individual level. These activities provide the structure for this chapter.

The chapter began with a description of the interview schedule developed to gather information on the services used to support individuals in the community. It is a comprehensive approach, spanning all the areas of community living which have cost implications: accommodation, employment, income, and use of generic and specialist health and social care services, including hospital services.

The activities described in the section on costing services provide a clear and consistent methodology which is a good compromise between economic ideals and the constraints imposed by the real world. The final section described the activities undertaken to manipulate service receipt and costs data to calculate the total, comprehensive costs of care packages for each individual in the study. It is only by maintaining the focus on the individual that the variation in costs of community care can be examined.

Note

* This chapter is based on two previously published chapters: Beecham and Knapp (1992); and Allen and Beecham (1993).

References

Allen, C. (1988) Average time spent by general practitioners on surgery consultations and home visits, Discussion Paper 592, Personal Social Services Research Unit, University of Kent at Canterbury.

Allen, C. and Beecham, J.K. (1993) Costing services: ideals and reality, in A. Netten and J.K. Beecham (eds) *Costing Community Care: Theory and Practice*, Ashgate, Aldershot.

Attkisson, C.C. and Zwick, R. (1985) The Client Satisfaction Questionnaire: psychometric properties and correlation with service utilization and psychotherapy outcome, *Evaluation and Program Planning*, 5, 233-7.

Bebbington, A.C. (1993) Calculating unit costs of a centre for people with AIDS/HIV, in A. Netten and J.K. Beecham (eds) *Costing Community Care: Theory and Practice*, Ashgate, Aldershot.

Bebbington, A.C. with Kelly, A. (1993) Area differentials in labour costs of personal social services and their relevance to Standard Spending Assessments, Discussion Paper 898, Personal Social Services Research Unit, University of Kent at Canterbury.

Beecham, J.K. and Knapp, M.R.J. (1992) Costing psychiatric interventions, in G. Thornicroft, C. Brewin and J. Wing (eds) *Measuring Mental Health Needs*, Oxford University Press, Oxford.

Beecham, J.K., Hallam, A., Knapp, M.R.J. and Cambridge, P. (1992) The costs of care for people with dual sensory impairment, Discussion Paper 891, Personal Social Services Research Unit, University of Kent at Canterbury.

Beecham, J.K., Cambridge, P., Hallam, A. and Knapp, M.R.J. (1993) The costs of Domus care, *International Journal of Geriatric Psychiatry*, 8, 10, 827-831.

Bromwich, M. (1976) *The Economics of Capital Budgeting*, Penguin, Harmondsworth.

Brugha, T., Bebbington, P., Tennant, C. and Hurry, J. (1985) The list of threatening experiences: a subset of twelve life event categories with considerable long-term contextual threat, *Psychological Medicine*, 15, 189-94.

Butler, J. and Calnan, M. (1987) *Too Many Doctors?*, Gower, Aldershot.

Cambridge, P., Hayes, L. and Knapp, M.R.J. (1994) *Care in the Community: Five Years On*, Arena, Aldershot.

Darton, R.A. and Knapp, M.R.J. (1984) The cost of residential care for the elderly: the effects of dependency, design and social environment, *Ageing and Society*, 4, 157-83.

Davies, B.P. and Challis, D.J. (1986) *Matching Resources to Needs in Community Care*, Gower, Aldershot.

Department of Health (1991) Memorandum laid before the Health Committee, House of Commons Paper 408, HMSO, London.

Department of Health and Social Security (1987) *General Medical Practitioners' Workload*, report prepared for Doctors and Dentists' Review Body, 1985-86, HMSO, London.

Derbyshire, M. (1987) Statistical rationale for grant related expenditure assessment (GREA) concerning personal social services, *Journal of the Royal Statistical Society*, 150, 309-33.

Donnelly, M., McGilloway, S., Mays, N., Perry, S., Knapp, M.R.J., Kavanagh, S., Beecham, J.K., Fenyo, A.J. and Astin, J. (1994) *Opening New Doors: An Evaluation of Community Care for People Discharged from Psychiatric and Mental Handicap Hospitals*, HMSO, London.

Dunnel, K. and Dobbs, J. (1983) *Nurses Working in the Comunity*, Office of Population Censuses and Surveys, Social Survey Division, HMSO, London.

Granzini, L., McFarland, B.H. and Cutler, D. (1990) Prevalence of mental disorders after catastrophic financial loss, *Journal of Nervous and Mental Disease*, 178, 680-85.

Haycox, A. and Wright, K.G. (1984) Public sector costs of caring for mentally handicapped persons in a large hospital, Discussion Paper 1, Centre for Health Economics, University of York.

H.M. Treasury (1989) Discount rates in the public sector, Press Office circular 32/89, 5 April.

Jenkins, R. (1985) Minor psychiatric morbidity in employed young men and women and its contribution to sickness absence, *British Journal of Industrial Medicine*, 42, 147-54.

Jones, R., Goldberg, D.P. and Hughes, H. (1980) A comparison of two different services treating schizophrenia: a cost-benefit approach, *Psychological Medicine*, 10, 493-505.

Kavanagh, S., Schneider, J., Knapp, M.R.J., Beecham, J.K. and Netten, A. (1993) Elderly people with cognitive impairment: costing possible changes in balance of care, *Health and Social Care in the Community*, 1, 69-80.

Kirk, J. and Miller, M.L. (1986) Reliability and validity in qualitative research, *Qualitive Research Methods*, Volume 1, Sage Publications, Beverly Hills, California.

Knapp, M.R.J. and Beecham, J.K. (1990) Costing mental health services, *Psychological Medicine*, 20, 893-908.

Knapp, M.R.J. and Robertson, E. (1989) The cost of services, in B. Kahan (ed.) *Child Care Research, Policy and Practice*, Open University Press, Buckingham.

Knapp, M.R.J., Beecham, J.K., Anderson, J., Dayson, D., Leff, J., Margolius, O., O'Driscoll, C. and Wills, W. (1990) Predicting the community costs of closing psychiatric hospitals, *British Journal of Psychiatry*, 157, 661-70.

Knapp, M.R.J., Cambridge, P., Thomason, C., Beecham, J.K., Allen, C. and Darton, R.A. (1992) *Care in the Community: Challenge and Demonstration*, Ashgate, Aldershot.

Larsen, D.H., Attkisson, C.C., Hargreaves, W.A. and Ngeyen, T.D. (1979) Assessment of client/patient satisfaction: development of a general scale, *Evaluation and Program Planning*, 2, 197-207.

Leff, J. (ed.) (1993) *Evaluating Community Placement of Long-Stay Psychiatric Patients, British Journal of Psychiatry*, 162, Supplement 19.

McCrone, P., Beecham, J.K. and Knapp, M.R.J. (1994) Community psychiatric nurse teams: cost effectiveness of intensive support versus generic care, *British Journal of Psychiatry*, 165, 218-21.

Mangen, S.P., Paykel. E.S., Griffith, J.H., Burchall, A. and Mancini, P. (1983) Cost-effectiveness of community psychiatric nurse or out-patient psychiatrist care of neurotic patients, *Psychological Medicine*, 13, 407-16.

Marks, I., Connolly, J. and Muijen, M. (1988) The Maudsley Daily Living Programme: a controlled cost-effectiveness study of community-based versus standard in-patient care of serious mental illness, *Bulletin of the Royal College of Psychiatrists*, 12, 22-3.

Mayston, D. (1990) NHS resourcing: a financial and economic analysis, in A.J. Culyer, A.K. Maynard and J.W. Posnett (eds) *Competition in Health Care: Reforming the NHS*, Macmillan, Basingstoke.

Melzer, D., Hale, A.S., Malik, S.J., Hogman, G.A. and Wood, S. (1991) Community care for patients with schizophrenia one year after hospital discharge, *British Medical Journal*, 303, 1023-6.

Renshaw, J., Hampson, R., Thomason, C., Darton, R.A., Judge, K. and Knapp, M.R.J. (1988) *Care in the Community: The First Steps*, Gower, Aldershot.

Secretaries of State (1989) *Caring for People: Community Care in the Next Decade and Beyond*, Cm 849, HMSO, London.

Thompson, D. and Pudney, M. (1990) *Mental Illness: The Fundamental Facts*, Mental Health Foundation, London.

Weisbrod, B.A., Stein, L.I. and Test, M.A. (1980) Alternatives to mental hospital treatment. II: Economic benefit — cost analysis, *Archives of General Psychiatry*, 37, 400-405.

Wright, K.G. (1987) *Cost-Effectiveness in Community Care*, Centre for Health Economics, University of York.

4 Costs and Outcomes: Variations and Comparisons

Martin Knapp

4.1 Variations in principle

No two individuals are identical. Although there may often be a core of similarity, no two mental health service users of a given facility or programme are likely to present exactly the same symptoms, circumstances, needs or preferences. Service responses may show less variability than are to be found for individual characteristics of health or quality of life, because they are constrained by resource availability, professional norms, the weight of accumulated evidence on effectiveness or efficacy, and perhaps the simple desire for consistency. Nevertheless, variations in service use and cost between users, facilities, providers and locations will usually be quite marked — as will be illustrated later in the chapter — and the health, behavioural and quality of life consequences of service use will also vary.

The starting point for this chapter is that cost and outcome variations of this kind should not be ignored. They warrant comment, analysis and interpretation. They can and should be explored for policy and practice insights, both short-term and longer-term, and they can offer assistance when seeking to make generalisations or extrapolations from existing evidence to other groups of users, facilities or services.

What causes costs and outcomes to vary? Service or treatment types and levels are responses to individual needs, albeit imperfect responses in any real mental health system. Because needs vary, so too will costs. And because individual circumstances and service responses vary, so too — usually — will outcomes. The key to recognition of these variations and their sources

— if it is not already obvious — is the set of linkages between needs, resources and outcomes, located within contexts where external factors can also have an influence. The production of welfare framework, introduced in Chapter 1, offers one way to identify these linkages or to organise them conceptually. The framework thus helps us to hypothesise reasons for cost and outcome variations.

Cost variations. Unless the organisation of mental health care is so completely routinised or inflexible that it utterly disregards individual needs, direct service costs will partly reflect client differences. But health and social care decision-making is inevitably influenced by service availability and service characteristics, and so these direct costs will also be influenced by the preferences and perspectives of professionals and agencies, organisational scale, and the characteristics of local communities and economies. Another source of service cost variations could be provider efficiency. In addition, users' own circumstances, characteristics, experiences and preferences will be likely to push up or pull down the *indirect* costs associated with mental health problems and their treatment: assistance with housing may be needed; a user may need carer support and a carer may need agency support; employment may have been lost or a supported work programme recently started; offending may have become a problem warranting police intervention.

Outcome variations. Individual users of mental health services or general medical services may perhaps display similar clinical symptoms or behavioural traits, but their personalities, social and economic circumstances, previous care experiences, and family or household compositions will differ. Although psychiatric and other services will be working to help all of these people regain full health, the achievements will not be uniform. Moreover, the differences in health status (broadly defined) between the beginning and end of care or treatment — which is how *outcomes* tend to be defined — will be likely to show even more variation. Outcome variations thus stem from a combination of influences: personal characteristics and preferences (of users, carers and staff members) , baseline needs, the quality and quantity of services offered and services used (hence the degree of compliance), agency efficiency, and a host of other factors.

The number of potential influences on the costs and outcomes of mental health interventions clearly makes interpretation difficult. Methodologically, this either necessitates a research design which removes or controls for all major sources of variation (known and unknown) bar one in order to reveal the influence of the exceptional factor which is permitted to vary — which is basically the approach used in the classic randomised controlled trial (RCT) — or it is necessary to use multivariate statistical methods to explore and seek to 'explain' multiple variations. In fact, the two are not mutually exclusive, and exploring multivariate influences on cost or outcome *within* a randomised controlled design is often feasible and should normally be informative. Both the randomised trial and the multivariate statistical analysis have their drawbacks, and there is always the possibility that using the two in combination could compound the problems or more than double the errors, but as a general rule the two should complement and cross-fertilise. Moreover, the multivariate interrogation of data is often the only sensible way to uncover the sources of differences in cost or outcome in the absence of a randomised design.

The aim of this chapter, therefore, is to introduce and illustrate frameworks within which to examine variations in cost and outcome. The chapter does not pretend to be an introduction to research design *per se*, nor would that be needed in a book of this kind. What *is* needed is appreciation on the part of people who undertake or utilise research that, first, cost and outcome variations are often — perhaps usually — immense; and, second, that these variations should, where possible, be understood through further analysis.

4.2 Ignore, override or explore?

Three options present themselves when faced with cost or outcome variations. The variations can be *ignored* (which is very common, often inevitable, but rarely advisable), or they can be *overridden* in a purposive and informed way (which is necessary or at least understandable in certain circumstances, but not always defensible), or they can be *explored* with a cost or production (outcome) function. The second and third of these — one through a randomised controlled trial, the other built on an estimated cost or production function (perhaps within an RCT: the two are not mutually exclusive) — allow variations to be *'partialled out'*. The randomised trial removes all but one of the hypothesised sources of variation — both the known and the unknown factors. Subject to the availability of data (and thus subject also to knowledge of likely cost-raising factors), the multivariate cost or production (outcome) function allows multiple marginal effects to be examined (after some straightforward differential calculus) to remove influences on cost or outcome which are not of primary interest. Because most mental health care interventions are neither monotechnic nor uniform (as are, for example, some surgical procedures), and because they are liable to be influenced by a number of factors extraneous to the interventions themselves, the RCT could be argued to be less than fully adequate in some contexts if it is not developed further.

In the next section, examples are given of two studies which have 'overridden' within-sample variations. Each offers a good illustration of how an economic evaluation can supplement a clinical evaluation, within a randomised design, at relatively little additional research cost. Both examples are drawn from PSSRU/CEMH research, but good illustrations could have been offered from elsewhere (such as the studies by Weisbrod et al., 1980; Burns et al., 1993; or those described in Chapter 2). The emphasis is then on the *exploration* option, with illustrations in section 4.4 of the benefits and uses of cost and production functions. (Most attention will be paid to cost functions.) However, it is important not to misunderstand the thrust of the argument. It is most certainly *not* correct to argue that the randomised trial is, in any new sense, 'wrong'. But it *is* valid to argue that many RCTs fail to exploit the opportunities offered by their data to address a wider set of policy and practice questions.

4.3 Overriding the variations

The RCT purposively overrides all but one source of (hypothesised) variation: the therapy, drug, practice or accommodation alternative which initiated or justified the trial. It will be recalled from Chapter 1 that making like-with-like comparisons is one of the core principles suggested for economic evaluations. Thus the need to avoid spurious comparisons is as great in economic research as in any clinical or social evaluation, and some of the methods employed to ensure like-with-like comparisons are similar. When circumstances allow, the randomised controlled design will ensure comparability. Quasi-experimental designs with matched or statistical controls can also be employed — as outlined in Chapter 2 — and the multivariate methods described later can be viewed as forms of statistical control.

Two examples are given here of economic evaluations conducted with an RCT design — one of a reorganised community psychiatric nursing service, the other of an intensive home-based alternative to standard hospital-based care. Both examples illustrate *both* the comparative ease with which an economic evaluation can supplement a clinical study *and* the need for further multivariate investigation.

Alternative community nursing arrangements

In 1989, the community psychiatric nursing (CPN) service was reorganised in Greenwich, with individual staff acting as care (case) managers and client advocates. This new arrangement was compared with the standard organisation of 'generic' CPN services in a randomised controlled study, with a focus on their activities, and the associated costs and effects. Eighty-two people referred to the specialist psychiatric services by consultant psychiatrists or ward teams at the point of discharge from hospital (usually after short stays) or during community residence at the point at which CPN support was considered to be necessary met the study criteria (psychotic disorder, duration of illness of more than two years, more than two hospital admissions during the previous two years, aged 18-64). They were randomly allocated to either the traditional, generic CPN team or a new community support team (CST). Tests revealed no significant differences between the two samples at entry to the study (Muijen et al., 1994).

Each person was assessed four times: at baseline, and after six, twelve and eighteen months. Data were gathered on clinical outcomes, social and behaviourial functioning, family burden and consumer satisfaction. At entry to the study, service use data were collected retrospectively for the previous three months. At subsequent interviews, service use data referred to the period since last interview. Data were also collected from case records on frequency and duration of CPN service receipt, including domiciliary and office visits, and medication received.

Muijen et al. (1994) report marked differences between the CST and generic CPN services in terms of the number and type of contacts, but no differences in numbers of admissions, length of stay, social functioning, psychopathology, or users' and relatives' satisfaction. (However, van Os et al., 1994, suggest that these negative findings may not be entirely justified.) The economic evaluation — reported by McCrone et al. (1994) — found a difference in comprehensive weekly cost between the two groups, with the generic (control) group costs being 39 per cent greater than the CST group costs, although the difference was only significant in the first six months of the evaluation period (Figure 4.1). In the longer term, there was a small but not significant difference: the 'care management' approach was thus no more nor less cost-effective, although client satisfaction was slightly higher in the short term. The overall level of input from CPNs was significantly higher and more costly for the

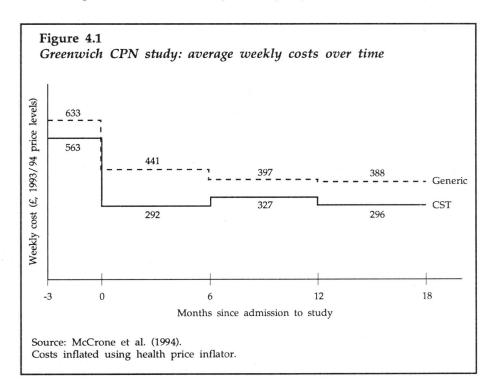

Figure 4.1
Greenwich CPN study: average weekly costs over time

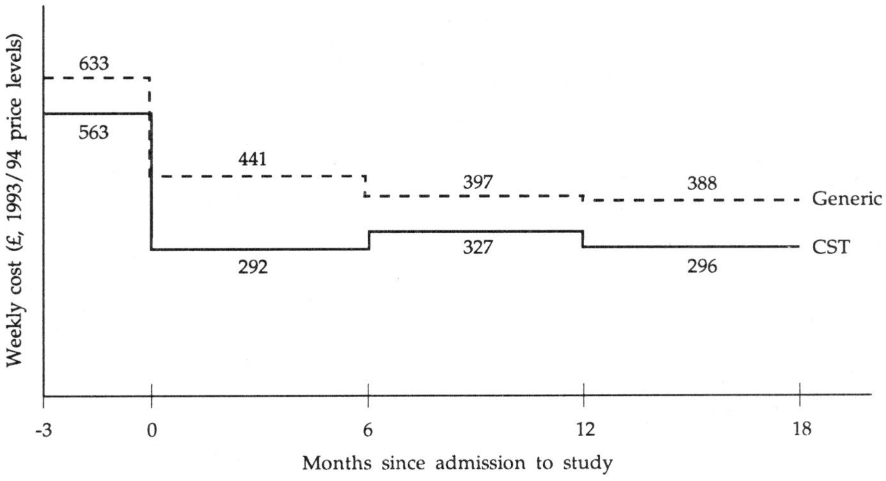

Source: McCrone et al. (1994).
Costs inflated using health price inflator.

CST group, and CPNs worked on a wider range of issues and areas. Although they received no additional training, encouraging CPNs to work with wider responsibilities and giving them more autonomy produced some short-term economic advantages and no medium-term disadvantages. The CST model reduced reliance on specialist residential accommodation.

Unfortunately, the Greenwich CST evaluation may not have been long enough to test the ramifications of nurse-based care management properly, nor was the sample of users large enough to permit exploration of inter-user outcome or cost variations (Table 4.1). Indeed, the sample has been argued to be on the small side even for an RCT (van Os et al., 1994). The study was nevertheless useful because its randomised design gave a certain power to the comparisons between the samples, and the findings warrant attention because they reflect on some of the proposals for the national development of community mental health services in the 1990s. The second illustration has similar relevance.

Table 4.1
Cost variations: the need for explanation

Study, sample and time period		Weekly costs (£, 1993-94 prices)				
		Mean	sd	Min.	Max.	N
Greenwich CPN study						
CST sample:	12-18 months	296	222	69	1200	32
	0-18 months	300	174	110	839	32
Generic sample:	12-18 months	388	280	99	1001	30
	0-18 months	415	283	112	1074	20
Maudsley DLP sample						
DLP sample:	12-20 months	224	156	45	1205	74
	0-20 months	254	126	98	810	55
Control sample:	12-20 months	329	337	41	1739	68
	0-20 months	464	313	81	1630	48

The Maudsley Daily Living Programme

The Daily Living Programme (DLP) offered home-based care for people with serious mental illness facing emergency admission to the Maudsley Hospital. The multidisciplinary DLP team (psychiatric nurses, a social worker for part of the time, a senior registrar in psychiatry, a part-time consultant psychiatrist and an occupational therapist) provided some direct services and liaised with other services on behalf of patients. Type and intensity of care were tailored to patient needs by keyworkers providing case management. Where possible, the DLP sought to substitute community care for standard inpatient treatment. The DLP was modelled on the experimental intensive community care services developed in Madison (Stein and Test, 1980) and Sydney (Hoult et al., 1983). The main evaluation of the DLP focused on processes and outcomes (Audini et al., 1994; Marks et al., 1994), and the economic evaluation on costs (Knapp et al., 1994, 1995), and provides the second example of this chapter.

People with serious mental illness facing emergency inpatient admission to the Maudsley were randomly allocated (equal probabilities) to DLP or standard inpatient care. The DLP supported 92 people, and the hospital-based control group 97. Once discharged from inpatient care, control group members attended outpatient services and received other community support services. The study was conducted over two phases; here we concentrate on the first. Assessments of patients were scheduled to be undertaken within 72 hours of trial entry, and three, nine and eighteen months later, although actual timings varied. Ratings of characteristics were conducted using the Global Assessment Scale (GAS; Endicott et al., 1976), the ninth edition of the Present State Examination (PSE; Wing et al., 1974), the Brief Psychiatric Rating Scale (BPRS; Overall and Gorham, 1962; Lukoff et al., 1986), the Social Adjustment Scale (SAS; Weissman et al., 1971, 1974), a daily living skills rating (Marks et al., 1994) and questions on patients' and relatives' satisfaction with the service (Larsen et al., 1979; Attkisson and Zwick, 1985; Lemmens and Donker, 1990). Service use, employment, sources of income and accommodation data were collected at entry and at subsequent assessments using a variant of the Client Service Receipt Interview (see Chapter 3). Complete CSRI data on admission were available for 91 DLP and 90 control patients (*not* a biased subsample of the 92 and 97 patients at randomisation). By the time of the 20-month rating, the available CSRI data had declined to 74 DLP and 70 control patients, and by 45 months the sample was 60 DLP and 70 control. Costs were measured comprehensively. There were few differences between people for whom costs were and were not missing, and none which supported any alteration of the main finding of the controlled evaluation (Knapp, 1995).

A wide range of services was accessed during treatment, although the two groups used services in different combinations and with different intensities (Knapp et al., 1994). The associated costs varied over time and between samples (Figure 4.2). The controlled evaluation found that home-based DLP care was significantly less costly than standard inpatient-based care over the first 20 months after admission/referral and during each of the component periods. Indeed, in cost-effectiveness terms the DLP was superior to standard hospital-based care during this period, for it slightly improved symptoms and social adjustment and enhanced patients' and relatives' satisfaction (Marks et al., 1994). The DLP did *not* appear to shift the burden of support and funded services from the health service to other agencies, or to patients and families.

In the longer term — from 30-45 months — there were, however, few advantages in symptoms or social adjustment in the DLP versus two control groups (the original control group, and a random subset of the original DLP group who returned to use the standard services), although patients' and

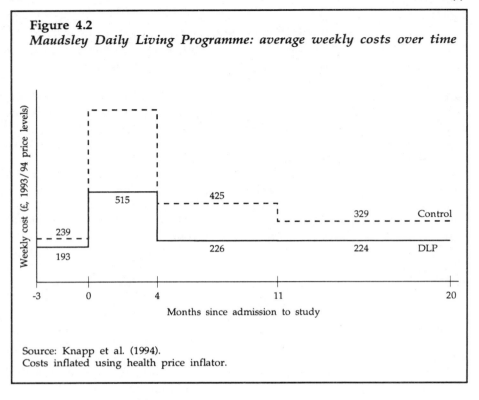

Figure 4.2
Maudsley Daily Living Programme: average weekly costs over time

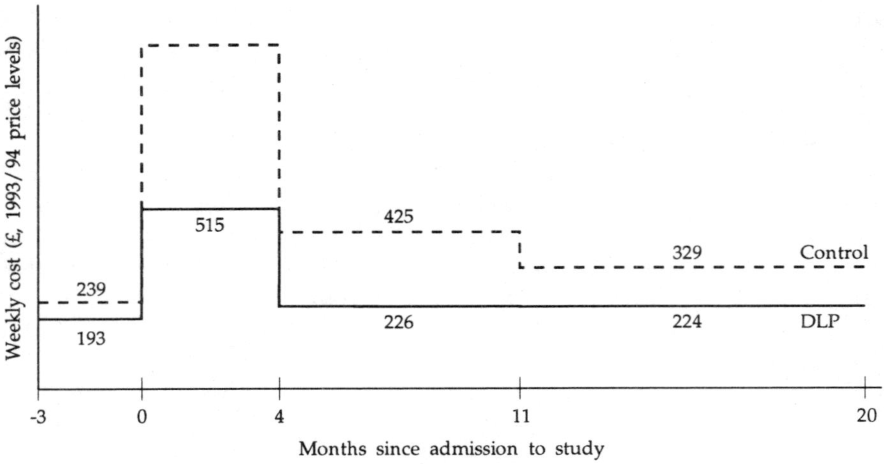

Source: Knapp et al. (1994).
Costs inflated using health price inflator.

relatives' satisfaction continued to be significantly superior (Audini et al., 1994). Comparisons revealed a small cost advantage to the DLP service (Knapp et al., 1995). These longer-term findings are not discussed further in this book.

4.4 Exploring the variations

It is not *standard* practice in UK health economics evaluations to explore within-sample cost or outcome variations. This is not because economics does not have the statistical armoury to conduct the exploration, for the subdiscipline of econometrics is many decades old and has developed and refined some excellent techniques. Nor should it be lack of familiarity, because introductory econometrics is a compulsory subject in most economics undergraduate courses. There is no doubt that the blame might occasionally be attributed to researcher idleness, and sometimes to an overcrowded work schedule. However, two other reasons have been more important: insufficient data, for many RCTs or quasi-experimental evaluations simply do not have samples large enough to permit sensible exploration of inter-user or inter-facility variations (as was the case in the Greenwich CPN study, for example); and a lack of appreciation of the advantages and insights that can flow from well-conducted multivariate analyses.

Two examples of the exploration of cost variations are offered here. The first extends the evaluation of the DLP described in the previous section to give an illustration of a user-level or micro cost function. The second looks at psychiatric hospitals, providing a facility-level or mezzo cost function. Other examples could have been given, such as the facility-level cost function study by Shiell et al. (1993) of residential services for adults with learning disabilities. At the system or macro level, cost functions might be estimated for authorities as a whole, which was effectively the approach in a recent look at the costs of mental health services for children (Beecham et al., 1994). Chapter 5 includes another example of user-level cost predictions and moves on to cost-outcome associations. Before giving these illustrations, it is necessary to introduce cost functions and their interpretation.

The cost function approach

Even a cursory examination of the costs of care in the Greenwich or DLP evaluations reveals sizeable variations in weekly average cost between users (Table 4.1). For example, the highest weekly cost among the Greenwich CST sample was ten times larger than the lowest cost over the full eighteen-month period, and the equivalent ratio was 8:1 in the DLP sample and 20:1 in the control group (see Table 4.1). Some of this variation is stochastic (random), being the consequence of temporary accounting glitches, short-term unplanned fluctuations in service use or provision, or perhaps (accidental) measurement errors. However, a part of the observed variation in cost may be predictable, linked to the characteristics of users, services or providers. An estimated cost function can be used to distinguish the random elements from the predictable, and — more importantly — to tease out the relative contributions of each of the latter ('predictable') reasons for the cost variations.

A *statistical cost function* is thus the estimated relationship between the cost of providing care or treatment, the characteristics of users, the outcomes for the user or others, the prices of the resources employed and other factors with hypothesised influences suggested by the context and purposes of the care mode under examination. The cost function approach has good theoretical credentials, for it follows directly from the economic theory of production, and it is based on assumptions which have been widely debated and refined in a variety of market and non-market contexts. In application in public health and social policy contexts, the approach has proved both manageable and informative. In the employment of the cost function approach, the analogy is being made between the economist's production model of inputs and outputs and the processes of delivering mental health services. The validity of the analogy is thus established by reference to the production of welfare approach.

The cost function was first estimated for production units or firms in the agricultural and manufacturing sectors. In health and social care contexts, cost functions were first estimated for treatment or care facilities. They can also be estimated for cross-section samples of users. In each case, multivariate rather than bivariate analyses are needed in order to investigate the simultaneous influences of different factors. Estimation is usually effected through multiple regression analysis, often in a series of ordinary least squares regression equations, taking average weekly cost as the dependent variable, and introducing client characteristics and other hypothesised influences as predictors. Not all such hypothesised predictors will remain in the cost function. The criteria for inclusion in the regression equations are usually statistical significance, interpretability of estimated effects and parsimony.

Variations in the DLP: patient and treatment effects

The DLP evaluation allows the cost difference between experimental and control groups to be 'unpacked' by exploring the sources of within-sample cost variations. There are two stages to this part of the evaluation. The first stage involves cost function examination of the links between characteristics at baseline (the point of referral or admission) and the comprehensive care costs 12-20 months after referral. The second stage is to conduct cross-predictions from these equations. The technique and underlying algebra were first used in this context in work on child care (Knapp, 1986).

Cost functions. The individual characteristics explored in the statistical analyses were constructed from assessments at entry to the study using the instruments described earlier (see section 4.3), and costs were measured using a version of the CSRI. Other characteristics examined in the multivariate analyses included age, Mental Health Act legal status and diagnosis. The DLP and control groups were examined separately.

The final forms of the two cost functions — strictly, they are cost prediction equations — are summarised in Table 4.2. It can be seen that both equations perform satisfactorily from a statistical viewpoint, and both reveal interesting cost-need linkages. For the control group, costs are higher in the medium term for people who scored higher on the specific neurotic syndrome subscore of the PSE, the BPRS and the SAS global score. The only exception to the general finding of a positive link between 'needs' at entry and costs between 12 and 20 months is the negative effect of the non-specific neurotic syndrome subscore of the PSE. For the DLP group, the links between characteristics at entry and later costs are less straightforward. The non-specific neurotic syndrome and delusions and hallucinations subscores of the PSE, and the SAS global score all exert curvilinear effects on average weekly cost. Greater needs at entry are *less likely* to be associated with higher costs for the DLP group than for the control group, which is probably an indication of the relative

Table 4.2
Cost prediction equations for the DLP and control group samples, 12-20 months[a]

	DLP sample		Control group	
Predictor variables	Coeff.	Sig.	Coeff.	Sig.
Constant	219.71	0.121	1195.43	0.039
Female[b]	-81.08	0.020		
Afro-Caribbean ethnic group[b]	128.93	0.003		
Lived with relatives at entry[b]	-112.37	0.002		
Duration of previous inpatient admission in days			8.66	0.053
Non-specific neurotic syndrome subscore[c] (PSE)	-19.25	0.012		
Non-specific neurotic syndrome subscore[c], squared	0.58	0.021	-0.52	0.011
Delusions and hallucinations subscore[c] (PSE)	-16.12	0.021		
Delusions and hallucinations subscore[c], squared	0.55	0.085		
Specific neurotic syndrome subscore[c] (PSE), squared			0.99	0.067
BPRS score[c]			-46.93	0.041
BPRS score[c], squared			0.48	0.027
SAS global adjustment score[c]	29.70	0.051		
SAS global adjustment score[c], squared	-0.78	0.039	0.56	0.004
R^2	0.41		0.34	
F-statistic	4.47	0.000	5.26	0.000
Sample size	68		68	

a Dependent variable is average weekly cost during the period 12-20 months after entry to the study (referral to the Maudsley), £, 1993/94 price levels.
b Dummy variable taking the value 1 if an individual has the named characteristic and the value 0 otherwise.
c Higher scores indicate more severe mental health problems.

success of the DLP team in addressing mental health symptoms during this period (Marks et al., 1994). Costs for the DLP group were also lower for females, lower for the 64 per cent of people who lived with relatives at entry (an indication, perhaps, of the DLP's ability to galvanise and support informal care), and higher for people in the Afro-Caribbean ethnic group.

These analyses are thus informative, for they provide an indication of the likely medium-term cost implications of people with different characteristics at entry (referral), and they hint at differences in the future.

Cross-predictions. The two multivariate equations in Table 4.2 standardise for differences *within* samples before drawing conclusions about cost-raising characteristics. We can also use them to make cost comparisons *between* treatment options having standardised for individual differences. The research question is whether or to what extent the cost differences between the DLP and control groups illustrated in Figure 4.2 reflect differences in the characteristics of individuals or the consequences of the two modes of care. Cross-predictions can be made from the estimated equation fitted for one group to the actual characteristics of the other group.

There is a general point to be illustrated here about variations and like-with-like comparisons. Costs vary with user or patient characteristics, although the nature and extent of variation need not be the same in different care settings. They can have a number of implications. Consider the two solid

Figure 4.3
Like-with-like cost comparisons

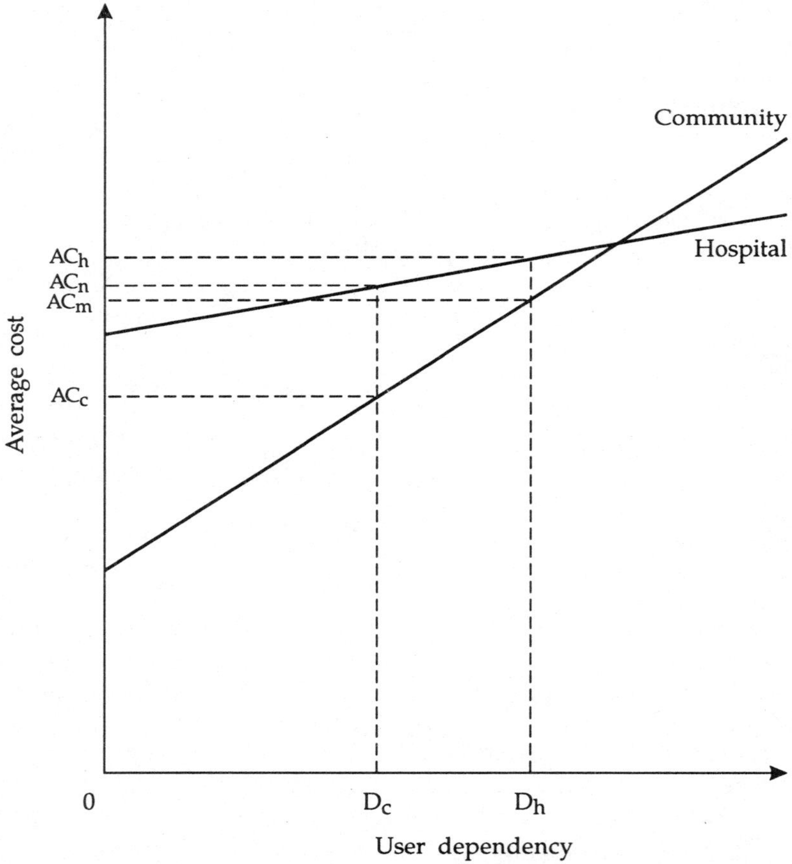

lines drawn on Figure 4.3, representing the relationship between cost and clinical, social and behavioural characteristics of users (called 'dependency' for short). One line is the cost-dependency relationship for people in hospital, and the other represents the relationship in the community. Movement from left to right along the horizontal axis represents an increase in user dependency. Thus the two cost lines or functions indicate that cost and dependency are positively correlated — it costs more to provide care for a more dependent user. The shape and position of the two cost lines reflect what is usually found in applied research: hospital tends to be more costly than community care for people whose mental health problems are less serious, but is probably *less* costly at the other end of the dependency or seriousness range. The points D_c and D_h are the average dependency levels in community and hospital settings, the assumption being that the 'average' or 'typical' hospital inpatient is more dependent than the 'average' community care service user.

The costs marked as AC_h and AC_c are then the observed average costs of hospital and community care — the averages reported by agencies or researchers. One obvious implication of the diagram — which has been built up from existing knowledge about today's services — is that the simple or observed difference between the two average cost measures (= $AC_h - AC_c$) exaggerates the *real* difference, for like is not being compared with like: dependency levels are not the same. The real cost difference is $AC_h - AC_m$. In consequence, a health authority or other agency which seeks to resettle the 'average' hospital patient will have to find funding, not at the level AC_c, but the larger sum AC_m. Thus the savings of, for example, a dehospitalisation programme will be exaggerated by today's observed average costs. There is consequently a danger of underfunding of the new community placements for the former hospital residents. (The danger is greater if the *full* costs of community care are missed because comprehensive measures have not been employed.)

Of course, the typical community care policy not only resettles the 'easiest' or less dependent hospital residents first, but also tends to move people who are more dependent than the community average. (On the diagram, this would be illustrated by the movement of someone of dependency D_c and D_h from hospital to community.) The result is that *both* average dependency and average cost will go up in *both* settings. Policy-makers will observe inflated costs in hospital and in the community, and may thus get anxious if they originally supported a policy of community care on the grounds of economy. (For example, cost per inpatient week in English non-teaching psychiatric hospitals was almost three times higher in real terms in 1984/85 than it was twenty years earlier, with the real cost inflation as high as 32 per cent in the last five years of that period. Not all of this inflation can be laid at the door of changes in patient 'dependency' — and part of the dependency change was due not to the discharge policy but to the ageing of the hospital population — but this has undoubtedly had a marked effect.) The policy of altering the balance of provision away from inpatient care is, in fact,

Table 4.3
Predicted weekly costs, DLP evaluation, 12-20 months

	Predicted costs for treatment types		
Sample	DLP £	Standard £	Significance p
DLP	AC_c = 231	AC_n = 397	0.001
Standard (control)	AC_m = 254	AC_h = 329	0.096
Significance	0.175	0.297	

economical because *total* expenditure is falling.

The estimated cost prediction equations in Table 4.2 are the multivariate representations of the lines in Figure 4.3. Using them we can therefore predict the costs if the individuals who received the standard inpatient treatment (control group service) had instead been supported by the DLP, or vice versa. Thus, if the hospital cost line in Figure 4.3 represents the control service (standard in/outpatient care) and the community cost line represents the DLP, we want to use the two prediction equations to compare AC_h with AC_m (the two alternatives — control and DLP, respectively — for the control sample) and to compare AC_c with AC_n (the two alternatives for the DLP sample).

The resultant predicted costs are given in Table 4.3. The figures in the first row of the table indicate the costs of the two treatment options for the DLP group members: £231 is the observed mean weekly cost of DLP for the people who were actually allocated to the DLP service, and £397 is the predicted cost for the same group if they had received standard inpatient treatment. The difference is statistically significant (p=0.001), confirming the finding reported in section 4.3. If we compare vertically rather than horizontally, the figures in the first column give the predicted costs of receiving DLP for each of the two groups. Vertical comparisons reflect differences in group characteristics. It can be seen that the differences are not statistically significant: the samples are not different, which is exactly what would be expected from randomisation.

The difference between the mean costs of each pair of groups/treatments can be decomposed into a treatment component and a patient characteristics component.

The DLP's simple cost advantage of £98 over standard inpatient treatment ($AC_h - AC_c$ = £329 – £231; 1993/94 price levels) decomposes into a patient effect of only £23 per week ($AC_m - AC_c$ = £254 – £231; p=0.175), and a treatment effect of £75 ($AC_h - AC_m$ = £329 – £254; p=0.096). Alternatively, if we use the standard inpatient treatment function as the basis for standardised comparison, we find a patient effect of £68 (p=0.297) and a (like-with-like) treatment effect indicating a cost advantage to DLP of £166 (p=0.001).

The examination of cost variations within each of the two samples has thus exposed a number of interesting connections between patient characteristics and costs, and has also given us a basis for comparisons between the samples. Along the way, we have illustrated how like-with-like comparisons can be made, even though in this case the RCT design has already ensured that valid comparisons could be made.

Psychiatric hospital cost variations

The second example of the exploration of cost variations differs from the first in a number of respects, notably the focus on *facilities* rather than users, the reliance on retrospective rather than prospectively-collected data, and the analysis of administrative rather than research data. There is also no RCT. (This analysis was described in Knapp and Beecham, 1990.)

One of the controversial features of the present emphasis on running down the number of hospital beds is the way in which money is or is not transferred from hospitals to community care provision. The transfers are intended to facilitate the development of community care provision so that discharged hospital patients can move into a system of support services which is at least as good as hospital. These transfers out of hospital budgets (so-called 'dowries') are tied to the permanent closure of hospital beds, and usually are based on some proportion of average hospital revenue cost. Hospital managers and consultant psychiatrists, among others, have argued that money is being transferred out of the hospital budgets faster than it is being saved as beds close, because, *inter alia*, there are overhead costs which are not saved until whole wards or whole establishments close. This issue can be examined by estimating a hospital cost function.

Using data for every psychiatric hospital in ten of the fourteen former English regional health authorities for each of three years in the mid-1980s, an average cost function was fitted in an attempt to estimate (after some simple differential calculus) the *marginal cost* of hospital inpatient care. The data were limited because they were taken from routine (administrative) collections — there were no patient profiles and no casemix information, for example — but it was possible to make some progress towards an understanding of the *average* speed with which hospital costs fall as inpatient numbers decline. Previous British studies of the costs of psychiatric hospital care do not generally permit a comparison with the results described below (Stern and Stern, 1963; Mercer, 1975; McKechnie et al., 1982). The only exception is the unpublished doctoral work of Casmas (1976), whose finding that average and marginal costs are similar in magnitude mirrors the finding from this study.

Table 4.4
Cost function for psychiatric hospitals, ten English regions, 1986/87

(Dependent variable = average cost per inpatient day in 1986/87 but inflated to 1993/94 prices)

Variable	Coefficient	Significance
Inverse of number of inpatient days in 1986/87	172182	<0.01
Change in occupancy percentage, 1986/87 minus 1985/86	-23.68	<0.01
Hospital located in Northern region	-21.02	<0.05
Hospital located in North-Western region	-32.02	<0.01
Constant term	76.07	<0.01

$\bar{R}^2 = 0.72$
F = 72.16<0.01
Sample size = 119

Multiple regression (ordinary least squares) estimation was used to fit a cost function with average revenue cost per inpatient day as the dependent variable. (Out- and day patient costs were omitted, as were all capital cost elements and any costs falling outside the hospital budget.) The explanatory variables were the number of inpatient days, the proportion of available beds occupied over the year and regional location (since regions have different policies for their long-stay hospital beds and face different labour supply prices). The best cost function is detailed in Table 4.4, where 'best' refers to the conventional criteria of parsimony, statistical significance and interpretability. From the function in the table we can derive the marginal cost (MC) (by multiplication and then differentiation by the number of inpatient days) which is equal to:

MC = 76.07 – 71.64 x (change in occupancy, 85/86 to 86/87) + regional effects.

Taking the mean change in occupancy across the 119 hospitals in the sample, marginal cost (averaged across regions) in 1986/87 was £71 per inpatient day, or £493 per week, at 1993/94 prices. Yet the mean average cost per inpatient day for these same hospitals was £609. On average across the full sample, marginal cost — the cost of one additional or one fewer inpatient — was 81 per cent of average revenue cost, and the estimated function indicates that this marginal cost will be higher in hospitals which are quicker to adjust their available beds to falling inpatient numbers. This is exactly as one would expect. Hospitals which 'closed' beds (or whole wards or wings) as patients have moved out or died have smaller year-on-year changes in their occupancy proportions and therefore higher marginal savings.

We conclude, therefore, that, *on average*, as much as 81 per cent of a hospital's revenue costs are saved in the short term as inpatient numbers decline. This is a higher proportion than hospital managers usually claim they can save. They argue that overheads, such as management and centralised catering, which cannot be run down at the same speed as patient numbers, make it impossible for them to save very much in the short run. Certainly the function assumes *smooth* cost adjustment when the reality is a stepped process, but many hospitals are running down bed numbers at a speed that easily allows the annual closure of a whole ward, should this be acceptable from a professional point of view and to users. Financial transfers should not proceed at a pace which leaves hospitals denuded of resources, for this can quickly result in poor-quality settings for remaining patients (and staff), but hospitals should not be holding on to resources which they no longer need and which could be used to improve community mental health care.

Estimates of this kind give a perspective on the financial implications for hospitals as they move towards long-term inpatient targets. They also offer evidence on economies of scale, which are pervasive, if gentle. This perhaps suggests that the Victorians were practising sound financial management when they built the huge asylums, although then, as today, patient welfare and other non-monetary considerations were at least as important in shaping services.

4.5 From principles to practice

Chapters 1 to 4 have set out the basic frameworks and concepts needed for economic evaluations of mental health services, giving illustrations along the way. In this chapter the emphasis has been on appropriate comparisons and the examination of variations for the insights they might offer. Neither topic has been explored in full, but the examples should have demonstrated the value of more searching multivariate analyses where data, time and research budgets allow.

The remaining chapters of the book build on the methods set out in these first four chapters, sometimes developing or enhancing the methodology, and sometimes constrained from exploiting the methods fully. Economic evaluations need to adapt flexibly to policy contexts, practice circumstances and data availabilities, not so far as to compromise on basic principles but not so little as to lose opportunities to offer valuable insights to policy-makers and practitioners.

References

Attkisson, C.C. and Zwick, R. (1985) The Client Satisfaction Questionnaire: psychometric properties and correlation with service utilization and psychotherapy outcome, *Evaluation and Program Planning*, 5, 233-7.

Audini, B., Marks, I.M., Lawrence, R.E., Connolly, J. and Watts, V. (1994) Home-based versus out-patient/in-patient care for people with serious mental illness. Phase II of a controlled study, *British Journal of Psychiatry*, 165, 204-10.

Beecham, J.K., Knapp, M.R.J. and Asbury, M. (1994) A national review of mental health services for children and young people: the cost dimension, Discussion Paper 1049, Personal Social Services Research Unit, University of Kent at Canterbury.

Burns, T., Raftery, J., Beadsmoore, A., McGuigan, S. and Dickson, M. (1993) A controlled trial of home-based acute psychiatric services. II: Treatment patterns and costs, *British Journal of Psychiatry*, 163, 55-61.

Casmas, S.T. (1976) Inter-hospital and inter-local variation in patterns of provision for the mentally disordered, PhD thesis, University of Manchester Institute of Science and Technology, Manchester.

Dunn, M., O'Driscoll, C., Dayson, D., Wills, W. and Leff, J. (1990) An observational study of the social life of long-stay patients, *British Journal of Psychiatry*, 157, 842-8.

Endicott, J., Spitzer, R.L., Fleiss, J.L. and Cohen, J. (1976) The Global Assessment Scale. A procedure for measuring overall severity of psychiatric disturbance, *Archives of General Psychiatry*, 33, 766-71.

Hoult, J., Reynolds, I., Charbonneau-Powis, M., Weekes, P. and Briggs, J. (1983) Psychiatric hospital versus community treatment: the results of a randomised trial, *Australian and New Zealand Journal of Psychiatry*, 17, 160-67.

Knapp, M.R.J. (1984) *The Economics of Social Care*, Macmillan, London.

Knapp, M.R.J. (1986) The relative cost-effectiveness of public, voluntary and private providers of residential child care, in A. Culyer and B. Jönsson (eds) *Public and Private Health Services*, Basil Blackwell, Oxford.

Knapp, M.R.J. (1995) Home- v. hospital-based care for people with serious mental illness (letter), *British Journal of Psychiatry*, 166, 120-21.

Knapp, M.R.J. and Beecham, J.K. (1990) Costing mental health services, *Psychological Medicine*, 20, 893-908.

Knapp, M.R.J., Beecham, J.K., Koutsogeorgopoulou, V., Hallam, A., Fenyo, A.J., Marks, I.M., Connolly, J., Audini, B. and Muijen, M. (1994) Service use and costs of home-based care versus hospital-based care for people with serious mental illness, *British Journal of Psychiatry*, 165, 195-203.

Knapp, M.R.J., Wolstenholme, J., Marks, I., Beecham, J.K., Astin, J., Audini, B. and Connolly, J. (1995) Cost-effectiveness over four years of home-based versus hospital-based care for people with serious mental illness, Working Paper 41, Centre for the Economics of Mental Health, Institute of Psychiatry, London.

Larsen, D.H., Attkisson, C.C., Hargreaves, W.A. and Ngeyen, T.D. (1979) Assessment of client/patient satisfaction: development of a general scale, *Evaluation and Program Planning*, 2, 197-207.

Lemmens, F. and Donker, M. (1990) Kwaliteitsbeoordeling door clienten, Utrecht, Nederlands Centrum Geestelijke Volksgezondheid.

Lukoff, D., Liberman, R.P. and Neuchterlein, K.H. (1986) Symptom monitoring in the rehabilitation of schizophrenic patients, *Schizophrenia Bulletin*, 12, 578-602.

McCrone, P., Beecham, J.K. and Knapp, M.R.J. (1994) Community psychiatric nurse teams: cost-effectiveness of intensive support versus generic care, *British Journal of Psychiatry*, 165, 218-21.

McKechnie, A.A., Rae, D. and May, J. (1982) A comparison of in-patient costs of treatment and care in a Scottish psychiatric hospital, *British Journal of Psychiatry*, 140, 602-7.

Marks, I.M., Connolly, J., Muijen, M., McNamee, G., Audini, B. and Lawrence, R.E. (1994) Home-based versus hospital-based care for people with serious mental illness, *British Journal of Psychiatry*, 165, 179-94.

Mercer, A.D. (1975) A model for nursing cost, *Hospital and Health Services Review*, 71, 194-5.

Muijen, M., Cooney, M., Strathdee, G., Bell, R. and Hudson, A. (1994) Community psychiatric nurse teams: intensive support versus generic care, *British Journal of Psychiatry*, 165, 211-17.

Overall, J.E. and Gorham, D.R. (1962) Impact of treatment intervention on the relationship between dimensions of clinical psychopathology, social dysfunction and burden on the family of psychiatric patients, *British Journal of Psychiatry*, 12, 651-8.

Shiell, A., Pettipher, C., Raynes, N. and Wright, K.G. (1993) A cost function analysis of residential services for adults with a learning disability, *Health Economics*, 2, 3, 247-56.

Stein, L.I. and Test, M.A. (1980) Alternative to mental hospital treatment. I: Conceptual model, treatment program, and clinical evaluation, *Archives of General Psychiatry*, 37, 392-7.

Stern, B. and Stern, E.S. (1963) Efficiency of mental hospitals, *British Journal of Preventive and Social Medicine*, 17, 111-20.

van Os, J., McKenzie, K., Gilvarry, K. and Fahy, T. (1994) Community psychiatric nurse teams (letter), *British Journal of Psychiatry*, 165, 839-40.

Weisbrod, B.A., Stein, M.A. and Test, L.I. (1980) Alternatives to mental hospital treatment. II: Economic benefit – cost analysis, *Archives of General Psychiatry*, 37, 400-405.

Weissman, M.M., Paykel, E.S., Siegel, R. and Klerman, G. (1971) The social role performance of depressed women: comparisons with a normal group, *American Journal of Orthopsychiatry*, 41, 390-405.

Weissman, M.M., Klerman, G.L., Paykel, E.S., Prusoff, B. and Hanson, B. (1974) Treatment effects on the social adjustment of depressed patients, *Archives of General Psychiatry*, 30, 771-8.

Wing, J.K., Cooper, J.E. and Sartorius, N. (1974) *The Description and Classification of Psychiatric Symptoms*, Cambridge University Press, Cambridge.

5 *Eight Years of Psychiatric Reprovision: An Economic Evaluation*

Angela Hallam, Martin Knapp, Jennifer Beecham and Andrew Fenyo

5.1 Introduction

The question of cost is central to the British government's policy of substituting community care for hospital residence for people with long-term mental health problems. In a report to the Department of Health's Mental Health Task Force in 1993, it was estimated that the actual number of places in homes and hospitals specialising in mental health care has remained relatively unchanged at around 80,000 over the past decade. However, the number of facilities themselves has increased from 1,000 to 2,500. This figure includes local authority accommodation and privately-run homes; the level of provision in housing schemes remains unmeasured (Davidge et al., 1993).

The relocation to community-based care is being accomplished in increasingly cost-conscious policy and practice environments, compelling service providers to ask about the resource implications of any care or treatment decisions. There is a growing need for accurate cost information at almost every stage as community care services are planned, commissioned and, once in operation, evaluated.

In 1983 the (then) North East Thames Regional Health Authority affirmed their commitment to the national policy of service relocation. The decision was taken to concentrate capital and revenue resources on developing services that would allow the closure of Friern and Claybury hospitals. Advances in medication and changes in attitude towards institutionalised care during the 1960s and 1970s meant that the numbers of beds in these two large Victorian institutions had already declined quite sharply from their peak in the early

1950s. However, by 1985, when preparations were being made for the first group of patients to move to the community, Friern still had 945 beds and Claybury 870. The closure was planned to take ten years (Leff et al., 1993) and, in fact, the last patients left Friern in March 1993. It is estimated that Claybury will close in 1996.

The economic evaluation conducted by the Personal Social Services Research Unit (PSSRU) was funded from 1986 to 1994 as part of the regional research programme monitoring the impact of the move from hospital to community care. The reprovision of hospital-based services presents a rigorous challenge to planners and purchasers, for they are attempting to coordinate the social and health care needs of users, now that this is no longer the responsibility of the hospital. Our original remit was to describe *services* used by former inpatients, to cost this *psychiatric reprovision* and to examine *cost-outcome links*. However, as reported in this paper, the size and comprehensiveness of the dataset have made it possible to examine other cost associations and to explore a number of policy issues.

The Team for the Assessment of Psychiatric Services (TAPS), under the direction of Professor Julian Leff, is undertaking the detailed assessment of patients before they leave hospital and the follow-up appraisal of leavers in the community, one, two and five years after the index discharge. Information collected by the TAPS team includes personal characteristics such as gender, age, marital status and original diagnosis; and detailed clinical, behavioural and social characteristics (O'Driscoll and Leff, 1993; further details are given below). We work closely with TAPS at the one- and five-year follow-ups.

5.2 Description of the study population

The criteria for entry to the study described in this chapter ensure that people have been inpatients for a minimum of one year and, if over 65 years old, do not have a diagnosis of dementia. For convenience, we distinguish and describe groups of leavers in terms of annual cohorts, each cohort running from September to August. Other parts of our research programme are looking at acute provision and services for elderly people with dementia.

The comprehensive costs sample

Our costs information currently relates to the service packages received by members of the first seven cohorts during the twelfth month after discharge. The total number of people in these groups who moved from hospital to community was 630 and we have detailed service receipt information, obtained at interview, for 428 study members.

It was not possible to interview hospital leavers who were re-admitted to hospital for long periods, or who refused permission. Community costs have, therefore, been interpolated for 138 people, using our existing costs data. A further eighteen people who were transferred from Friern to other hospitals were included in the costs sample, as costs could be calculated from hospital accounts. Although such hospital transfers are not community placements, the clients are 'leavers' in the sense of moving out of the hospitals monitored by the evaluation. Future work will examine the total cost of hospital rundown and closure, so it is important to include this group. (Details of the methodology used to interpolate community costs are given in Hallam et al., 1994a.)

Individual characteristics

Fifty-four per cent of the hospital leavers for whom we have community costs data are male. When they were interviewed in hospital, their ages ranged between 21 and 98 (around a mean of 55 years). At that time, 68 per cent of the patients were single, 12 per cent divorced and 7 per cent widowed. Schizophrenia was the primary diagnosis for 79 per cent of the sample. Other diagnoses were affective disorder (9 per cent), neurosis and personality disorder (8 per cent), and organic disorders (4 per cent). However, diagnosis was not recorded for 76 people. Length of the most recent hospital admission ranged between one and 62 years, around a mean of fifteen years.

The numbers leaving Friern and Claybury Hospitals each year have varied, and at cohort 6 the Claybury follow-up was discontinued to allow research time to focus on the early leavers after five years in the community. Up to and including the fifth cohort, 56 per cent of the people in our sample came from Friern.

Relative dependency of successive cohorts

Clearly, the development of efficient community services to replace long-term hospital inpatient care takes time and involves professional and political risks. Risks during the transitional period will be reduced if patients whose service needs are comparatively easily met are the earliest to leave hospital, since this group presents fewer challenges to purchasers and providers (Knapp, 1995b). After three cohorts of leavers had moved to community placements, the discharge practice was investigated and it was found that there were significant differences in characteristics between these clients and the people who were, at that time, still in hospital. Leavers in the first three cohorts were younger, had spent less time in psychiatric hospitals, were less likely to have a diagnosis of schizophrenia, had larger social networks and had expressed more positive views about leaving hospital than patients remaining after these three groups had left (Jones, 1993).

During the reprovision programme, each succeeding cohort has been shown to have greater needs and become more similar to the remaining hospital population, with cohort 5 no different from the overall hospital average at the start of the closure programme in terms of personal, clinical, behavioural and social characteristics (Knapp et al., 1993). Inevitably, the more severe mental health problems of the later leavers put increasing pressure on community resources, with implications for the cost of providing community-based care for this client group.

Box 5.1
Freddie

Freddie left hospital quite late in the reprovision programme, moving to an accommodation unit owned by a housing association and managed by a consortium arrangement between the health authority and a voluntary organisation. He was one of nine residents whose care needs were judged by staff to be 'medium'. Twenty-four hour cover within the unit was provided by a team of six staff.

An occupational therapist made regular visits to all residents and case reviews, conducted within the home every six months, involved a community psychiatrist and general practitioner. Freddie also had regular contact with a social worker and with police officers on several occasions when he caused a disturbance in the street.

The total weekly cost of Freddie's care during his first year after leaving Friern was £1796.22 (at 1993/94 price levels), the most expensive service package we have costed to date. Unusually, only 28 per cent of this total relates to community accommodation facility costs. Freddie spent long periods as an inpatient in a large teaching hospital in central London, at a cost of almost £348 per day. His community place was kept for him each time he was re-admitted to hospital and, although this was another cost-raising factor we had to take into consideration, it also meant that he did not return to hospital on a permanent basis.

5.3 Service receipt

Data collection

The Client Service Receipt Interview (CSRI, see Chapter 3) is used to collect the client-specific data which allow us to describe and cost individual packages of care. Our aim is to reflect living arrangements, service use and client income and expenditure in the twelfth month after the index discharge, adjusting for regularly but infrequently used services over the previous year.

Accommodation arrangements

We give accommodation arrangements particularly close attention. The accommodation offered to former hospital inpatients is an important element in the description of community care practices and accounts for approximately 85 per cent of the cost of care in the community (see below). Many inpatients moved from hospital under special financial arrangements — 'dowries' — where a sum of money, equal to the average revenue cost of a hospital bed, was transferred from the hospital budget to the relevant district health authority and thence to the community services provider. Most people moved to accommodation within the eight district health authorities (DHAs) and nine local authorities in London for which the two hospitals have provided inpatient facilities.

To facilitate analysis we use standardised definitions of accommodation types, distinguished by levels of staffing and numbers of places. In other contexts the terms used by the PSSRU might have different or more nebulous meanings, so it is important to emphasise exactly how we interpret them.

A *residential or nursing home* is defined as a unit which has continuous staff cover by day, and waking night staff, while a *hostel* has sleeping-in or on-call staff during the night and continuous or regular staffing by day. In both cases the number of client places is six or more. *Sheltered housing* units (individual flats or bed-sits as part of a larger complex) have continuous or regular staff cover by day and waking, sleeping or on-call staff at night. A *staffed group home* has similar staffing arrangements but is a single living unit which provides between two and six resident places. Although an *unstaffed group home* also has fewer than six places, it has ad hoc or no day staff and on-call or no night cover. A client in an *adult foster placement* moves into an established household and has regular foster family support by day and on-call night support. Finally, most clients in *independent accommodation* (usually rented public sector housing) will be looking after themselves, or supported by informal carers; in some cases ad hoc day staffing and on-call night cover are provided by outreach services.

Thirty-seven per cent of the people in the costed sample were living in residential or nursing homes one year after leaving hospital (Table 5.1). This high number is not surprising as, by definition, homes in this category provide a high level of support on-site and are more similar to inpatient care than any other of our community accommodation categories. However, there are as many differences as similarities. A community-based unit with 24-hour staff cover for twenty clients provides a very different living environment from a long-stay psychiatric hospital with several hundred patients living in large wards.

A variety of agencies manage the accommodation units (Table 5.1). It can be seen that DHAs accommodate a greater number of people than any other agency; however, in addition to directly managed units, they are also involved in joint arrangements with voluntary organisations (listed under the

Table 5.1
Clients' accommodation arrangements — one year after discharge

	Managing agency for accommodation[a]						
Type of accommodation	DHA	SSD	VOL	PRIV	HSG	CON	All
Residential home	113	38	42	34	0	4	231
Hostel	16	22	53	4	0	17	112
Sheltered housing	0	3	6	0	0	6	15
Staffed group home	0	5	16	10	0	13	44
Unstaffed group home	9	2	15	0	0	3	29
Foster care	0	16	0	0	0	0	16
Independent living	1	1	6	6	77	1	92
Hospital	45	0	0	0	0	0	45
Total	184	87	138	54	77	44	584

a Abbreviations are DHA = district health authority; SSD = local authority social services department; VOL = voluntary organisation; PRIV = private sector agency; HSG = local authority housing department; CON = consortium arrangement, jointly managed but led by voluntary organisation.

consortium category). By transferring the responsibility for care between DHAs, the dowry finances remain within the public sector National Health Service. DHAs also continue to provide hospital-based care for members of the study population: 45 people had either been transferred directly to other hospitals or were resident in Friern or Claybury at the time when the one-year interview should have taken place.

Nine per cent of clients moved into privately managed units. Private sector (for-profit) provision for study members is concentrated around units with 24-hour staff cover, due in part to regulations which governed clients' social security entitlements and funded these placements. At the other end of the spectrum, 15 per cent of people were living independently, usually in domestic housing rented from the local authority.

Social services departments (SSDs) and voluntary (non-profit) organisations provide accommodation facilities across a range of categories. As Table 5.1 shows, voluntary organisations have direct responsibility for managing accommodation facilities used by 22 per cent of our sample, as well as a further 7 per cent as part of consortium arrangements, which have only recently been separately identified in our costs work. Linking with voluntary organisations and obtaining registered charity status allows DHAs to access funds from multiple sources. Although a large part of consortium income is derived from health authorities, access to a higher rate of social security benefits is also possible. Under consortium management arrangements there is a trend towards smaller and less highly staffed units than DHAs otherwise provide.

Box 5.2
Della

Della was one of the early hospital leavers. A local authority flat was rented for her to share with a friend (another former patient from Friern), but this involved Della sleeping permanently in the living room and was not an ideal arrangement.

During the year after she moved from Friern, Della had regular contact with a social worker and general practitioner and saw a psychiatrist on two occasions. No other service was used and her service package was the least expensive we have costed (£75.30 per week at 1993/94 price levels). Although she had no hospital inpatient stays during the year, she was subsequently re-admitted to Friern and stayed long enough to enter the study again. Her second move to the community took her to a residential unit with 24-hour waking staff cover but, although she was living in a more highly supported environment than before, she was nevertheless re-admitted to hospital and remained another year, meeting the entry requirements for the study a third time.

Use of other services

Services based outside the accommodation unit provide small but usually vital components of a community care package (Table 5.2). It is unnecessary to comment at length on the details, but some key findings can be emphasised. Most notably, a large number of agencies, departments and services are involved in supporting people with long-term mental health problems in the community. Although a high proportion of total cost is accounted for by the accommodation budget, there are implications for a range of other services and budgets.

With a multiplicity of client needs and agency responsibilities, there are dangers of overlaps and gaps in service provision; care management and care programming aim to address these potential problems. Note that Table 5.2 reports whether services have been used, not the intensity of use or the contribution to total weekly cost. For example, most people had some contact with a GP, although the contribution of GP services to total reprovision cost averaged less than half of one per cent across the sample.

An examination of the changes in service use over time allows us to monitor how individual community services are responding to the demands of the developing mixed economy of care. For example, the number of people using day care (in particular day services provided by social services) has been falling as succeeding cohorts have moved to the community. Also noticeable is the steady decline in field social worker involvement. More than half of the people in the first cohort had contact with a social worker; by cohorts 3 and 4 numbers had fallen to 20 per cent and by cohort 6 to 4 per cent. It is

Table 5.2
Service utilisation by cohort in year since discharge[a]

	Percentage of each cohort using service						
	1	2	3	4	5	6	7
Service	%	%	%	%	%	%	%
Accommodation facility	100	100	100	100	100	100	100
Hospital inpatient	18	22	5	17	21	21	20
Hospital outpatient	39	15	25	40	22	46	41
Hospital day patient	50	21	20	19	25	27	15
Community psychiatry	39	54	76	45	70	65	41
Nursing services	37	31	21	28	34	50	31
Chiropody	37	30	40	28	63	58	36
Psychology	3	1	35	2	26	2	13
Physiotherapy	3	0	5	0	2	0	10
Occupational therapy	0	7	27	4	5	2	0
GP	76	69	96	79	80	88	85
Dentist	21	21	29	15	28	15	28
Optician	24	9	18	15	24	21	15
Pharmacy	16	0	7	0	2	0	0
Social services day care	26	34	20	23	9	8	15
Field social work	55	41	21	23	16	4	26
Voluntary organisation day care	5	23	21	13	24	21	8
Social club	0	2	11	0	11	15	10
Volunteer inputs	0	3	6	2	0	0	0
Education classes	5	14	2	0	3	2	0
Police	5	2	2	0	17	6	13
Client's travel	16	30	37	28	9	60	54
Miscellaneous services	11	8	10	21	11	19	33
Sample size	38	87	82	47	87	48	39

a For people for whom we have completed CSRIs. The sample is therefore biased against those people re-admitted to hospital (for whom, generally, inpatient utilisation is higher and other utilisation lower).

likely that the fall in service use reflects scarcity of resources rather than reduction in client need, so it is perhaps surprising that a quarter of all cohort 7 members saw a social worker during their first year in the community. As Table 5.2 shows, use of day care facilities provided by social services also rose sharply for this group of leavers. We are currently examining these trends and apparent anomalies in greater detail.

Some changes in service use over time appear to be influenced by accommodation arrangements. For example, a number of purpose-built, highly staffed DHA units, planned at the beginning of the reprovision programme, came on-stream for cohort 3 leavers. Use of these new-build units with on-site nursing staff may have contributed to a fall in the number of people using inpatient hospital services in cohort 3, a figure which has otherwise remained constant.

5.4 The costs of community care

Methodology

In calculating and interpreting the costs of community care, we are guided by four basic principles. Briefly (a) costs should be measured comprehensively to include all service components; (b) differences in cost between individual clients should not be overlooked but examined and explained for policy insights, although (c) comparisons drawn from these examinations should be on a like-with-like basis. Finally, (d) cost information is of most use when combined with outcome evidence (Knapp and Beecham, 1990; and see Chapters 1 and 4). The basic principles of economic theory and the realities of community care policy lead us to use long-run marginal opportunity costs, which are calculated according to the methodologies set out in Chapter 3.

Costs descriptions

The comprehensive costs of community care for succeeding cohorts of leavers are laid out in Table 5.3. The average total cost of community care across the whole sample is £537 per week (expressed at 1993/94 prices). Costs include those absorbed by accommodation-related services and the provision of *all* service components that make up clients' individual care packages. The general trend shows that successive cohorts are more expensive to support in a community setting (after adjusting for inflation). Cohort 4 appears to be an exception, but when the influences on costs of the (hospital-assessed) needs and other characteristics of cohort members were checked statistically, we found that cohort 4 members were not, on average, as dependent as cohorts 3 or 5. In addition, the service packages for cohort 3 clients were relatively expensive, since these leavers benefited from a number of new accommodation units built at the height of the property price boom of the mid-1980s.

Costs relating to cohort 7 members appear to be lower on average than for cohort 6. Certainly, the rate of increase has levelled out, but it should be borne in mind that we have yet to interpolate costs for people we were unable to interview in cohort 7. Eleven clients in this group were transferred from Friern to other inpatient facilities and a further seven clients were re-admitted to hospital from their community placements. Therefore, the average cost of caring for *all* cohort 7 members will be higher than we have reported here.

Table 5.3
Cohorts of leavers and their costs after one year in the community

Cohort	Year of leaving	Year of costing	Cost per week (£)[a]	Sample size	Full population of leavers
1	1985/86	1986/87	313	43	44
2	1986/87	1987/88	467	110	118
3	1987/88	1988/89	538	115	119
4	1988/89	1989/90	456	74	78
5	1989/90	1990/91	595	148	140 (+ 21 'transfers')
6	1990/91	1991/92	704	55	69 (+3 'transfers')
7	1991/92	1992/93	686	39	62 (+ 11 'transfers')
Sample size	–	–	537	584	630[b] (+ 35 'transfers')

a At 1993/94 prices, inflating 1989/90 prices using the Department of Health general PSS inflator. Includes 428 people for whom costs were calculated from completed CSRIs and associated data and 156 people for whom costs were interpolated.
b Includes 20 people who died before the one-year interview; also 11 members of cohort 6, and 20 people in cohort 7 for whom costs will be interpolated.

Table 5.3 makes it clear that community care is not a cheap alternative to hospital inpatient services. Inevitably, the more dependent people who left hospital later in the closure programme require higher levels of support in their community units. However, there are many study clients, particularly in the early cohorts of leavers, who did not need the 24-hour nursing arrangements of a hospital and were able to move to much less formal care environments. This element of flexibility in service provision is a vitally important part of a successful reprovision programme:

> Community care is a matter of marshalling resources, sharing responsibilities and combining skills to achieve good quality modern services to meet the actual needs of real people, in ways those people find acceptable and in places which encourage rather than prevent normal living. ... A good quality community-orientated service may well be more expensive than a poor quality institutional one. ... The aim is not to save money: but to use it responsibly (Secretary of State for Social Services, 1985, pp.1-2).

It comes as no surprise that the most expensive care packages are received by those people in residential or nursing homes or that, for clients in these facilities, accommodation costs make up approximately 90 per cent of the total costs of care. Generally, as the level of support provided on site diminishes, so does the proportion of total cost which is absorbed by accommodation facility costs. Independent accommodation, where clients usually live in low-cost housing with little on-site support, is the least costly of the arrangements. There would be cause for concern if outside service receipt did not make a substantial contribution to the total cost of these clients' packages, since this could indicate lack of access to services rather than lack of need.

Funding arrangements

Several sources of funding contribute to the provision of community care. Money from the Department of Health reaches DHAs and family health service authorities (FHSAs) by way of separate national or regional routes. The former have traditionally held responsibility for mental health services, although the National Health Service and Community Care Act 1990 encourages local authorities to play a greater part. SSDs receive funding from central government departments and local taxes; voluntary organisations and housing associations are funded from SSDs or DHAs, central grants, donations and users' fees (usually paid from social security entitlements). Local authority housing departments bear some accommodation costs through provision of rented accommodation and housing benefit, and an amount equal to local taxes forgone is included where clients are exempt from payment. (For more details of funding routes, see Beecham et al., 1995.)

These agencies all provide funding for the support of the study population. Under the reprovision arrangements, the money from hospital budgets was 'protected' for use on community mental health services for these clients. More of this money went into the provision of specialised accommodation placements and less into other support services. Table 5.4, therefore, concentrates on the funding of the community-based accommodation. Although DHAs make a substantial input into four of the six agencies which manage accommodation units, their percentage share of funding is now less than when they funded long-stay hospital placements. Other agencies, therefore, bear a greater part of that burden and are not always reimbursed by the NHS (or specifically from the savings resulting from hospital rundown) for provision of these services.

Private sector residential accommodation relies almost entirely on client contributions for funding, a fact which emphasises the relationship between social security entitlements and proprietors' income prior to the changes introduced by the 1990 Act. The breakdown of agencies funding voluntary sector accommodation is similar to that of consortium arrangements, which might be expected considering the charitable status of these consortia. The table shows that only a small percentage of the funding burden of these agencies is met by the voluntary sector (which includes housing associations); both rely heavily on the public sector and client contributions (Hallam et al., 1994b).

A key feature of community care policy in England in the 1990s is the development of a mixed economy, introducing an internal market within the health service. (For details and discussions of these reforms see, for example, Wistow et al., 1994.) Although the formal care systems are still heavily dominated by public expenditure, it is likely that there will soon be moves to shift

Table 5.4
Funding of community accommodation[a]

Sources of funding	Managing agency for accommodation[b] DHA %	SSD %	VOL %	PRIV %	HSG %	CON %
District health authority	92.3	39.2	50.2	11.6	0.0	47.3
Local authority social services department	0.0	37.9	2.1	1.9	0.0	0.7
Voluntary organisation	0.0	0.0	3.5	0.0	0.0	0.0
Local authority housing department	0.1	0.2	0.2	0.2	30.4	0.1
Housing association	0.5	0.0	4.8	0.0	0.0	12.3
Local authority forgone local taxes	0.8	1.7	1.6	1.8	4.0	1.9
Housing benefit	0.1	1.3	0.5	0.7	13.3	1.9
Client contribution	6.3	19.8	37.2	84.0	52.3	35.7

a Relates to accommodation facility costs only; not total cost of care.
b Abbreviations are DHA = district health authority; SSD = local authority social services department; VOL = voluntary organisation; PRIV = private sector agency; HSG = local authority housing department; CON = consortium arrangement.

more of the financial responsibility for purchasing health and social care onto patients and users, and away from taxpayers (Knapp, 1995a).

5.5 Explaining cost variations

Planning to meet the costs of community care

We examined the associations between costs in the community and the assessed characteristics of inpatients prior to hospital discharge. Our aim was to build up a prediction equation which might assist service planners in structuring community support for people with long-term mental health problems. Using the TAPS database we were able to include data relating to clinical status, behaviour, size of social networks, and physical health as potential explanatory predictors. (Full details of the schedules used to collect these data can be found in O'Driscoll and Leff, 1993.) Multivariate statistical analyses were used to tease out the simultaneous influences of these predictors. (See Chapter 4 for background and theoretical bases for these analyses.) Data on the comprehensively costed sample from the first five cohorts were used in this work: a sample of 341 former long-stay patients. We examined the links between the baseline (hospital) characteristics and the subsequent costs of support in the community.

Average cost per week of community support for each individual was taken as the dependent variable in a series of multiple regression analyses, using the baseline data to generate the potential explanatory factors. Ordinary least squares estimation was employed. Clinical and other characteristics were introduced into the regression equations singly and in multiplicative combinations (including higher powers) to capture possible non-linear effects. The 'best' prediction equation is given in Table 5.5. The sample size has fallen to 217 because we do not have social network data on all inpatients (due to their inability or unwillingness to be interviewed). We also examined the relationship between cost and diagnosis after the effects of other factors had been included, but found no significant effect (see base of Table 5.5). The main equation in Table 5.5 'explains' 35 per cent of the observed variation in community cost. This is a slightly lower percentage of variance explained than the 39 per cent achieved with a smaller sample of early leavers (Knapp et al., 1990). This small reduction in predictive power is not surprising given the increase in sample size, increased heterogeneity of inpatient characteristics among leavers, and changes in local policy and practice, all of which have left their mark on service responses to presented needs.

The prediction equation. We give only a brief interpretation of the estimated prediction equation here (for full details see Knapp et al., 1995). *Other things being equal,* the costs of community care are influenced by the following factors:

- Costs are higher for people who never married and also for the 6 per cent of the sample who are divorced or separated men. These groups are less likely to receive informal support from family members, so they look to staff to meet their day-to-day care needs.
- Age has a negative effect on cost: older people appear to receive fewer non-accommodation services such as employment programmes, industrial therapy or further education. There is no evidence to suggest that their outcomes after one year are worse than those of younger clients.
- Costs are higher for males, although the effects are mediated through other factors.
- It might be expected that longer residence in psychiatric hospitals produces the kind of institutionalisation which would need more attention in the community. In fact, people who have spent longer periods in psychiatric hospitals seem to receive less support than others, perhaps because it is expected that the concentration of scarce resources on those whose hospital stays have been shorter will produce greater results in terms of health gain. However, it should be stressed that this effect is actually very small.
- People who have spent greater proportions of their lives in hospital receive service support packages which are more costly (although the effect is non-linear).

Table 5.5
Regression of community cost on client characteristics in hospital prior to discharge

	Coefficient	Significance
Constant	215.07	0.001
Male, divorced or separated[a]	182.70	0.009
Single[a]	95.843	0.007
Age in years, squared	-0.01633	0.093
Total previous time in mental hospital, in months squared[b]	$-7.52x10^{-4}$	0.047
Percentage of life in hospital	690.03	0.005
Percentage of life in hospital, squared	-569.96	0.084
Non-specific neurotic syndrome (PSE)	7.8388	0.003
If male,[a] delusions & hallucinations (PSE)	-5.3603	0.073
Negative symptoms (PSE)	29.296	0.011
Total Social Behaviour Schedule (SBS) score	36.192	0.003
Total SBS score, squared	-2.1733	0.009
If male,[a] daily nursing care, squared	98.425	0.020
No. of ex-patients named and seen (SNS)	-19.235	0.089
No. of hospital staff named and seen	8.8097	0.090
If male,[a] total persons named and seen	-6.6465	0.001
R^2	0.35	
F-statistic	7.27	0.00
Marginal impact of adding diagnostic group variables		
Organic[a]	1.2730	0.989
Schizophrenia[a]	–	–
Affective disorder[a]	-26.932	0.599
Neurosis/personality disorder[a]	-89.819	0.096
Learning disability[a]	6.0493	0.956
R^2	0.36	
F-statistic	5.86	0.00

a Dummy variables taking the value 1 if an individual had the named characteristic or diagnosis, and the value 0 otherwise.
b Excludes current admission.
Sample size = 217
Source: Knapp et al. (1995).

The influences of the clinical factors on cost are also interesting:

- Three constructed measures from the Present State Examination (PSE) were significant cost predictors: non-specific neurotic syndrome, negative symptoms, and delusions and hallucinations. The first and second exerted positive effects, and the third a negative effect, though only for males.
- Higher scores on the Social Behaviour Schedule (greater staff-reported ratings of abnormal behaviours) indicate higher needs and imply higher costs.
- The greater the number of areas in which daily nursing care is required the higher are costs, though interestingly again only for males.
- The instrument used to gather data on social networks (the SNS) requires an interview with each patient, so schedules could not be completed for everyone. Higher SNS scores mean more social contacts and our equation suggests that more communicative and gregarious people are less costly. An exception is that hospital inpatients who saw more hospital staff later cost more in the community (although the effect is modest).

Diagnosis has no obvious effect on cost once the above factors have been taken into account. Perhaps this should not come as a surprise, since these data were taken from case notes at admission, and many years have often elapsed since the diagnoses were made. The underlying psychiatric, behavioural and other characteristics of patients better predict downstream costs, not the diagnostic label. Diagnostic-related groups would therefore be of little predictive value for former long-stay hospital residents.

Costs, needs and outcomes

Reporting on the first 475 leavers (cohorts 1-5) one year after leaving hospital, the outcomes evaluation could find no adverse effects of relocation on clients on clinical and social measures, when compared to similar data for the matched stayers. Moreover, statistically significant differences between leavers and their 'matches' over time were revealed in terms of positive attitudes to present accommodation and a reduction in the restrictiveness of the environment (Anderson et al., 1993). In other words, the levels of expenditure described earlier produced encouraging outcomes for clients.

It is important to examine whether there is a statistical association between costs, needs and outcomes. In an earlier series of analyses employing data for members of just the first three cohorts of leavers, we examined the factors which together best explained the observed variation in weekly cost of community care one year after discharge from hospital (Beecham et al., 1991). The assessments originally undertaken while clients were resident in hospital were repeated one year after discharge, giving us a measure of needs in the community. Outcomes were calculated as the differences between these two scores.

Table 5.6
Estimated cost functions

	Equation A		Equation B	
	Coeff.	Sig.[a]	Coeff.	Sig.[a]
Constant term	57.72		204.7	<0.01
Client never married[b]	84.7	<0.01	83.3	<0.01
Length of stay in hospital (months)	0.329	<0.01	0.184	<0.05
Community skills (BELS[c])	29.6	<0.05		
Community skills, squared	-2.12	<0.01	-0.600	<0.01
Activity and social relationships (BELS)	13.40	<0.01	12.20	<0.01
Blunting of affect (PSE)	92.2	<0.01	83.3	<0.01
Incontinent (PHI)[b]	113.4	<0.01	112.0	<0.01
Impaired mobility (PHI)[b]	130.6	<0.05	115.6	<0.05
Social network — patients (SNS) squared	2.14	<0.01	1.81	<0.01
Expressed desire to move (PAQ)	85.2	<0.05	69.9	<0.05
Absolute difference in negative symptoms (PSE)	-34.8	<0.01	-22.3	<0.05
Relative difference in general anxiety squared (PSE)	21.8	<0.01	19.0	<0.01
Relative difference in delusions, hallucinations (PSE)	-0.192	<0.01	-0.12	<0.10
Reduced need for care (PHI)[b]	234	<0.01	182	<0.05
Absolute difference in non-professional network (SBS)	5.54	<0.05	5.21	<0.01
Relative difference in relatives network (SNS)	-0.562	<0.01	-0.434	<0.05
Relative difference in patient network (SNS)	-0.322	<0.05		
Improved helpfulness of medication (PAQ)	113.4	<0.05	109.5	<0.05
Health authority accommodation			91.7	<0.01
Voluntary or private sector accommodation			-69.9	<0.05
R^2	0.568	<0.01	0.642	<0.01
Adjusted R^2	0.499		0.585	

a Significance levels from t-tests on individual coefficients and F-test on R^2.
b Dummy variable taking the value 1 if the condition is satisfied, 0 otherwise.
c The mnemonics refer to the following instruments: BELS = Basic Everyday Living Skills; PSE = Present State Examination; PHI = Physical Health Index; SNS = Social Network Schedule; PAQ = Patient Attitude Questionnaire; SBS = Social Behaviour Schedule. See O'Driscoll and Leff (1993) for further details.

Sample size = 132 (Cohorts 1-3)
Source: Beecham et al. (1991).

Cost functions were estimated using ordinary least squares multiple regression, the final representation being selected on the usual criteria of statistical significance, interpretability and parsimony (Table 5.6). In fact, two estimated cost functions are reported, one of them excluding the dummy variables for sector of accommodation (private, voluntary, local authority, health authority). They explain 57 and 64 per cent of the observed community cost variation.

It is not necessary to discuss every one of the factors shown to have a significant effect on costs, but some key findings should be emphasised. First, there is an encouragingly strong link between costs and outcomes. Higher community care costs (higher levels of spending) were associated with greater improvements in the health and welfare of former hospital inpatients. In particular, improvements in negative symptoms, delusions and hallucinations, social networks (broadening) and the need for physical health care are all associated with higher costs.

A second key finding is that costs are sensitive to client characteristics and needs, as assessed in the community. Costs are higher for people with blunting of affect, incontinence, mobility problems and difficulties with community living skills. The estimated cost function also suggests that the private and voluntary sectors provide community care services for former long-stay inpatients more cost-effectively than local authorities, which in turn are more cost-effective than health authorities, although these inter-sector differences need further examination (Beecham et al., 1991).

5.6 The long-term cost consequences of psychiatric reprovision

The design of the North London reprovision study allows us to examine the longer-term service use patterns and their associated costs. Alongside the outcomes research by TAPS, we have costed the care packages received by the first three cohorts of leavers in their fifth year after leaving Friern and Claybury. A comparison of data relating to 72 people in cohorts 1 and 2 revealed an average increase of £56 per week ($p=0.02$) between the two points in time when this group was interviewed. It may be that the early, and more independent, leavers will have more contact with services over the years, if only because of the health problems generally associated with advancing age. The needs of later cohorts, known to be greater from the start, have been associated with higher costs during the first year in community placements. However, it is possible that any increase in care needs over time will be met by existing resources within their accommodation facilities and, consequently, the costs of care may not be greatly affected. This certainly appears to be the case with cohort 3 members. The average cost of caring for these study members actually *fell* by £5 per week between their first and fifth year in the community, although the difference is not significant.

Figure 5.1
Service use and cost after one and five years

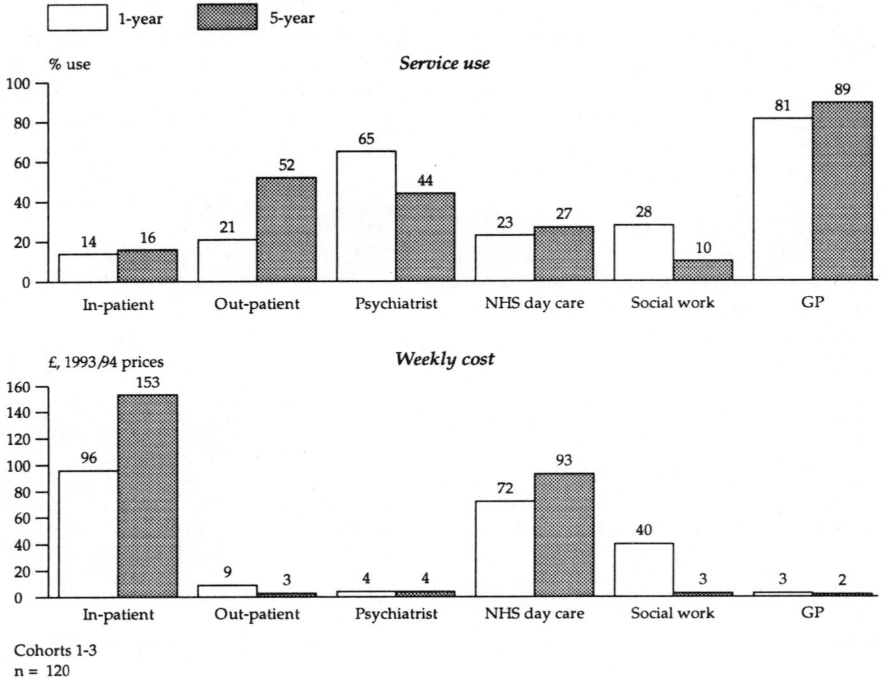

Figure 5.1 shows the percentage of people who used certain key services during their first and fifth year after leaving hospital. The fall in contact with field social workers appears to be as marked between the two interview points as it was with successive cohorts, but there may be an explanation for this. During the earliest years of the closure programme, it was part of discharge practice to allocate six months' follow-up social work to clients leaving hospital. It is possible that not everyone needed this service: certainly, as we see from Figure 5.1, not everyone received it, or the decrease in contact over time would be much more dramatic.

Although hospital inpatient services have been used by fewer people in the fifth year than in the first, they are being used, on average, more *intensively*: when they occur, inpatient stays are now longer. We can tell this from the increase in cost per week of the inpatient component of users' packages of care: from £96 to £153. This increase in cost also reflects the move from Friern and Claybury's acute facilities to those of more expensive general hospitals.

Box 5.3
Marjorie

Marjorie left hospital early in the reprovision programme and moved to a residential home owned and managed by the district health authority. She was in her early sixties at the time, considerably younger than the other six residents. The health of the unit's occupants was monitored during regular visits by a psychiatrist, social worker and chiropodist: the routine nature of the service contact and its domiciliary basis indicate the age and frailty of most of the residents. In addition to these services, Marjorie attended a DHA day unit once or twice a week. The total weekly cost of her package of care was £1027.83 (at 1993/94 price levels), reflecting a three-month inpatient hospital stay, after which she returned to the same accommodation unit in the community.

When we visited Marjorie five years after her initial discharge from hospital, we found that she had remained in the same residential home. However, during the time since the first interview, the property had been leased by the DHA to a housing association, which had taken over the management of the unit.

A psychiatrist was still making regular, though less frequent, visits to residents, but the social worker was no longer involved. An occupational therapist and a speech therapist had begun coming to see the residents on a weekly basis. The cost of Marjorie's care in the fifth year was £640 per week. There were no hospital inpatient stays and attendance at the day unit had stopped, but she was going to a social club occasionally and had made friends in the nearby shops. She had got into the habit of collecting the prescriptions for the whole house and the pharmacist sent her a present at Christmas.

Early findings from the long-term outcomes research suggest there are improvements in clients' neurotic symptoms, verbal and non-verbal behaviour and, most notably, in a reduction of negative symptoms after five years. During their first year after leaving hospital, clients reported an increasing number of friends and, although these social networks had not expanded further by the time of the five-year interview, an increase in the number of confidants was recorded, so relationships appear to be deepening (Leff et al., 1994).

5.7 Discussion

This research has produced encouraging findings at a time when many countries are committed to a policy of developing comprehensive community care for people with mental health problems while reducing dependence on inpatient hospital beds. However, the relocation of care from Friern and Claybury has certainly not eliminated the need for the hospitals and the services they provide. From a service perspective, even though the long-stay 'hotel' services of hospitals have been replaced in community-based units, we have shown that there is a continuing need for clinical, social and other support provided by day patient, outpatient and short-stay inpatient facilities. To provide adequate and appropriate community-based care for people with high support needs, it is vital that all services which long-stay hospitals provide are relocated appropriately, in sufficient number, and can be accessed when needed.

Moreover, although most people appear to be stable and enjoy living in their new homes, a few are reported to be grieving for the hospital, and some people attempt to return when life in the community becomes too demanding. Maintaining some form of contact with old friends, staff and familiar surroundings has been important to the continuity of most leavers' lives: closure of the hospitals means another major adjustment, and structures should be put in place in recognition of these needs.

The variety of accommodation types used by members of this study reflects their different demands and needs but, over and above these facilities, a range of other services is required to provide comprehensive support. Even in the most highly staffed accommodation units, not all the components of care packages can be provided in-house: psychiatry, psychology, chiropody and social work services are usually supplied on a peripatetic basis; recreational and leisure activities are still required. The CSRI asks carers whether there are any services the client needs but does not receive: lack of suitable day care and advocacy services are often mentioned. However, shortage of personal money is the most common and major problem. Despite efforts to allow residents to choose their own room furnishings or be involved in the running of the home, it is difficult to encourage integration into community life if a cinema ticket or snack meal takes nearly half their weekly income.

The reprovision of long-stay hospital services from Friern and Claybury is a well-planned and well-financed programme: two factors which have undoubtedly contributed to its success. In addition to general medical and nursing care, supervision of medication, monitoring and assessment, the two hospitals provided residents with hotel services, day activities and social support. In the community, these services are supplied by a range of agencies in a variety of settings. Adequate funding is obviously crucial to enable replacements for all these service areas, not just in the long-term but *before* patients move out of hospital.

Importantly, our data highlight the *distribution* of funding between providing agencies: the burden no longer falls to the health authority in the same way as it did when hospitals provided care for this client group and, at present, the load is far from evenly distributed between agencies or services (Knapp et al., 1992). The implementation of the National Health Service and Community Care Act 1990 has brought about organisational changes as well as those designed to shift the onus of financial responsibility; however, even in the fast-changing world of care policy, implementation and practice, the research evidence points to a successful approach that can be transferred to other closure programmes.

References

Anderson, J., Dayson, D., Wills, W., Gooch, C., Margolius, O., O'Driscoll, C. and Leff, J. (1993) Clinical and social outcomes of long-stay psychiatric patients after one year in the community, *British Journal of Psychiatry*, 162, Supplement 19, 45-56.

Beecham, J.K., Knapp, M.R.J. and Fenyo, A.J. (1991) Costs, needs and outcomes: community care for people with long-term mental health problems, *Schizophrenia Bulletin*, 17, 3, 427-39.

Beecham, J.K., Knapp, M.R.J. and Schneider, J. (1995) Policy and finance for community care: the new mixed economy, in M. Watkins, N. Hervey, S. Ritter and J. Carson (eds) *Collaborative Community Mental Health Care*, Edward Arnold, Sevenoaks.

Davidge, M., Elias, S., Jayes, B., Wood, K. and Yates, J. (1993) Survey of English mental illness hospitals, report prepared for the Mental Health Task Force, Department of Health, London.

Hallam, A., Beecham, J.K., Fenyo, A.J. and Knapp, M.R.J. (1994a) Reprovision costs: comparing a detailed approach with interpolations, Discussion Paper 1029, Personal Social Services Research Unit, University of Kent at Canterbury.

Hallam, A., Beecham, J.K., Knapp, M.R.J. and Fenyo, A.J. (1994b) The costs of accommodation and care: community provision for former long-stay psychiatric hospital patients, *European Archives of Psychiatry and Clinical Neuroscience*, 243, 6, 304-10.

Jones, D. (1993) The selection of patients for reprovision, in J. Leff (ed.) *Evaluating Community Placement of Long-Stay Psychiatric Patients, British Journal of Psychiatry*, 162, Supplement 19, 36-9.

Knapp, M.R.J. (1995a) From psychiatric hospital to community care: reflections on the English experience, in M. Moscarelli (ed.) *The Economics of Schizophrenia*, Wiley and Sons, New York.

Knapp, M.R.J. (1995b) Community mental health services: towards an understanding of cost-effectiveness, in P. Tyrer and F. Creed (eds) *Community Psychiatry in Action*, Cambridge University Press, Cambridge.

Knapp, M.R.J. and Beecham, J.K. (1990) Costing mental health services, *Psychological Medicine*, 20, 893-908.

Knapp, M.R.J., Beecham, J.K., Anderson, J., Dayson, D., Leff, J., Margolius, O., O'Driscoll, C. and Wills, W. (1990) Predicting the community costs of closing psychiatric hospitals, *British Journal of Psychiatry*, 157, 661-70.

Knapp, M.R.J., Beecham, J.K. and Gordon, K. (1992) Predicting the community cost of closing psychiatric hospitals: national extrapolations, *Journal of Mental Health*, 1, 315-26.

Knapp, M.R.J., Beecham, J.K., Hallam, A. and Fenyo, A.J. (1993) The costs of community care for former long-stay psychiatric hospital patients, *Health and Social Care in the Community*, 1, 193-201.

Knapp, M.R.J., Beecham, J.K., Fenyo, A.J. and Hallam, A. (1995) Community mental health care for former hospital inpatients: predicting costs from needs and diagnoses, *British Journal of Psychiatry*, 166, supplement 27, 10-18.

Leff, J., Dayson, D., Gooch, C., Thornicroft, G. and Wills, W. (1993) A matched case-control follow-up study of long-stay patients discharged from two psychiatric institutions, TAPS Paper 19, Team for the Assessment of Psychiatric Servicess, Royal Free Hospital, London.

Leff, J., Thornicroft, G., Coxhead, N. and Crawford, C. (1994) A five year follow-up of long-stay psychiatric patients discharged to the community, *British Journal of Psychiatry*, 165, supplement 25, 13-17.

O'Driscoll, C. and Leff, J. (1993) Design of the research study on the long-stay patients, in J. Leff (ed.) *Evaluating Community Placement of Long-Stay Psychiatric Patients, British Journal of Psychiatry*, 162, Supplement 19, 18-24.

Secretary of State for Social Services (1985) *Community Care: Government Response to the Second Report from the Social Services Committee*, Cmnd 9674, HMSO, London.

Wistow, G., Knapp, M.R.J., Hardy, B. and Allen, C. (1994) *Social Care in a Mixed Economy*, Open University Press, Buckingham.

6 Elderly People with Dementia: Costs, Effectiveness and Balance of Care

*Shane Kavanagh, Justine Schneider, Martin Knapp, Jennifer Beecham and Ann Netten**

6.1 Introduction

The projected increase in the number of people of retirement age and above is particularly marked for those aged 85 and over: the Office of Population Censuses and Surveys (OPCS, 1991) estimates an increase of 31 per cent, from 761,000 persons in 1991 to 998,000 persons in 2001. The 'greying' of the population, along with technological advances in medical treatments, is placing an increasing burden on the public purse and on carers.

Particular financial pressure built up in the 1980s due to the social security funding of places in independent residential and nursing homes (growing from £10 million for 12,000 claimants in 1979 to £1,625 million for 220,000 claimants in 1991), fuelled by open-ended entitlements and incentives to managers in health and local authorities to minimise the drain on their own budgets. This spending on residential care has been reined in by the community care reforms which placed funding for care places with local authorities. The 1990 National Health Service and Community Care Act — along with subsequent guidance documents — has placed considerable emphasis on the reduction of long-stay hospital places and delayed admission to residential or nursing homes. In addition, the place of 'continuing care' beds within the NHS is a contentious issue. However, the ageing population and the demand for long-overdue improvements in the support provided to carers means that formal care services continue to face financial pressures.

One of the main public health and economic challenges is the extensive prevalence of mental health problems in old age, particularly dementia. The prevalence of dementia increases significantly with age, and the expected number of cases therefore rises markedly as the proportion aged over 85 increases. In this chapter we describe the balance of care and support for elderly people with cognitive impairment, focusing on service utilisation in each mode of care and the accompanying resource consequences, and then explore and cost a number of possible changes to the balance of provision as central government policies are implemented. Of particular interest in relation to very dependent elderly people with dementia is reduced reliance on institutional care and enhanced support for unpaid carers in the community. Although cost containment and the desire to improve cost-effectiveness in the delivery of services were considerations in the reform of health and social care in the UK, and rightly remain relevant as criteria for policy and practice, it is fundamentally important that potential changes to the balance of care are discussed in the light of evidence on quality and effectiveness of each option.

6.2 The prevalence of mental health problems in old age

A variety of mental health problems affect people in old age, dementia being particularly serious because it is clinically irreversible. The American Psychiatric Association (1980) describes dementia as memory impairment, associated with impairment in abstract thinking, impaired judgement, other disturbances of cortical function, or personality change, affecting work, social activities and relationships with others. The DSM III classification distinguishes between mild, moderate and severe dementia in the following ways: *mild* — although work or social activities are significantly impaired, the capacity for independent living remains, with adequate personal hygiene and relatively intact judgement; *moderate* — independent living is hazardous and some degree of support is necessary; *severe* — activities of daily living are so impaired that continuous support is required: for example, the person is unable to maintain minimal personal hygiene, is largely incoherent or mute (American Psychiatric Association, 1980). Alzheimer's disease and arteriosclerotic dementia (multiple-infarct) are the most common causes of dementia.

A number of surveys have estimated the prevalence of dementia in the UK (Gurland et al., 1983; Maule et al., 1984; Clark et al., 1986; Brayne and Calloway, 1989; Livingston et al., 1990). The meta-analysis of prevalence data by Hofman et al. (1991) provides a satisfactory summary. Age and sex-specific prevalence rates were provided by pooling the results of twelve population-based European surveys, with the studies screened to ensure that they were representative by controlling for factors such as sample size, diagnosis equivalent to DSM III, and inclusion of people resident in institutions as well as those living in private households. Figure 6.1 illustrates the age and sex-specific rates. These estimated prevalence rates were combined with population estimates for England (OPCS, 1993) to produce figures for expected numbers of cases (see Table 6.1). About two-thirds of those cases presented will have 'mild' dementia and about one-third moderate or severe dementia.

However, it could be argued that focusing on just a narrow clinical definition of dementia may underestimate the requirement for care services. Many older people have other mental health problems and neurological disorders, and co-morbidity is common. All of these people may have considerable levels of dependency and require similar health and social care services. A

Table 6.1
Prevalence of dementia in the population

Age group	Population of England, 1992 (million)	Prevalence (rate per 1000)	Expected cases (000)
65-69	2.272	16	36.4
70-74	1.988	42	83.5
75-79	1.525	60	91.5
80-84	1.070	130	139.1
85-89	0.563	216	121.6
90 +	0.230	336	77.3
Total	7.648	71	549.3

Sources: Hofman et al. (1991), OPCS (1993).

Figure 6.1
Age and sex-specific prevalence rates for dementia (meta-analysis of European studies)

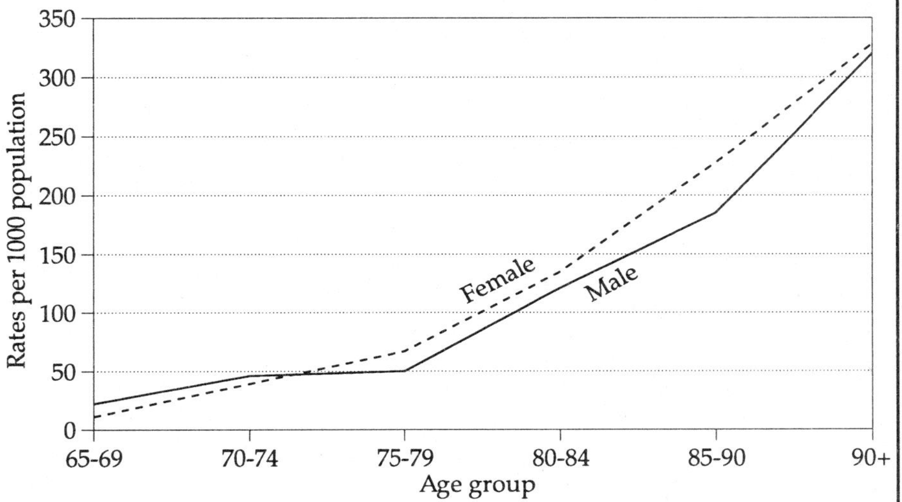

Source: Hofman et al. (1991).

more inclusive approach is to include all people over the age of 65 who have impaired intellectual functioning.

This approach allowed us to access the data contained in the OPCS Surveys of Disabilities in Great Britain which provide useful information on place of accommodation, utilisation of health and social care services (therefore providing the basis for estimating costs), as well as prevalence estimates. Two surveys were conducted: the first related to adults living in private households (conducted in 1985) and the second related to adults living in communal establishments such as residential care homes, nursing homes and hospitals (1986). Details of the survey methods are provided by Martin et al. (1988). An eleven-point inventory was employed to assess the degree of impairment with respect to intellectual functioning (see Box 6.1).

The surveys provide weightings that allowed us to obtain gross estimates of the number of people with cognitive impairment by age and sex within the population in Great Britain in 1986. Prevalence rates were obtained by

Box 6.1
OPCS intellectual functioning scale

Number of problems from the following:
Often forgets what he/she was supposed to be doing before finishing it
Often loses track of what is being said in the middle of a conversation
Thoughts tend to be muddled or slow
Often gets confused about what time of day it is
Cannot watch a half-hour TV programme all the way through and tell someone what it was about
Cannot remember and pass on a message correctly
Often forgets to turn off things such as fires, cookers or taps
Often forgets the name of people in the family or friends seen regularly
Cannot read a short article in the newspaper
Cannot write a short letter to someone without help
Cannot count well enough to handle money

Severity score	Number of problems identified from above
13.0	11
12.0	10
10.5	9
9.5	8
8.0	7
7.0	6
6.0	5
4.5	4
3.5	3
2.0	2
1.0	1

Table 6.2
Overall prevalence of cognitive impairment as measured by the OPCS Disability Surveys, estimated for 1992

Age group	Population of England, 1992 (million)	'Advanced' impairment		All impairment	
		Prevalence rate (per 1000)	Expected cases (000)	Prevalence rate (per 1000)	Expected cases (000)
65-69	2.272	14	32.9	35	102.1
70-74	1.988	16	32.8	45	101.9
75-79	1.525	37	56.8	82	142.4
80-84	1.070	68	72.9	137	163.5
85+	0.793	162	126.5	264	224.6
Total	7.648	42	321.8	96	734.6

Sources: OPCS (1989a,b, 1993).

dividing the projected number of people with cognitive impairment by the estimated population for 1986. These rates were then combined with the population of England in 1992 (OPCS, 1993) to estimate the number of people with cognitive impairment[1] (see Table 6.2).

The broader definition employed by the OPCS disability surveys produces an estimated prevalence of cognitive impairment of 9.6 per cent (score on intellectual impairment scale greater than 2) for the population aged over 65, equivalent to three-quarters of a million people. This compares to the Hofman et al. (1991) estimate of just over half a million expected cases, or 7.1 per cent. In the remainder of this chapter we will concentrate on the approximately 320,000 people aged over 65 with scores greater than 7 on the cognitive impairment scale, and refer to these people as having *advanced cognitive impairment*. The clinical complaints which the elderly people or their proxies[2] reported as the underlying causes of disability were senile dementia (62.5 per cent), stroke (13.7 per cent), depression (4.6 per cent) and schizophrenia (2.6 per cent). Further investigation of the pathological causes of cognitive impairment was not considered fruitful for two reasons: the OPCS survey complaint questions do not provide clinical information robust enough to yield accurate epidemiological estimates for such small numbers of cases; and cognitive impairment or dementia are terms which encompass a wide variety of pathological complaints (Gilleard, 1984), for example thyroid disease, drug toxicity and alcoholism. Although there are problems in relying on self-reported diagnoses, senile dementia was the most commonly reported cause of cognitive impairment, and there was significant correlation between intellectual impairment scores and scores on other relevant impairment scales, such as continence, communication, behaviour and ability for self-care: symptoms that commonly affect people with dementia (Kitwood, 1990).

6.3 The balance of care

Place of accommodation in 1986

The OPCS surveys allow a description of where people with advanced cognitive impairment were resident (Table 6.3) in 1986. Thirteen per cent were living alone in private households, despite the greater risks involved (Taylor et al., 1983). Informal care may have been received, but generally the same level of supervision as that offered by co-residents could not be provided. Half of the elderly people with advanced cognitive impairment were living in households with other people, which provided them with a better chance of informal support, but simultaneously increased the likelihood of carer stress (Greene et al., 1982; Brodaty and Hadzi-Pavlovic, 1990). The OPCS survey information suggests the mean age of carers is 63, disguising a bi-modal distribution between younger carers and older spouse-carers.

The remaining 37 per cent of elderly people with advanced cognitive impairment lived in institutions (defined as having been continuously resident for six months). The OPCS survey classified accommodation into *residential services only*, taken to mean residential homes run by local authorities, private or voluntary organisations, and *residential services with medical or nursing support*, taken to mean private or voluntary nursing homes, high dependency local authority homes, and hospitals. It would be misleading to draw a sharp distinction between these two groups on the basis of care provided, for there are numerous overlaps in level and style of care, and many homes now carry dual registration (Darton and Wright, 1991). Approximately 10 per cent of people with advanced cognitive impairment were resident in NHS hospitals. The majority were in geriatric, psychogeriatric and psychiatric beds (see Appendix 6.1 for a full description of the balance between different settings in 1986).

Table 6.3
Where people reside

Place of residence	Estimated number, 1992 (000)	%
Households — living alone	40.6	12.6
Households — living with others	152.6	47.4
Local authority residential homes	26.7	8.3
Independent sector residential homes	21.4	6.6
Independent sector nursing homes	58.8	18.3
NHS hospitals	21.9	6.8
Total	321.8	100

Sources: OPCS (1989a,b), see Appendix 6.1 for further details.

It is interesting to see how the degree of cognitive impairment was associated with where people lived (see Figure 6.2a). The change in the balance between households and institutional care was most marked for those people whose impairment was rated 7 or above on the intellectual functioning scale, particularly for those with the highest ratings of 12 and 13. People with higher scores on the intellectual impairment scale were much less likely to live alone in households, but many of those with higher impairment scores still lived in households with others. This finding using cross-sectional data tends to support longitudinal studies that illustrate that people living with others are less likely to be admitted to long-term supported accommodation (Bergmann et al., 1978; Reddy and Pitt, 1993) and emphasises the key role of carers within the process of community care. The use of different forms of supported accommodation appears to be relatively insensitive to the degree of intellectual impairment (Figure 6.2b).

Other factors appear to influence the use of supported accommodation, such as the ability for self-care and incontinence. The balance between care in households and care in supported accommodation appeared to be more sensitive to the rating of overall disability (Figure 6.3a).[3] The degree of disability again had a greater effect on the proportion of people living alone in households compared to the proportion living with others. The use of hospital accommodation was more likely for the highest two categories of impairment, and the use of residential accommodation was more common at lower levels of impairment (Figure 6.3b). (Appendix 6.2 provides estimates of the actual number of people in Great Britain at each level of impairment.)

Changes since 1986

The OPCS data allow us to estimate the relative proportions of people with advanced cognitive impairment in each care environment at the time of the surveys in 1985 and 1986. However, changes in the population aged 65 and over between then and 1992 have been taken into account. The increase in the number of people aged 65 and over — particularly the growth in the number of people in older age groups — means that the absolute number of people with cognitive impairment has increased. In addition, the distribution of people between care settings may also have changed. There was continued growth in the private and voluntary sectors due to the incentives offered by social security financing arrangements (Darton and Wright, 1993), and the long-term policy of de-institutionalisation reduced the number of beds in psychiatric and geriatric wards. In addition, the policies embodied in the 1990 National Health Service and Community Care Act have reduced the numbers of places in local authority homes. Overall, there was an increase in places provided by independent sector residential and nursing homes and a decrease in the places available in NHS hospitals and local authority homes.

Unfortunately, we lack the necessary information to document precisely

Figure 6.2

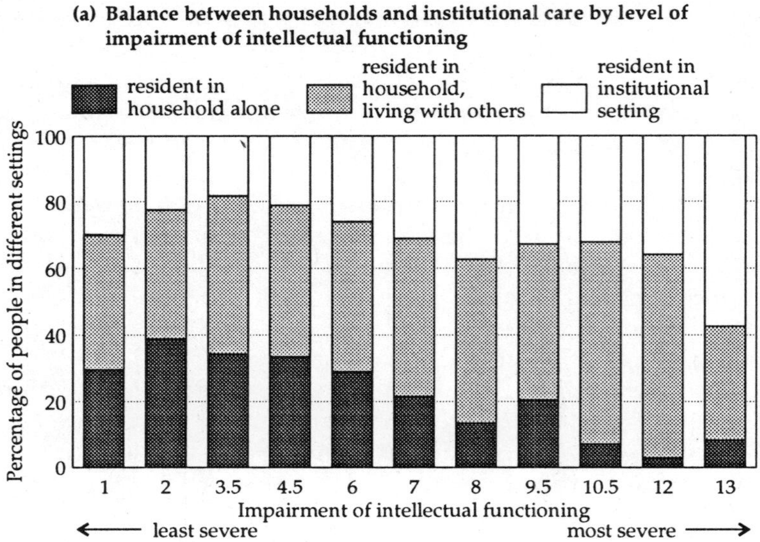

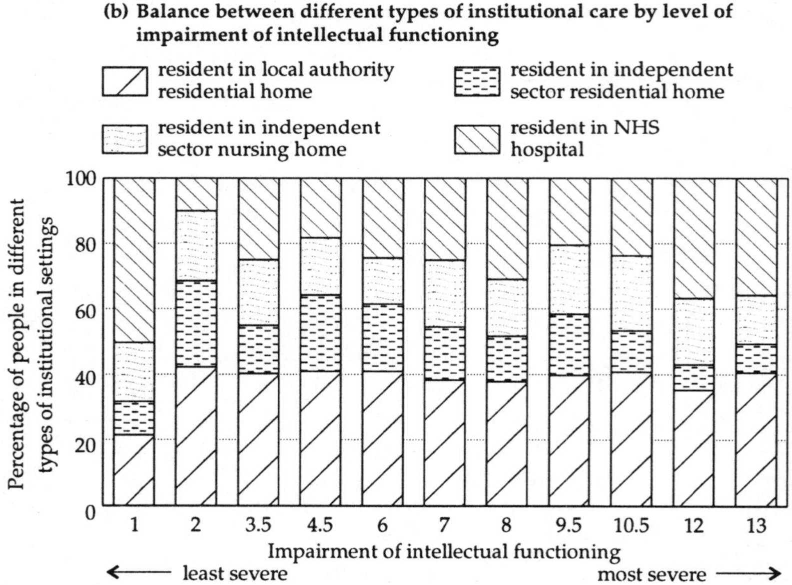

Source: OPCS (1989a,b); see Appendix 6.2 for further details.

Figure 6.3

(a) Balance between households and institutional care by overall rating of disability

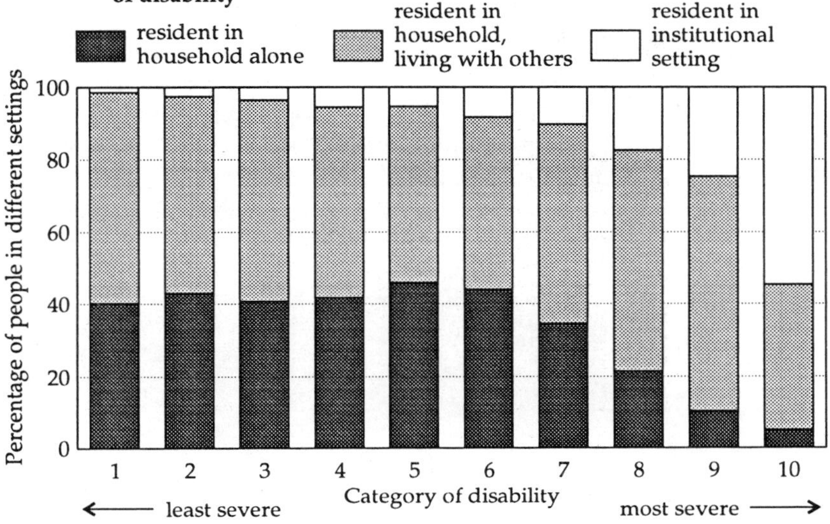

(b) Balance between different types of institutional care by overall rating of disability

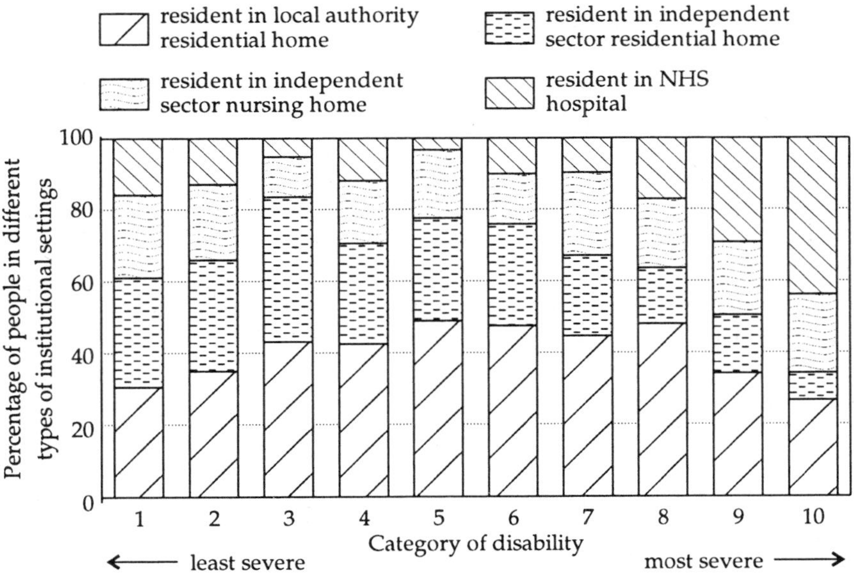

Source: OPCS (1989a, b); see Appendix 6.2 for further details.

the effect of these changes on the balance of care for people with advanced cognitive impairment, but we can provide an indicative estimate based on certain assumptions. First, we assume that the prevalence rate remained unaltered, and applied the age and sex specific rates to the population in England in 1992. Second, we assume that, although the number of places in different forms of supported accommodation has altered, the dependency profile with respect to cognitive impairment has remained unchanged. This allowed us to estimate the likely number of people with advanced cognitive impairment in institutional care in 1992. We were then able to estimate the numbers of people resident in households by subtracting our estimate of the numbers in institutional care from our overall estimate of the prevalence of advanced cognitive impairment. The estimated balance of care using these assumptions is shown in Table 6.3, and a detailed description of the calculations and methods employed is contained in Appendix 6.1.

Service utilisation and costs

Information on service receipt was gathered in the OPCS surveys, although it was incomplete and needed to be supplemented with data collected in other research (Davies et al., 1990; Knapp et al., 1992). As far as possible, we attached estimated figures for long-run marginal opportunity costs to all services used by elderly people (see Chapter 3). We had to employ different strategies for costing each of the three main groups of accommodation settings.

For people living in *private households,* we include the costs of housing, personal consumption and informal care. Housing has an opportunity cost in that if the person moves into an alternative care setting the accommodation becomes available for someone else to use. We estimated this cost by up-rating to 1992/93 prices the figures calculated by Challis and Davies (1986).[4]

For people living in a hospital or care home, items such as food and heating form part of the 'hotel' cost of care, and people in these settings also purchase personal requisites such as toiletries. In costing the care provided to people in private households, all these items therefore need to be included to ensure valid comparison. These personal living expenses, or personal consumption, were estimated using the 1990 *Family Expenditure Survey* (Central Statistical Office, 1991).

In the case of informal care, where relatives or friends provide help with self-care when the person is living in a private household, a similar argument applies. Should the person move to an alternative care setting, this role is performed by the staff of the facility. It is therefore necessary to place a monetary value on the opportunities forgone by friends and relatives in their caring role. We costed this using the approach developed by Netten (1990).

The proportions of people using most health and social care services were small, the one notable exception being contacts with general practitioners. Estimates of service contact rates for people living in private households are

Table 6.4
Percentage of elderly people with advanced cognitive impairment in private households receiving services in past year

Service	Persons with advanced cognitive impairment receiving service %
Hospital inpatient	16
Psychiatrist	12
Community nurse	36
Auxiliary nurse	11
Community psychiatric nurse	2
Chiropodist	16
Health visitor	12
Meals on wheels	8
Home help	24
Social worker	14
Day care	12
General practitioner	91
Respite — hospital	3
Respite — nursing home	3
Respite — local authority	5

Source: OPCS (1989a).

provided in Table 6.4,[5] while the costing methodology is described by Netten (1992b) and in Chapter 3. Table 6.5 summarises the average weekly costs by funder.

For *residential and nursing homes*, cost information came from a variety of sources. We estimated the cost of local authority homes using the figures cited in the DH Memorandum laid before the House of Commons Select Committee on Health[6] (Department of Health, 1991). Because these refer to *all* residents, we added an element related to the higher dependency of people with advanced cognitive impairment derived from earlier cost function analyses (Darton and Knapp, 1984)[7] to produce an estimate of £338.22 per week (1992/93 prices). Private and voluntary residential and nursing home costs were based on figures calculated by Laing and Buisson (1993) giving an average charge of £218 for private residential homes, and £338 for private nursing home agency was calculated on the basis of the arrangements for funding after 1 April 1993.[8] To these direct costs for the various sectors we added two elements: the indirect financial responsibilities falling to other parts of the local authority or to other agencies, estimated in previous research to be 5 per cent of direct cost (Knapp et al., 1992); and the 'pocket money' DSS allowance (£12.20 per week) paid to residents, which we use as a proxy measure of the cost of personal consumption.

Table 6.5
Average weekly costs for people living in private households, 1992/93 prices

Funders	Living alone £	Living with others £
District health authorities	17.46	33.21
Social services department	27.26	20.13
Family health services authorities	3.03	3.19
DSS clients and their families		
Informal care	49.23	69.14
Personal consumption	74.90	77.67
Accommodation costs	40.17	40.17
Total	212.05	243.51

Source: OPCS (1989b).

We based *hospital* costs on the summary specialty costs per inpatient day in Financial Return FR12 to the Department of Health, supplemented to take account of 'hotel' services (laundry, meals), administration, some other treatments (pathology, for example) and capital.[9] The resultant cost of continuing care hospital provision was £110 per patient day at 1992/93 prices, including external services funded by social services and other agencies.

The results of these various cost calculations are summarised in the first six rows of Table 6.6; the care packages in the remaining four rows are explained below.

6.4 Policy options for the future balance of care

The policy prescriptions for health and social care suggested by the two White Papers of 1989 (Secretaries of State, 1989a,b) were predicated on assumptions about the relative effectiveness of alternative care settings, some of those assumptions being backed by research evidence. Among the possible changes to the balance of care given prominence in the White Papers, and also in the 1990 National Health Service and Community Care Act and subsequent government guidance documents, were a reduction in the use of long-stay hospital accommodation, delayed admission to residential care from private households, and better support for carers.

Below we set out a number of broad policy options for changing, and hopefully improving, the balance of care services for elderly people with advanced cognitive impairment. Unfortunately, evidence on the effectiveness and cost-effectiveness of different care settings is scarce (Melzer et al., 1991).

Table 6.6
Summary of average weekly care package costs, 1992/93 prices

	DHA[a] £	FHSA[a] £	SSD[a] £	DSS[a]/Clients £	Total £
Living alone in private household	17.46	3.03	27.26	164.30	212.05
Living with others in private household	33.21	3.19	20.13	186.98	243.51
Local authority residential home	8.15	8.15	326.02	12.20	354.52
Private and voluntary residential home	5.30	5.30	65.72	164.19	240.51
Private and voluntary nursing home	7.77	7.77	143.52	178.64	337.70
Long-stay hospital	739.95	0.00	21.94	11.20	773.09
Living with others in private household with improved respite support	57.94	3.19	41.60	186.98	289.71
Living alone in private household with improved home care	41.52	3.03	58.61	164.30	267.46
NHS nursing home	420.95	0.00	0.00	12.20	433.15
Enhanced local authority home provision	5.78	2.60	402.65	12.20	423.23

a Abbreviations are: DHA = district health authority; FHSA = family health service authority; SSD = social services department; DSS = Department of Social Services.
See text for sources and details of costs.

The policy options chosen are defined in terms of combinations of different packages of care, the latter selected on the basis either that they are already commonly found in England today, or because they have been shown to be effective in pilot experiments. Each is costed on the basis of best available evidence, although the assumptions that we have been forced to make should not be overlooked. As well as the overall cost implications, we consider the distribution of the cost burden between agencies under the funding arrangements and boundaries which came into effect in April 1993. The projected numbers of people in the different care settings for each policy option are given in Table 6.7. Of course, given the nature and breadth of this national balance of care mapping and analysis, we cannot examine or project with any ease the micro-targeting of community and other support services.

Table 6.7
Distribution of elderly people with advanced cognitive impairment by accommodation type, Options I-VIII, England, 1992

Package	Numbers of elderly people (000s) by Option							
	I	II	III	IV	V	VI	VII	VIII
Living alone in private household	40.6	40.6	0	40.6	40.6	40.6	0	0
Living with others in private household	152.6	0	152.6	152.6	152.6	152.6	0	0
Local authority home	26.7	26.7	26.7	32.2	26.7	0	0	0
Private and voluntary residential home	21.4	21.4	21.4	25.8	21.4	21.4	21.4	21.4
Private and voluntary nursing home	58.8	58.8	58.8	70.8	58.8	58.8	58.8	58.8
Long-stay hospital	21.9	21.9	21.9	0	0	21.9	0	10.95
Living with others in private household with improved respite support	0	152.6	0	0	0	0	152.6	152.6
Living alone in private household with improved home care	0	0	40.6	0	0	0	40.6	40.6
NHS nursing home	0	0	0	0	21.9	0	21.9	10.95
Enhanced local authority home provision	0	0	0	0	0	26.7	26.7	26.7

See text for sources and further details.

Option I: Baseline provision

The first policy option is *the status quo*: to remain with baseline provision for elderly people with advanced cognitive impairment as revealed by the OPCS surveys. We can cost this option as described in the previous section, giving a comprehensive annual cost of approximately £5,067 million, having adjusted the numbers of people in each care setting in line with changes in the size of the elderly population since the surveys were undertaken. This option obviously would not improve the amount or quality of support for anyone. Total and component costs by agency are set out in the first row of Table 6.8.

Option II: Improved community support with respite care

A second policy option would be to extend considerably the availability of respite care to the carers of the approximately 153,000 elderly people with advanced cognitive impairment living in shared private households, so as to lessen the burdens of informal care and allow elderly people to remain in the community longer before entering institutional care. A number of studies have found positive benefits for caregivers flowing from respite care and support programmes (for example, Brodaty and Gresham, 1989; Drummond et al., 1991; Levin and Moriarty, 1994), although a recent review of available research concluded that the effects on carer stress might be modest, and may be gained at the expense of worsened outcomes for clients (Melzer et al., 1991).

Donaldson and Gregson (1988) evaluated a specialist family support unit (FSU) which offered tailor-made packages of respite care with a mix of other community services. They found that fewer people in the FSU group died while resident in the community and that people could be supported satisfactorily in the community for a longer period when compared to community care without this form of support, though at higher cost (because of the FSU itself and increased service utilisation). If time spent at home is considered to be at least as desirable as long-term hospital care, then the FSU may be viewed as cost-effective, given its lower cost in comparison to hospital provision for each of these additional days. The Donaldson and Gregson evaluation had incomplete measures of costs and outcomes, for example omitting the costs of several community health services, capital cost elements, costs to carers and the impact of respite services on carer stress. Nevertheless, the FSU is a good service arrangement to include in the options for changing the balance of care, and the evaluation provides a helpful starting point for costing it. Missing costs were therefore imputed (costs for accommodation, personal expenditure and informal care were estimated as before), and the whole uprated to 1992/93 price levels.[10] We assume that the cost of informal care remains constant, although over time the FSU could reduce the informal

Table 6.8
Annual cost of policy Options I-VIII, 1992/93 prices

	DHA £m	FHSA £m	SSD £m	DSS/Clients £m	Total £m
Option I: Baseline provision	1187	73	1210	2596	5067
Option II: Improved community support with respite care	1384	73	1381	2596	5434
Option III: Community support with enhanced home care	1238	73	1277	2596	5184
Option IV: Reducing long-stay hospital provision, replacing with combination of different institutional care	351	81	1386	2737	4556
Option V: Reducing long-stay hospital provision, replacing with NHS nursing home provision	823	73	1185	2597	4678
Option VI: Higher quality residential care	1184	65	1317	2596	5162
Option VII: Universal changes in provision, reducing long-stay hospital provision by 100%	1067	65	1529	2597	5259
Option VIII: Universal changes in provision, reducing long-stay hospital provision by 50%	1250	65	1542	2597	5453

For details of abbreviations, see note on Table 6.1.
See text for sources and details of costs.
Totals may not exactly match the sum of agency costs due to rounding.

care input needed. The comprehensive weekly costs for the FSU-type respite care package are given in the seventh row of Table 6.6, and total £289.71.

The second policy option, therefore, is simply to substitute supported for unsupported informal care for elderly people living with others in private households. The 'static' cost implications of this policy option are shown in Table 6.8, representing an additional £367 million per year at a national level compared to the baseline option. Just under half of this additional expenditure (£171 million) would fall to local authorities if the FSU model were replicated exactly, and the remainder would fall to health authorities. Over time, of course, it would be expected that admissions to communal establishments could be reduced, with consequent cost savings, but we have not costed these dynamic changes here.

Option III: Community support with enhanced home care

Provision of enhanced home support to the 41,000 people living alone in the community may enable them to remain in their own homes longer and improve their quality of life. Challis and Davies (1986) found that elderly people, some with dementia, entered institutional care somewhat later when given case-managed support services in the community, although O'Connor et al. (1991) reached a different conclusion, finding that early intervention increased the likelihood of admission for people with dementia living alone. Askham and Thompson (1990) examined home support schemes in Ipswich and Newham that stressed the coordination of existing services — similar in some respects to care management — and additionally provided two development workers and 'home support workers' who supplied practical assistance, care and sitting services. The service was targeted at people living alone as well as those with carers, and may be representative of numerous home care schemes being implemented to support frail elderly people at home. We costed the Askham and Thompson service using information recorded by the evaluation team, uprated using NHS and PSS pay and prices indexes (see the eighth row of costs in Table 6.6).

If the third policy option is delivery of enhanced home care along the lines of service in Ipswich[11] to every elderly person with advanced cognitive impairment living alone, the additional cost over and above today's expenditure levels (option I) would amount to £117 million, falling to local and health authorities, but there may be a lower burden for informal carers (not living with the client). Other enhanced home care arrangements might be chosen, but probably with only slightly different cost implications.

Options IV and V: Reducing long-stay hospital provision

At the heart of central government and much local policy is reduction of the number of people in long-stay or continuing care hospital accommodation. The number of NHS long-stay beds for geriatric and psychogeriatric patients has been declining in recent years, and evidence from a survey by Laing and Buisson (1992) suggests that the number will continue to decline for a few years. Two illustrative possibilities for the estimated 22,000 inpatients with advanced cognitive impairment would be: to move them to a combination of local authority residential homes (25 per cent), voluntary or private residential homes (20 per cent), and private and voluntary nursing homes (55 per cent) based on the current distribution of people in those settings; or to move hospital residents to NHS nursing homes similar to the three evaluated by Bond and colleagues (1989), and shown to be preferred by relatives, to produce improved resident performance in the activities of daily living, and to reduce costs when compared to hospital (Bond and Donaldson, 1989). These we call policy options IV and V, respectively.

The cost implications of these two policy options are given in Table 6.8. There is insufficient evidence to comment on the likely effectiveness of option IV in terms of client outcomes, although the potential cost savings are large (£511 million). These savings would accrue to health authorities, at the cost of increased financial pressure on local authorities, social security budgets and families.[12] Option V would bring an overall resource saving of £389 million, mostly accruing to health authorities. Many of the 22,000 hospital inpatients will have physical health needs in addition to cognitive impairment, so it could prove a major challenge to move them all to community settings.

Option VI: Higher quality residential care

A further option would be to provide specialist residential care for the estimated 27,000 elderly people with advanced cognitive impairment currently in local authority homes by altering certain environmental characteristics (Netten, 1992a). One such model of provision could be the specialist unit established in West Cumbria, which offered a high level of therapeutic input based on 'reality orientation' (which has been shown to be effective in community settings elsewhere; see Greene et al., 1983). The West Cumbria service was established and evaluated as part of the Care in the Community demonstration programme (Knapp et al., 1992, 1994), and shown to be a cost-effective alternative to hospital. Quality of life was not inferior to and in some respects was better than in hospital, and costs were markedly lower. The costs are given in the bottom row of Table 6.6. The costs of substituting this higher quality residential service for standard local authority care are £95 million per year greater than today's arrangements (Table 6.8). Again, over time there might be knock-on cost savings, but we have restricted our attention to static changes here.

Options VII and VIII: Universal changes in provision

We could take any number of combinations of these hypothetical policy options. If we sought (near) universal improvements, so that people living alone received enhanced home care (option III), carers of people living in shared households received respite care support (option II), those in local authority homes enjoyed a different care regime (option VI), and those in hospital were resettled in NHS nursing homes (option V), approximately

242,000 elderly people with advanced cognitive impairment would be affected, and the net cost would appear to be £192 million per year. The only people not affected by this final option would be those in private and voluntary accommodation. This we label option VII. Another combined option (VIII) could be to move only half of the hospital residents to other care settings, recognising that some of these people are very dependent and could require continuing hospital care. The additional cost of this option would be £386 million per year. Of course, other permutations can be calculated by combining the relevant numbers of people and costs from Table 6.6.

The eight options described and costed here obviously do not span the full range of policy alternatives available at national or local level. For example, the consultations to assess the needs of all people aged 75 or over stipulated in the new GP contracts might raise case-finding and hence systems effectiveness.[13] We have also not costed changes to day care services, although previous research has produced mixed views on their effectiveness. For example, Turner et al. (1984) found that day hospitals were more costly but not more effective than other forms of rehabilitation, and Woods and Phanjoo (1991) found that attendance at a day hospital had little positive effect on eventual needs for residential care. In contrast, the findings of Macdonald et al. (1982) suggested that day centres performed better in bringing about reductions in user dependency when compared to local authority homes, day hospitals and hospital wards.

Our consideration of these options has not included analysis of the *transition* from one arrangement to another, although it is widely recognised that resources are needed early enough to lubricate change.

6.5 Conclusions

What is suggested by these analyses is that widespread improvements in provision could be achieved with comparatively modest injections of additional resources if long-stay hospital provision were reduced. However, as shown by option VII, Table 6.8, even if there were no long-stay hospital provision, and assuming the finance could be redirected, the amount saved would be insufficient to fund universal improvements. It could be argued that such changes improve horizontal equity targets (increasing the resource provision to most people with advanced cognitive impairment) by trading off some vertical equity, in that resource provision for the most impaired — some of those in hospital — is reduced. However, if the desired maximand is client outcomes rather than resources expended, then community alternatives to hospital can be less costly and improve the wellbeing of less dependent elderly people in hospital (Bond and Donaldson, 1989; Bond et al., 1989; Knapp et al., 1992), thus improving rather than compromising vertical equity.

There are clearly limitations on the implementation of these and other policy options. Various factors may influence the development or continued availability of particular supply-side resources. Projections by the Department of Employment (1990) suggest that the proportion of women aged 45 and over in paid employment will remain relatively stable. But if an increasing number of middle-aged women choose to remain in paid employment, then the potential number of carers could fall markedly, implying greater demands for domiciliary support and other community health and social care services. Further expansion of the independent residential and nursing home sector, as suggested by option V, may not be possible. Private care homes are usually highly geared,[14] so that a return to high interest rates may put a brake on expansion of the sector, as could declining numbers entering the nursing profession in the next decade, which will increase competition for staff, and costs. Local authority long-term care provision may decline further due to the new funding arrangements, with some homes transferred or sold to private or voluntary providers or taken over by not-for-profit trusts (Wistow et al., 1994). Local wage bargaining in the NHS may mean cost increases in areas facing staff shortages.

Such supply-side constraints, coupled with the possible adverse consequences of moving frail elderly people, will inevitably mean that any policy changes would need to be implemented gradually, ideally targeted at particular groups of people on the basis of need. Supply constraints could alter the costs of some of the service inputs to the various policy options, as could some of the secondary (knock-on) effects posited above. If the diversification of service provision and funding introduced in the mixed economy of community care continues to develop over the next few years, this too could considerably alter the comparative costs of different services and options. Because any balance of care changes will inevitably be gradual, their evaluation could ensure that information on changing cost implications (and hopefully also on service effectiveness) is fed back into the policy process.

Our costings of the various policy options are the best that can be obtained with available information; even these estimates required considerable data and policy analysis. In addition, the lack of reliable information on the current dependency profiles of people in different care settings forced us to assume constant dependency profiles despite the widespread changes in provision between 1986 and 1992. (See Darton, 1994, for a comprehensive review of the available literature.) Moreover, the absence of national data on receipt of health and social services has compelled us to make a number of assumptions. The findings are therefore tentative, and to some extent illustrative. New or better population estimates, a different distribution of accommodation used by elderly people with cognitive impairment, and new care packages could all be incorporated with comparative ease in the framework we have presented. Purchasers, planners and those with regulatory responsiblity can use this analysis to explore the implications of policy changes. It will also be of interest to families affected by cognitive impairment and to the taxpayer at large. As public sector agencies attempt to make their resource allocation decisions more explicit and to alter the balance of provision within the newly emerging health and social care systems, analyses of the kind presented here will increasingly be needed.

Appendix 6.1: Estimating the balance of care

The OPCS surveys of disability among adults were conducted in the mid-1980s. The first survey of disabled adults living in private households took place in 1985. A large sample of the general population was screened using a postal questionnaire to identify people with some form of disability. People identified as having a disability were then interviewed about the extent of their disability, personal circumstances, employment status, use of care services, and so on (see Martin et al., 1988). A second survey of disabled adults in communal establishments was conducted in 1986. A sample of homes, hospitals and hostels was selected, and residents (or a staff member acting as their proxy) were interviewed. Sample weights for both surveys were calculated to allow for selection, non-response and ineligibility (due to a lack of disability) so that 'grossing' weights could be calculated. These weights allow the estimation of the number of cases at a national level.

Table A6.1 provides an estimate of the number of people who meet the criterion for advanced cognitive impairment (scoring 7 or more on the intel-

Table A6.1
The balance of care in 1986

		Projected cases	
Type of accommodation	Great Britain (000)	%	Estimate for England (000)
Household — living alone	44.4	13.5	38.4
Household — living with others	166.9	50.7	144.3
Local authority residential home	4.5	13.8	39.2
Voluntary residential home	3.0	0.9	2.6
Voluntary nursing home	5.6	1.7	4.8
Private residential home	12.5	3.8	10.8
Private nursing home	17.2	5.2	14.9
NHS geriatric	20.3	6.2	17.5
NHS psychiatric	12.1	3.7	10.4
NHS mental handicap	1.9	0.6	1.7
NHS miscellaneous	0.3	0.1	0.3
Total	329.4	100	284.8

Sources: OPCS (1989a,b).

Table A6.2
Estimates of the proportion of residents with advanced cognitive impairment in different care settings in 1986

Type of accommodation	Estimated no. of people with advanced cognitive impairment, England[a] (000)	Total no. of residents (000)	Residents with advanced cognitive impairment %
Household — living alone	38.4	–	–
Household — living with others	144.3	–	–
Local authority residential home	39.2	108.7[b]	36.0
Voluntary residential home	2.6	26.0[b]	10.1
Private residential home	10.8	81.6[b]	13.2
Independent nursing homes	19.7	38.7[c]	51.0
NHS geriatric	17.5	49.5[d]	35.4
NHS psychiatric	10.4	64.8[d]	16.1
NHS mental handicap	1.7	35.1[d]	4.7
NHS miscellaneous	0.3	–	–
Total	284.8		

a OPCS (1989a,b).
b Estimates of the number of residents from Department of Health and Social Security (1986).
c Estimates of the number of available places from Department of Health and Social Security (1988). Estimated occupancy rate of 93 per cent from Darton and Wright (1990).
d Estimates of the number of places from Department of Health (1991). We assumed an occupancy rate of 90 per cent.

lectual impairment scale; see Box 6.1) in Great Britain in 1986, by their place of accommodation. Age- and sex-specific prevalence rates were calculated by dividing the projected number of cases by the relevant population figures for Great Britain in 1986 (OPCS, 1991) (rates are reported in Table 6.2 in the main text). In order to obtain an estimate of the number of people with advanced cognitive impairment in England in 1986, two assumptions were employed: first, that the age- and sex-specific prevalence rates in England were similar to those estimated for Great Britain; and second, that the distribution of people between accommodation settings was also similar. Applying these assumptions to population estimates for England in 1986 (OPCS, 1991) yields the estimated balance of care (see the fourth column of Table A6.1).

However, many changes have taken place between 1986 and 1992. The number of elderly people — particularly in the older age groups — has increased considerably. If the age- and sex-specific prevalence rates for cognitive impairment remained constant between 1986 and 1992, the absolute number

Table A6.3
Estimate of the balance of care in England in 1992

Type of accommodation	Total no. of residents (000)	Residents with advanced cognitive impairment[e] %	Estimated no. of people with advanced cognitive impairment, England (000)
Household — living alone	–	–	40.6
Household — living with others	–	–	152.5
Local authority residential home	74.0[a]	36.0	26.6
Voluntary residential home	34.6[a]	10.1	3.5
Private residential home	135.4[a]	13.2	17.9
Independent nursing home	115.3[b]	51.0	58.8
NHS geriatric	37.8[c]	35.4	13.4
NHS psychiatric	45.1[d]	16.1	7.3
NHS mental handicap	19.6[c]	4.7	0.9
NHS miscellaneous	–	–	0.3
Total			321.8

a Estimates of the number of residents from Department of Health (1993a)
b Estimates of the number of available places from Department of Health (1993b). Estimated occupancy rate of 93 per cent from Darton and Wright (1990).
c Estimates of the number of places from Department of Health (1993c). We assumed an occupancy rate of 90 per cent.
d Number of residents estimated from the number of unfinished inpatient episodes reported in House of Commons (1992)
e Estimated from Table A6.2.
Numbers in Table A6.3 do not identically match those in Table 6.3 due to rounding.

of cases will have increased. In addition, the balance of care has altered due to the decline in hospital and local authority home provision and the rapid increase in the provision of residential and nursing home places by private and voluntary providers. It is difficult to estimate exactly how these changes have affected the balance of care for people with advanced cognitive impairment. Data on the dependency of people with respect to confusion or dementia in different settings in the early 1990s are limited (Darton, 1994). However, employing a series of basic assumptions allows us to produce an indicative estimate of the balance of care in the absence of more robust information.

We assumed that the age- and sex-specific prevalence rates remained unaltered between 1986 and 1992. Applying these rates to the 1992 population estimates for England (OPCS, 1993) yields an estimate of 320,000 (Table A6.3) compared to 285,000 in 1986 (Table A6.2).

We estimated the proportion of people in different types of communal establishment who had advanced cognitive impairment in 1986. Estimates of

Table A6.4

The degree of cognitive impairment among the over 65s in different residential settings, Great Britain, 1986

Degree of cognitive impairment	Household — living alone (000)	%	Household — living with others (000)	%	LA residential home (000)	%	Ind. sector residential home (000)	%	Ind. sector nursing home (000)	%	NHS hospitals (000)	%
0	1133.0	85.6	1621.4	82.0	43.4	34.4	28.3	44.7	23.5	36.0	13.8	18.0
1	28.3	2.1	38.8	2.0	6.2	4.9	2.9	4.7	5.2	7.9	14.5	18.9
2	40.6	3.1	40.6	2.1	9.9	7.9	6.2	9.8	5.1	7.8	2.3	3.0
3.5	27.4	2.1	38.1	1.9	5.9	4.7	2.1	3.4	2.9	4.5	3.6	4.8
4.5	25.5	1.9	34.8	1.8	6.6	5.2	3.7	5.9	2.8	4.3	2.9	3.8
6	24.0	1.8	37.5	1.9	8.8	7.0	4.5	7.1	3.0	4.7	5.3	6.9
7	16.4	1.3	36.4	1.8	9.1	7.2	3.9	6.1	4.9	7.4	6.0	7.8
8	10.7	0.8	38.9	2.0	11.1	8.8	4.0	6.4	5.2	7.9	9.1	11.9
9.5	10.2	0.8	23.4	1.2	6.5	5.1	3.0	4.8	3.4	5.3	3.3	4.4
10.5	3.1	0.2	25.9	1.3	5.6	4.4	1.7	2.7	3.1	4.8	3.2	4.2
12	1.7	0.1	33.4	1.7	6.9	5.5	1.5	2.4	4.0	6.1	7.2	9.4
13	2.2	0.2	8.9	0.5	6.1	4.8	1.3	2.1	2.2	3.4	5.4	7.0
Total	1323.2	100	1978.1	100	126.1	100	63.2	100	65.4	100	76.7	100

Sources: OPCS (1989a, 1989b).

Table A6.5

The degree of disability among the over 65s in different residential settings, Great Britain, 1986

Degree of cognitive impairment	Household — living alone (000)	%	Household — living with others (000)	%	LA residential home (000)	%	Ind. sector residential home (000)	%	Ind. sector nursing home (000)	%	NHS hospitals (000)	%
1	246.9	18.7	358.4	18.1	2.5	2.0	2.5	4.0	19	3.0	1.3	1.7
2	214.4	16.2	269.3	13.6	4.4	3.5	3.9	6.1	2.6	4.0	1.6	2.1
3	173.3	13.1	235.8	11.9	6.6	5.2	6.2	9.8	1.7	2.6	0.8	1.1
4	158.9	12.0	199.5	10.1	8.9	7.1	5.9	9.3	3.6	5.6	2.5	3.3
5	188.1	14.2	197.2	10.0	10.5	8.4	6.2	9.8	4.2	6.4	0.7	0.9
6	144.9	11.0	155.4	7.9	13.0	10.3	7.7	12.2	3.9	5.9	2.7	3.6
7	108.6	8.2	174.9	8.8	14.4	11.4	7.2	11.4	7.5	11.5	3.1	4.1
8	54.4	4.1	155.3	7.9	21.3	16.9	6.9	10.9	8.5	13.0	7.6	10.0
9	26.4	2.0	169.5	8.6	22.0	17.4	10.4	16.5	13.1	20.0	18.8	24.6
10	7.7	0.6	62.9	3.2	22.5	17.9	6.4	10.1	18.3	28.1	36.9	48.5
Total	1323.5	100	1978.1	100	126.1	100	63.2	100	65.4	100	76.1	100

Sources: OPCS (1989a, 1989b).

the number of places available in different settings were combined with estimates of the occupancy rates in order to calculate the typical number of residents in each setting (see Table A6.2 and the accompanying notes for details). The projected number of people with advanced cognitive impairment were divided by the estimated number of residents to calculate the proportion of residents with advanced cognitive impairment.

In order to estimate the number of people in each of the different settings in 1992, we assumed that, although the number of places (residents) in different types of communal establishment had altered, the dependency profile of residents with respect to cognitive impairment remained unchanged. The number of residents in each type of communal establishment were estimated by again applying estimated occupancy rates to estimates of the number of places (see Table A6.3). The number of people with advanced cognitive impairment was calculated by applying the 1986 proportions to the 1992 estimates of the number of residents.

The number of people in private households was estimated by subtracting the estimated number of people in communal establishments with advanced cognitive impairment from the overall estimate of the total number of people with advanced cognitive impairment. The number living alone and the number living with others was estimated by applying the relative proportions from 1986 (13.5:50.7).

It should be stressed that these estimates are based on a considerable number of assumptions. In the absence of better data they are the best that we can provide. However, they are at best indicative and should not be considered as being precise. Alternative assumptions would produce a very different estimate of the balance of care.

Appendix 6.2

Tables A6.4 and A6.5 provide estimates of the number of people with intellectual impairment or some form of disability (broadly defined) by their degree of impairment and place of accommodation for Great Britain in 1986.

Notes

* This chapter pulls together material originally presented in Kavanagh et al. (1993) and Schneider et al. (1993), although statistical estimates have been updated. We would like to thank Robin Darton and Lou Opit (University of Kent at Canterbury) and David Melzer (Cambridge Health Authority) for their very helpful advice. We would also like to thank OPCS and the ESRC data archive for making data from the OPCS Surveys of Disability available for secondary analysis. This research was funded by the

Department of Health. Any errors are our own.

1 We assumed that the prevalence rates for Great Britain were applicable to England and that the actual age- and sex-specific rates remained unchanged between 1986 and 1992.

2 The proportion of people who required a proxy to answer for them increased markedly with the degree of cognitive impairment: 16 per cent of people with a score of 1 on the intellectual impairment scale required a proxy, by score 7 this had risen to 57 per cent, and by score 13 had increased to 100 per cent. These figures relate to the survey of people in private households.

3 The OPCS disability surveys collected information about the following types of disability: locomotion, reaching and stretching, dexterity, personal care, continence, seeing, hearing, communication, behaviour, intellectual functioning, consciousness, eating, drinking, digesting and disfigurement. A severity rating was calculated for each area. The overall disability rating was then calculated using the following formula: worst severity rating + 0.4 *x* (second worst) + 0.3 *x* (third worst) = overall rating of disability. This overall rating of disability was then classified within ten categories on the following basis:

Severity category	Weighted severity score
10 (most severe)	19-21.40
9	17-18.95
8	15-16.95
7	13-14.95
6	11-12.95
5	9-10.95
4	7-8.95
3	5-6.95
2	3-4.95
1 (least severe)	0.5-2.95

4 The estimation of housing cost by Challis and Davies (1986) used an experienced valuer to make a market assessment of the elderly person's housing. Replacement values were discounted over a period of 60 years at 7 per cent. We inflated the Challis and Davies figures to 1992/93 prices using the Department of the Environment 'output price index for private housing'. This gives a weekly opportunity cost of housing of £40.17.

5 No adjustment has been made for changes in rates of service utilisation since 1985.

6 The annual cost of residential care for the elderly is presented in this Memorandum as £9,529 per resident at 1989/90 prices, which we inflated to 1992/93 prices using the Personal Social Services pay and prices index to arrive at £11,698 (£224.35 per resident week). This is only the revenue cost. An estimated capital cost of £45.60 per resident week (for buildings, equipment, etc.) was based on capital cost recommendations for new homes, suitably discounted, as previously calculated for the PSSRU's evaluation of the

Care in the Community demonstration programme (Knapp et al., 1992), this having been inflated using the Department of the Environment construction cost and price index, 'output price index for other new work: public'.

7 The estimated cost function suggests that high dependency (which would include advanced cognitive impairment) imposes an extra care cost of 25 per cent. This means that the additional revenue cost is approximately £56.09 per week at 1992/93 prices. Thus the 'standard' cost of a local authority place can be set at £282.13, and a high dependency place at £338.08.

8 We use the following assumptions based on the work of Darton and Wright (1991): in the residential home sector, 40 per cent of residents pay the entire charge themselves and the remaining 60 per cent receive statutory funding; in nursing homes, 30 per cent of residents fund themselves and the remainder receive statutory funding.

9 An examination of hospital cost data in five English health regions suggests that general services account for 28.5 per cent of hospital revenue costs, and the remaining 71.5 per cent is accounted for by patient treatment services (the FR12 specialty costs account for 88 per cent of this) (see Beecham, 1994). Services provided by other agencies account for a further 4.2 per cent, and the cost of hospital capital was taken as approximately 16 per cent of total costs (Knapp et al., 1992). Costs were inflated to 1992/93 prices using the NHS pay and prices index.

10 The FSU was jointly funded by the health authority and the local authority, but because financial responsibility was likely to be devolved to the local authority in the longer term, costs have been attributed to the local authority.

11 Two schemes were evaluated by Askham and Thompson (1990): one in London and the other in Ipswich. Due to the difference in costs between London and elsewhere in England, we based our costs on the project in Ipswich.

12 Supply-side constraints are such that people leaving long-stay hospital care are most likely to obtain a place in private or voluntary nursing homes. The potential resource savings are significant. A *gradual* change in hospital rundown would not yield produce *pro rata* savings, for average hospital costs decline only slowly because of fixed inputs (including administrative and capital resources) and the tendency to transfer less dependent hospital residents in the early stages of rundown.

13 This has been questioned by Freer (1990), who argued that it would be more cost-effective to record the necessary information during patient-initiated consultations, and O'Connor et al. (1991), who found that early detection of dementia did not delay permanent admission to long-term care but in fact may have — beneficially — increased the rate of admission among those living alone).

14 A relatively high proportion of the financing of private care homes comes from loans rather than shareholders (a high debt to equity ratio).

References

American Psychiatric Association (1980) *Diagnostic and Statistical Manual of Mental Disorders*, 3rd edition (revised), APA, Washington, DC.

Askham, J. and Thompson, C. (1990) *Dementia and Home Care: A Research Report on a Home Support Scheme for Dementia Sufferers*, Age Concern, Mitcham.

Beecham, J.K. (1994) Estimating costs, Discussion Paper 844, Personal Social Services Research Unit, University of Kent at Canterbury.

Bergmann, K., Foster, E.M., Justice, A.W. and Matthews, V. (1978) Management of the demented elderly patient in the community, *British Journal of Psychiatry*, 132, 441-9.

Bond, J. and Donaldson, C. (1989) *Evaluation of Continuing Care Accommodation for Elderly People, Volume 5, A Cost Study of Continuing Care Institutions for Very Frail Elderly People*, School of Health Care Sciences, University of Newcastle-upon-Tyne.

Bond, J., Gregson, B. and Atkinson, A. (1989) Measurement of outcomes within a multi-centred RCT in the evaluation of the experimental NHS nursing homes, *Age and Ageing*, 18, 292-302.

Brayne, C. and Calloway, P. (1989) An epidemiological study of dementia in a rural population of elderly women, *British Journal of Psychiatry*, 155, 214-19.

Brodaty, H. and Gresham, M. (1989) Effect of a training programme to reduce stress in carers of patients with dementia, *British Medical Journal*, 299, 1375-9.

Brodaty, H. and Hadzi-Pavlovic, D. (1990) Psychosocial effects on carers living with persons with dementia, *Australia and New Zealand Journal of Psychiatry*, 24, 351-61.

Central Statistical Office (1991) *Family Expenditure Survey*, HMSO, London.

Challis, D.J. and Davies, B.P. (1986) *Case Management in Community Care*, Gower, Aldershot.

Clark, M., Lowry, R. and Clarke, S. (1986) Cognitive impairment in the elderly: a community survey, *Age and Ageing*, 15, 278-84.

Darton, R.A. (1994) Review of recent research on elderly people in residential care and nursing homes, with specific reference to dependency, Discussion Paper 1082, Personal Social Services Research Unit, University of Kent at Canterbury.

Darton, R.A. and Knapp, M.R.J. (1984) The cost of residential care for the elderly: the effects of dependency, design and social environment, *Ageing and Society*, 4, 157-83.

Darton, R.A. and Wright, K.G. (1990) The characteristics of non-statutory residential and nursing homes, in R. Parry (ed.) *Research Findings in Social Work 18: Privatisation*, Jessica Kingsley, London.

Darton, R.A. and Wright, K.G. (1991) PSSRU/CHE survey of residential and nursing homes: residential and nursing homes for elderly people: one sector or two?, Discussion Paper 725/2, Personal Social Services Research Unit, University of Kent at Canterbury.

Darton, R.A. and Wright, K.G. (1993) Changes in the provision of long-stay care, 1970-1990, *Health and Social Care in the Community*, 1, 11-26.

Davies, B.P., Bebbington, A.C. and Charnley, H. with Baines, B., Ferlie, E.B., Hughes, M. and Twigg, J. (1990) *Resources, Needs and Outcomes in Community-Based Care*, Avebury, Aldershot.

Department of Employment (1990) Labour force outlook to the year 2001, *Employment Gazette*, April.

Department of Health (1991a) Memorandum laid before the Health Committee, House of Commons Paper 408, HMSO, London.

Department of Health (1991b) *Health and Personal Social Services Statistics for England*, HMSO, London.

Department of Health (1993a) *Residential Accommodation for Elderly and for Younger Physically Handicapped People: All Residents in Local Authority, Voluntary and Private Homes. Year Ending 31 March 1992, England*, RA/86/2, Government Statistical Service, London.

Department of Health (1993b) *Private Hospitals, Homes and Clinics Registered Under Section 23 of the Registered Homes Act 1984: England — Position at 31 March 1992*, Government Statistical Service, London.

Department of Health (1993c) *Health and Personal Social Services Statistics for England*, HMSO, London.

Department of Health and Social Security (1986) *Residential Accommodation for Elderly and for Younger Physically Handicapped People: All Residents in Local Authority, Voluntary and Private Homes. Year Ending 31 March 1986 England*, RA/86/2, Government Statistical Service, London.

Department of Health and Social Security (1988) *Private Hospitals, Homes and Clinics Registered Under Section 23 of the Registered Homes Act 1984, 31 December 1986, National Regional and District Summaries*, HMSO, London.

Donaldson, C. and Gregson, B. (1988) Prolonging life at home: what is the cost? *Community Medicine*, 3, 200-209.

Drummond, M.F., Mohide, E.A., Tew, M., Streiner, D.L., Pringle, D.M. and Gilbert, R.J. (1991) Economic evaluation of a support program for caregivers of demented elderly, *International Journal of Technology Assessment in Health Care*, 7, 2, 209-19.

Freer, C.B. (1990) Screening the elderly, *British Medical Journal*, 300, 1447-8.

Gilleard, C.J. (1984) *Living with Dementia: Community Care of the Elderly Mentally Infirm*, Croom Helm, London.

Greene, J.G., Smith, R., Gardiner, M. and Timbury, G.C. (1982) Measuring behavioural disturbance of elderly demented patients in the community and the effect on relatives: a factor analytic study, *Age and Ageing*, 11, 121-6.

Greene, J.G., Timbury, G.C., Smith, R. and Gardiner, M. (1983) Reality orientation with elderly patients in the community, *Age and Ageing*, 12, 38-43.

Gurland, B., Copeland, J., Kuriansky, J., Kelleher, M., Sharpe, L. and Lee Dean, L. (1983) *The Mind and Mood of Ageing: Mental Health Problems of the Community Elderly in London and New York*, Croom Helm, London.

Hofman, A., Rocca, W., Brayne, C., Breteler, M., Clarke, M., Cooper, B., Copeland, J., Dartiques, J., da Silva Droux, A., Hagnell, O., Heeren, T., Engedal, K., Jonker, C., Lindsay, J., Lobo, A., Mann, A., Molsa, P., Morgan, K., O'Connor, D., Sulkava, R., Kay, D. and Amaducci, L. (1991) The prevalence of dementia in Europe: a collaborative study, *International Journal of Epidemiology*, 20, 736-45.

House of Commons (1992) *Development of Services for People with Learning Disabilities (Mental Handicap) or Mental Illness in England, Fourth Report Prepared Pursuant to Section 11 of the Disabled Persons (Services, Consultation and Representation) Act 1986*, House of Commons Paper 342, HMSO, London.

Kavanagh, S., Schneider, J., Knapp, M.R.J., Beecham, J.K. and Netten, A. (1993) Elderly people with cognitive impairment: costing possible changes in the balance of care, *Health and Social Care in the Community*, 1, 69-80.

Kitwood, T. (1990) The dialectics of dementia: with particular reference to Alzheimer's disease, *Ageing and Society*, 10, 177-96.

Knapp, M.R.J., Cambridge, P., Thomason, C., Beecham, J.K., Allen, C. and Darton, R.A. (1992) *Care in the Community: Challenge and Demonstration*, Ashgate, Aldershot.

Knapp, M.R.J., Cambridge, P., Thomason, C., Beecham, J.K., Allen, C. and Darton, R.A. (1994) Residential care as an alternative to long-stay hospital: a cost effectiveness evaluation of two pilot projects, *International Journal of Geriatric Psychiatry*, 9, 297-304.

Laing and Buisson (1992) *Laing's Review of Private Health Care 1992*, Laing and Buisson, London.

Laing and Buisson (1993) *Care of Elderly People: Market Survey 1992/93*, Laing and Buisson, London.

Levin, E. and Moriarty, J. (1994) *Better for the Break*, HMSO, Norwich.

Livingston, G., Hawkins, A., Graham, N., Blizard, B. and Mann, A. (1990) Gospel Oak study: prevalence rates of dementia, depression and activity limitation among elderly residents in Inner London, *Psychological Medicine*, 20, 137-46.

MacDonald, A.J.D., Mann, A.H., Jenkins, R., Richard, L., Godlove, C. and Rodwell, R. (1982) An attempt to determine the impact of four types of care upon the elderly in London by the study of matched groups, *Age and Ageing*, 11, 193-200.

Martin, J., Meltzer, H. and Elliot, D. (1988) *Report 1 — The Prevalence of Disability Among Adults*, Office of Population Censuses and Surveys, Social Survey Division, HMSO, London.

Maule, M.M., Milne, J.S. and Williamson, J. (1984) Mental illness and physical health in older people, *Age and Ageing*, 13, 239-56.

Melzer, D., Hopkins, S., Pencheon, D., Brayne, C. and Williams, R. (1991) *Epidemiologically Based Needs Assessment of Dementia Services*, report to the Department of Health, London.

Netten, A. (1990) An approach to costing informal care, Discussion Paper 637, Personal Social Services Research Unit, University of Kent at Canterbury.

Netten, A. (1992a) *A Positive Environment? The Residential Care of People with Severe Dementia*, Ashgate, Aldershot.

Netten, A. (1992b) Some cost implications of 'caring for people', Discussion Paper 809, Personal Social Services Research Unit, University of Kent at Canterbury.

O'Connor, D.W., Pollitt, P.A., Brook, C.P.B., Reiss, B.B. and Roth, M. (1991) Does early intervention reduce the number of elderly people with dementia admitted to institutions?, *British Medical Journal*, 302, 871-4.

Office of Population Censuses and Surveys (OPCS) (1989a) *Survey of Disability among Adults in Communal Establishments, 1986* [computer file], ESRC Data Archive, Colchester.

Office of Population Censuses and Surveys (OPCS) (1989b) *Survey of Disability among Adults in Private Households, 1985* [computer file], ESRC Data Archive, Colchester.

Office of Population Censuses and Surveys (OPCS) (1991) *National Population Projections, Number 17* (1989-based), HMSO, London.

Office of Population Censuses and Surveys (OPCS) (1993) *National Population Projections, Series PP2 Number 18* (1991-based), HMSO, London.

Reddy, S. and Pitt, B. (1993) What becomes of demented patients referred to a psychogeriatric unit? An approach to audit, *International Journal of Geriatric Psychiatry*, 8, 175-80.

Schneider, J., Kavanagh, S., Knapp, M.R.J., Beecham, J.K. and Netten, A. (1993) Elderly people with advanced cognitive impairment in England: resource use and cost, *Ageing and Society*, 13, 27-50.

Secretaries of State (1989a) *Working for Patients*, Cm 555, HMSO, London.

Secretaries of State (1989b) *Caring for People: Community Care in the Next Decade and Beyond*, Cm 849, HMSO, London.

Taylor, R., Ford, G. and Barber, H. (1983) *Research Perspectives on Ageing 6: The Elderly at Risk*, Age Concern Research Unit, Mitcham.

Turner, M.A., Davidson, J.G. and Ogle, S.T. (1984) Day hospital rehabilitation effectiveness and cost in the elderly: a randomised control trial, *British Medical Journal*, 289, 1209-12.

Wistow, G., Knapp, M.R.J., Hardy, B. and Allen, C. (1994) *Social Care in the Mixed Economy*, Open University Press, Buckingham.

Woods, J.P. and Phanjoo, A.L. (1991) A follow-up study of psychogeriatric day hospital patients with dementia, *International Journal of Geriatric Psychiatry*, 6, 183-8.

7 Costing the Care Programme Approach

Justine Schneider

Costing, no matter how scrupulously carried out, is a political activity undertaken to make a case for or against a given programme (World Health Organization, 1991, p.14).

7.1 Introduction

Community care for people with mental health problems is complex and fraught with difficulties. The care programme approach was introduced to reduce the risk that people with severe and enduring mental health problems would fail to have their needs met by community-based services. Cost information can add to or detract from the confidence with which care programming is implemented. This chapter will illustrate some of the applications and limitations of cost information with respect to the care programme approach.

Heralded by *Caring for People* (Secretaries of State, 1989, §7), the Circular on the Care Programme Approach (Department of Health, 1990) stated that, by April 1991, all patients accepted by specialist psychiatric services should have a systematic assessment of need, effective monitoring of service delivery, the appointment of a named keyworker, and regular reviews. These are not revolutionary ideas; they reflect widely-recognised good practice, yet to achieve this universal standard many mental health services have had to take a close look at existing provision and evaluate their current performance in relation to the care programme approach.

The question of cost is immediately raised by any changes in service systems. The demands of the care programme approach were expected to be met from existing resources, but it is clear that close coordination and more frequent contacts with service users can have both direct and indirect impacts on service costs, and that the review of individual needs on a regular basis seems likely to highlight shortfalls in provision, leading to demands for more services. Alternatively, better coordination could lead to lower needs and lower costs in the longer term, with a reduced number of public scandals due to inadequate monitoring. For existing providers, therefore, depending upon their starting point, the introduction of the care programme approach appears to imply a measure of change in the way services are organised, together with costs attributable to various causes:

- growing workloads, with a broader range of service users made eligible for formal provision by the care programme criteria;
- existing users consuming services more intensively because their needs are scrutinised more closely than before; and
- greater demands on limited resources because care programmes can be analysed at an aggregate level to reveal shortfalls in local provision.

Possible benefits would need to be proven, and weighed against the probable costs of implementation. This chapter looks at one aspect of costs: the services consumed by people admitted to the care programme approach. It does this by analysing the care packages of 60 service users in three health districts. First, we describe briefly the policy and legislative background to the Circular and the immediate circumstances affecting its introduction; then we go on to explain the methodology, review the findings, and discuss the implications of the research.

7.2 Policy and practice background

To encourage coordination between health and social services, *Caring for People* first proposed joint 'care programmes' to support people leaving hospital. The 1990 National Health Service and Community Care Act gave further impetus to the closure of outmoded psychiatric hospitals and the development of new forms of social support, and introduced the Mental Illness Specific Grant to fund initiatives in social care for people with mental health problems. In October 1991, the Royal College of Psychiatrists, at the recommendation of the Spokes Inquiry, published guidelines on after-care, emphasising coordination between responsible medical officers and other carers, and stressing the role of the psychiatrist in orchestrating care. These guidelines 'reflect the philosophy behind the care programme approach' (Royal College of Psychiatrists, 1991, p.2). *The Health of the Nation* White Paper (Secretary of State for Health, 1992) sets mental illness as a priority, and the *Health of the Nation: Mental Illness Handbook* (Department of Health, 1993) complements the original Circular by clarifying many of the details of implementing care programming.

For those people compulsorily admitted to hospital, the Mental Health Act 1983 makes after-care the joint responsibility of the health authority and the local authority social services department 'in cooperation with the relevant voluntary agencies' (§ 117), but this only applies to patients who have been detained under the Act. Not only was Section 117 inconsistently implemented, it was sometimes evaded by transferring patients to sections of the Act to which Section 117 did not apply (Secretary of State for Social Services, 1987). Thus the majority of people returning to the community after receiving psychiatric inpatient treatment are not assured of statutory after-care. The care programme approach is not enforced by law: like the Highway Code, it has the status of good practice.

The success of community-based alternatives to inpatient psychiatric treatment in the United States, Australia and Canada (Stein and Test, 1980; Fenton et al., 1982; Hoult et al., 1984) led to replications in the United Kingdom, with similar results (Dick et al., 1985; Dean and Gadd, 1990; Muijen et al., 1992; Burns et al., 1993; Marks et al., 1994). To summarise the impact of this research, it led to the widely-held conviction that cost-effective care for people with severe mental health problems can be achieved in non-hospital settings, provided certain conditions are met. Yet beyond the trials, in the generality of mental health services, breakdowns in support for people with mental health problems in the community still notoriously occur, as in the cases of Ben Silcock and Christopher Clunis. Failures have been attributed to lack of accountability, lack of planning, poor coordination between health and social services, a failure to involve informal carers and service users, and inadequate systems for service provision. Research in various settings, including mental health, indicates that care management can remedy such gaps in provision (Challis, 1993). It is no coincidence, therefore, that the principles of the care programme approach are essentially those of care management (Schneider, 1993).

At the same time, driven by concerns about public safety and homelessness among people with mental health problems, there is an acceptance that, where adequate community provision is not available, hospital provision will be required. This principle is expressed in *Caring for People*, as well as in the care programme Circular (Annex, para. 6):

> If a patient's minimum needs for treatment in the community — both in terms of continuing health care and any necessary social care — cannot be met, inpatient treatment should be offered or continued, although (except for patients detained under the Mental Health Act) it is for individual patients to decide whether to accept treatment as an inpatient. Health authorities will need to ensure that any reduction in the number of hospital beds does not outpace the development of alternative community services.

Therefore it would be erroneous to see care programming as a substitute for asylum, or hospital care. Rather, it is a more structured form of care in the community for those whose most appropriate place of residence is not hospital.

For a number of reasons, initial implementation of the care programme approach was far from uniform. Its introduction coincided with the major National Health Service reforms in 1991, with their resultant uncertainty and insecurity. Social services reforms were a further distraction: care management for elderly people became a priority because this group was often seen to require costly residential care; and the Children Act absorbed the remainder of social services' attention. Only the introduction of the Mental Illness Specific Grant stopped mental health from dropping off the agenda altogether. The mechanics of care programming were slow to be established in some districts and encountered numerous obstacles (North and Ritchie, 1993). Moreover, the effectiveness of care programming as such has not yet been established, but relies on the reputation built up by case management in mental health and elsewhere, since the core elements of the two systems (assessment, keyworker, monitoring and review) are practically identical.

The principal objections voiced by those required to implement care programming are the additional costs entailed by the relatively high levels of provision which it requires for people with severe and enduring mental health problems. Here we look in detail at the costs of care programmes for individuals in three health districts.

7.3 Methodology

The production of welfare model (see Chapter 1) provides a conceptual framework in which to locate the care programme approach in systems of mental health care. In terms of this model, the care programme approach is seen as a non-resource input which has a causal relationship with resource inputs and client outcomes. The model also shows that the nature of this relationship is not determined by the care programme approach itself. Rather, it is one of many factors which bring about change in the service user's wellbeing. Without controlling for these other factors, or taking them into account in some way, the effectiveness of the care programme approach cannot be properly assessed.

The research was carried out in three health districts where care programming had been adopted in 1992. The districts were not selected at random because we sought areas which were fairly well advanced in the approach. They did, however, differ widely: Area A being a northern metropolitan borough, Area B a southern coastal town, and Area C a large Midlands town with a wide rural catchment. With the cooperation of those responsible for care programming in each area, we sampled 60 service users (20 in Area C, 21 in Area B and 19 in Area A). We interviewed keyworkers for our sample of service users and gathered detailed information about each individual's care package, using the Client Service Receipt Interview (see Chapter 3) comprehensively to cost services, personal expenditure and accommodation.

The costing methodology employed in this research is described earlier in this book. The complexity of the estimation process is not treated fully in this chapter, but some of the assumptions made when using each source are discussed below to indicate the potential problems and how these affect the validity of the costs data produced. There were four main sources for the costs applied in this study:

- a managing agency's own unit costs estimates ('off the peg' costs);
- a compendium of previous PSSRU work which produced national estimates ('generic costs');
- costs calculated for this study using managing agencies' accounts, capital valuations and occupancy levels ('actuals'); and
- estimates based on other information, such as Statistical Information Service data ('third party').

Off the peg costs. It is a mixed blessing that some agencies produce their own unit costs, since they are not always devised in a manner which is consistent with our methodology. An example of problems arising from 'off-the-peg' unit costs was that devised for a day centre in Area C, which included a 'nominal rent' rather than referring to the capital value of the property. Since capital is often an important element in overall costs, in this case we declined the authority's unit cost in favour of one calculated by combining their revenue costs and an element for capital calculated from previous PSSRU work (Beecham, 1992).

Generic costs. We took most generic costs from previous PSSRU work (Beecham, 1992; Netten and Smart, 1993) which includes a compilation of nationwide average costs data for London, Outer London and other areas, and uprated them using the appropriate price index. The costs devised in this way included psychiatric outpatients appointments and domiciliary visits, and visits from general practitioners, dentists, opticians and local authority social workers (unless they were part of a mental health team which was costed separately).

Actuals. For many of the services and all the accommodation used by people on care programmes, we had to build up individual costs. For commercial residential homes and privately-rented accommodation, where we have no other information, we assumed that fees or rent covered both the revenue and the capital costs of the accommodation. In one district, costing of day care was complicated by the existence of an association of about twenty groups with a wide range of aims (support, self-help, leisure pursuits, social contact, skill acquisition) which were often linked with other community facilities and known collectively as the support network. Our costs represent an average per hour over all these groups, and the unusual nature of the network meant that capital costs could only be approximated.

A service which warranted its own costs was the mental health team with a base in the community and comprising staff from two or more agencies. Most costs of service provision were averaged out over actual attendances for 250 working days, unless we knew how often the facility was open. An important adjustment was made in costing community mental health workers. Most staff do not spend all their working time in face-to-face contact with service users, but the only information about service receipt which we collected concerned client contact with workers and (where relevant) the workers' travel. We therefore had to calculate the 'unseen' costs of administration, training, liaison with other agencies and so forth entailed in the job of community mental health worker. We drew here upon PSSRU colleagues' information about the distribution of mental health workers' time (von Abendorff et al., 1993). This shows that roughly 30 per cent of their time was spent in direct client/carer contact and client-related travel, and the remaining 70 per cent in non-contact activities. We therefore weighted our service costs by estimating that community mental health workers had on average 12 hours of client contact available per week (30 per cent of 40 hours). Group workers were assumed to have 20 hours per week available, and to work in pairs.

Third-party costs. These included services which were used by a small number of people and would contribute relatively little to total costs: day nurseries, legal services, laundry and informal care. For example, day nursery costs were calculated on the basis of national data for the authority in question (Statistical Information Service, 1992). Since English data were not readily available, a cost for legal advice was based on the *Annual Report of the Scottish Legal Aid Board, 1991/92*, but of course this is not entirely adequate because the Scottish legal system differs from that in England, where all our subjects lived. Laundry services were based on costs of hospital laundry in one region: 22p per item. We estimated that an elderly person who needed a laundry service, probably because of incontinence, would have at least 21 items per week to launder, costing £4.62 per week. The costs of informal care were based on the local rate of private domestic help with an element for travelling. This is probably a conservative estimate, since private cleaners might not take on the tasks that some neighbours and family undertake, and because this does not take into account many aspects of the opportunity costs to carers (Netten, 1990, 1993).

Accommodation costs

As discussed in Chapter 3, accurate estimation of housing and personal expenditure is important because accommodation is probably the greatest single cost for people with mental health problems who are not hospital inpatients. We found that most accommodation was either owner-occupied or rented from a local authority housing department, with a minority of people living in communal specialist settings, such as hostels or group homes. In costing owner-occupied accommodation, we relied upon the Halifax Building Society's *House Price Index*, which includes average regional house prices. In costing local authority accommodation we used figures for average subsidies, weekly rents and market values. For those people living in specialist settings, we sought details of capital valuations, revenue expenditure and occupancy from the managing agencies.

For people living in housing association accommodation, the Housing Association Group (HAG) allowances were used for maintenance, decoration, repairs and management. A range of current Total Cost Indicators (£30,000-£48,000 per bed space) was obtained from the housing association in question and, lacking more precise information, we took the median for hostels and the third quartile for accommodation catering for higher dependency. We calculated personnel costs on the basis of the staffing levels reported to us by a manager. More satisfactory estimates could have been made on the basis of the housing association's own accounts, but these were not available. Nevertheless, the estimates obtained in this way do reflect the differentials between the costs of living in specialist and in non-specialist accommodation.

As indicated by the need to add in staffing costs in specialist housing, accommodation sometimes provides much more than bed and board. Ideally, the support provided in certain settings should be disaggregated from housing costs and included with service costs, but it was not possible to make this distinction here.

The fact that the care programme approach is targeted at people being discharged from hospital makes it likely that, in the early stages of its implementation, people who have had brief periods of hospitalisation will be overrepresented among those on the care programme approach, since discharge from hospital is a trigger to care programme assessment. For this reason, the costs of time in hospital are treated separately here, since they are likely to be unrepresentative of longer-term hospital costs for these subjects. In addition, hospital costs vary widely throughout the country and between teaching and non-teaching hospitals. Moreover, in each case costs should be adjusted according to the use made by each person of the different aspects of hospital provision, such as pharmaceuticals, radiography, occupational therapy and surgery, so the costs given here are not as highly refined as they should be for comparisons to be viable. For these two reasons, hospital costs from this study should be treated with caution. There were four people in our sample who spent the whole study period in hospital. Although they did use some services outside the hospital, for the sake of clarity the data about their service use are presented separately in the findings.

We calculated personal expenditure (food, fuel, clothes, transport) for all those people who had not been in hospital throughout the study period. If people had admissions for shorter periods, their normal accommodation costs were assumed to be unaffected, but their personal expenditure was reduced to £12.20 (the Department of Social Security personal allowance) after six weeks in hospital. Benefits and grants which people received in addition to their social security entitlements were annuitised at 6 per cent over ten years and treated as income on the assumption that the lump sums would be spent on furniture and other durables (see Chapter 3).

Relatively few people in our sample had any income other than social security benefits and retirement pension. None was working, although one person was on sick pay, one occasionally earned about £8 by acting as treasurer for a voluntary organisation, and others living with parents or partners who were in employment presumably enjoyed a share of the household earnings in some form.

Personal expenditure included community charge (now council tax). People on social security benefits were assumed to receive community charge benefit and to pay one-fifth of the total, unless we knew from the keyworker that a person was considered exempt from the full amount by reason of mental incapacity. We also assumed that people living in specialised accommodation had been registered as exempt from community charge.

7.4 Expectations and evidence

Our analysis of the data was limited by the quality and size of the sample. Our aim was to describe and comprehensively cost the care programmes received by a sample of users. We also wanted to know whether certain subgroups differed significantly in their service receipt or costs. Here we present comparisons between people aged over and under 65, which reflects a common (but not universal) division in services for people with mental health problems. We were also particularly interested in the subset of people with a diagnosis of schizophrenia, of whom there were 35 in our sample of 60. A person with schizophrenia may have recurrent episodes of acute illness which can lead to hospitalisation, so systems of community mental health services which prevent relapses or unnecessary admissions to hospital are especially relevant for this group.

Sample characteristics

Keyworkers named a primary and secondary diagnosis for the subject of the care programme. Although some people were given more than one diagnosis, a principal diagnosis was not always clear. In Table 7.1, no distinction is made between primary and secondary diagnoses, so the total number of diagnoses is greater than the 60 subjects. Physical problems were also included. The greatest number of care programme subjects (58 per cent) were diagnosed as having schizophrenia. Fewer (35 per cent) had an affective disorder. Dementia was the third most prevalent diagnosis among our sample (18 per cent). Neuroses, personality disorders, substance abuse and other

Table 7.1
Analysis of sample by diagnosis[a]

Main diagnosis	No. of subjects	%
Schizophrenia	35	58
Affective disorder	22	37
Dementia	11	18
Neurosis or stress-related disorder	4	7
Personality disorder	4	7
Substance abuse	1	2
Other mental health problem	7	12
Disability or physical impairment	4	7

a There was more than one diagnosis in 47 per cent of cases.

problems affected smaller proportions of our sample. These findings confirm the relatively high prevalence of schizophrenia among people with severe and enduring mental health problems.

Costs of accommodation and personal expenditure

The overall costs of accommodation and personal expenditure were significantly higher in Area C (the coastal town), than in both other areas ($p<0.05$). This is probably due to the greater use in this town of staffed accommodation, including that provided by a housing association, for the people in our sample. While half of our subjects in the other two areas lived in privately-owned accommodation, only one-quarter of those in Area C lived in this type of housing. Nonetheless, a further factor contributing to the difference may be north-south variation in house prices.

Figure 7.1 illustrates the distribution of housing and expenditure costs between the various agencies which fund this provision. 'Forgone' community charge represents the amount which is waived due to low income or disability (80 or 100 per cent, depending upon the individual). Only one person's accommodation was funded by the social services department. The overall mean cost of housing and personal expenditure was £129 per week (median £108; range £38-£288) across the three areas.

Frequency of service receipt

We relied upon keyworkers to inform us about the services used by each individual, so the reliability of our findings depends on the accuracy of their records or powers of recall over the previous six months. All those people

Figure 7.1
All agencies' contributions to the costs of accommodation and personal expenditure

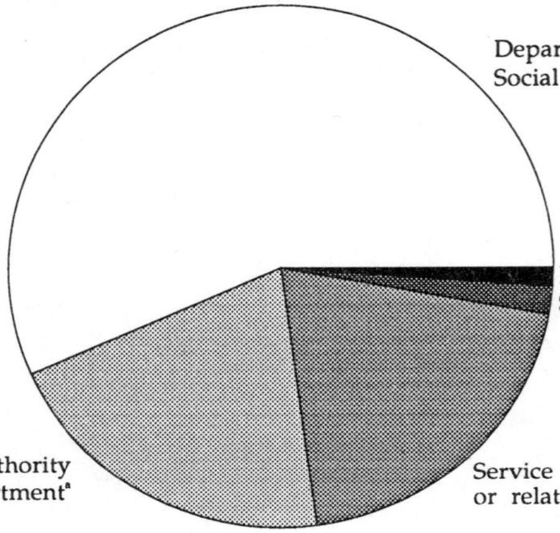

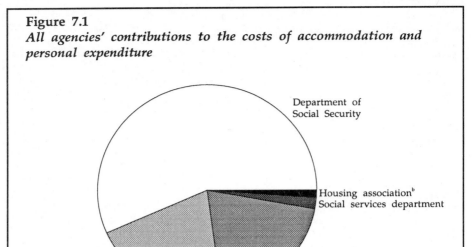

a Housing benefit, subsidies and community charge (now council tax) forgone.
b Although the housing associations provided accommodation for a number of people, they were funded largely by other sources, particularly the residential care grant (DSS) and housing benefit (local authority).

who were in hospital throughout the six-month study period used some outside services (day centres, employment rehabilitation, informal care and so forth). For three people the total costs of these services were £21, £24 and £51, but a fourth was estimated to cost £110 per week in day centre attendance alone. This person lived in halfway-house accommodation in the hospital grounds but also went out to other community resources. This illustrates that, just as it can be misleading to neglect temporary hospital admissions in measuring the costs of community care, people in hospital also use facilities not provided as part of the inpatient service, and a comprehensive costing of an inpatient episode should also include outside services.

We found that people with a diagnosis of schizophrenia did not differ in terms of costs from those with other diagnoses. The only service element which showed a statistically significant difference was, not surprisingly, the depot injections delivered by community psychiatric nurses. Overall costs for people with schizophrenia were not significantly higher in respect to accommodation, services or time in hospital.

We also looked at older and younger service users, of whom there were 21 and 39, respectively, in our sample. In Table 7.2 we show, for older and younger service users, the estimated mean number of contacts with the prin-

Table 7.2
Service receipt — frequency per year for all people in our sample

	Mean frequency of use per year		
Type of service	Under 65 years	65 years or older	Significance level[a]
Hospital inpatient days	28.1	34.5	ns
Outpatients appointments	3.6	2.5	<0.05
Day patient attendances	10.9	26.3	ns
CPN/community nurse visits	22.8	44.3	ns
Depot injections	8.0	3.8	ns
Psychiatrist — domiciliary visit	0.5	1.8	<0.02
Physiotherapist, chiropodist	3.2	10.6	ns
Psychologist	0.6	0.0	ns
General practitioner	6.8	7.5	ns
Dentist	1.6	0.2	ns
Social worker	12.7	17.6	ns
Day centre/rehabilitation	52.2	13.5	<0.01
Home help[b]	9.2	127.0	<0.02
Informal care visits	8.2	144.0	ns
All day hospital and day care	64.9	39.8	ns

a Pooled or separate variance estimates, as indicated by observed significance level.
b Private domestic and local authority home help taken together.
c Although the frequency of visits did not attain statistical significance, the cost of these visits was significantly higher for older people (p<0.02).

cipal services over *one year*. The services with most frequent contact with all our subjects appeared to be day centres (including day hospitals), community psychiatric nurses, home helps, social workers and informal carers.

Younger service users had significantly more day *centre* attendances, but the latter loses its significance when we take into account the use by older people of both general hospitals and psychiatric hospitals for day care. No older person in our sample saw a psychologist, and only a few younger people used this service.

The importance of informal care in terms of frequency of visits should be acknowledged since this number represents *extra* visits due to the subject's mental health problems, as compared to normal social contact. Other services used by our sample included: a leisure scheme for people with mental health problems supported by the city council (four); support workers employed by MIND (four); laundry and incontinence services (four); respite days or weekends in specialist accommodation, such as a local authority home or hostel (two); a dietician (one); church meetings and activities (one); a library volunteer (one); the probation service (one); environmental health (one); and a hospital nurse to give depot injections (one). Although many people were living in non-specialist settings, relatively few services fell outside the arena of formal care.

Costs of service receipt

To give a fuller picture of care programmes, information about frequency of service contacts needs to be interpreted in conjunction with information about costs. Costs reflect the amount of service input as well as the frequency of contact, and can be influenced according to whether people are seen alone or in a group and how much travelling and administration staff are required to do. For example, as shown in Table 7.2 (note c), although the difference in frequency of informal care for older and younger people was not statistically significant, the costs of informal care, which take into account the time and travelling entailed, were significantly higher for older service users.

In interpreting cost information, one should ideally control for factors (called non-resource inputs in the production of welfare model) which are not directly cost-related but which have a bearing on service quality, such as whether there is stability of staff or a high turnover, and what are the service user's and service provider's expectations and experiences of the contact. Finally, a full evaluation demands a measure of outcome. In this study we were only able to measure service frequency and costs, which are partial indicators of the inputs received by an individual but tell us little about the quality of those inputs or about the outcomes.

Table 7.3 gives the mean cost of services for older and younger people and for our sample as a whole, together with a range representing a 95 per cent confidence interval. In keeping with the higher frequencies shown in Table 7.2, costs for older service users were significantly higher than those for younger people for the following services: domiciliary visits from the psychiatrist and home help (private and local authority taken together). Table 7.4 summarises the service data and adds personal expenditure and accommodation, and inpatient costs.

In Table 7.5, service costs have been aggregated according to the agency responsible. In relation to individual agencies' responsibilities, while the health authority's costs for older people appeared to exceed its costs for younger service users, this only marginally achieved statistical significance in our small sample (p=0.06).. When the totals for all services were considered, there was no significant difference between costs for younger and older service users.

Table 7.3
Weekly service costs by agency (1992/93 prices), with 95% confidence interval (not including hospital inpatient costs)

Service	All service users £	Younger (95% c.i.) £	Older (95% c.i.) £
All services	84 (65-102)	73 (55-89)	103 (60-144)
Health authority services	42 (28-56)	32 (22-41)	58 (24-93)
FHSA services	2 (1-2)	1 (1-2)	2 (1-3)
Local authority services	28 (20-37)	28 (18-37)	30 (13-46)
Client/family/others contributions to services	12 (5-19)	11 (0.3-23)	13 (5-21)

a Includes private domestic help, respite, advice, legal representation, dentist, optician, police.

Table 7.4
Weekly global costs by age group and for all service users

Expenditure item	All subjects £	Younger (under 65) £	Older (65+) £
Accommodation and personal expenditure[a]	129	132	124
Total service costs	84	73	103
Cost of inpatient days	104	79	147
Total	317	284	374

a Includes dental services, optician services, private domestic care and informal care.

Hospital inpatient costs

Several of our subjects spent part of the time of the study in hospital. We found that there was no statistically significant difference either between the time spent in hospital by younger and older service users, or between the respective average costs. Mean weekly hospital costs for older people were £147, and for younger people £79, with an overall mean of £104. Virtually all of the hospital costs were borne by the health authority.

Table 7.5
The distribution of costs between agencies for five groups of care programme users, 1992/93 levels

Service user characteristics	All subjects	Younger (under 65)	Older (65+)
Total cost (£ per week)	317	284	374
Health authority[a] (%)	50	44	62
Family health services authority (%)	1	1	1
Social services[b] (%)	11	12	9
Client or relatives[c] (%)	10	8	12
DSS entitlements[d] (%)	15	19	9
Other source[e] (%)	3	5	1
Housing department[f] (%)	9	11	7

a Includes community services, outpatients, day patients and hospital inpatient care.
b E.g. day centres, social work, home help, meals, and a small element for accommodation.
c Mostly accommodation and personal expenditure, with a small element for services and informal care.
d This represents net DSS entitlements after payment of client contributions to services and accommodation.
e Includes housing association, police, legal aid and 'other' services named in the text.
f Comprising housing benefit, forgone community charge and local authority housing subsidy.

Global costs

For all subjects, the mean cost of services was £84 per week. This includes an amount which service users or their relatives contributed towards services. After subtracting this amount (£5) from their personal expenditure, we can add to the cost of services a weekly net amount of £124 for accommodation and other personal expenditure and £104 for inpatient treatment, making a total cost of looking after one person with a care programme of about £308 per week, or about £16,000 per year. Table 7.5 shows the distribution between various funders of the global costs of caring for different groups of service users. We found that, for all service users, the health authority met half the comprehensive costs of care programming, the client met 25 per cent (15 per cent being the user's entitlements to social security benefits, including state pension), social services met 11 per cent and housing met 9 per cent. This highlights the fact that local authority housing departments are an important element in support for people with mental health problems. As mentioned above, the health authority bears a higher proportion of the care for older than for younger service users. This is probably related to their higher levels of physical need.

7.5 Implications

The care programme approach, or its equivalent, is fundamental to community mental health care. It embodies widely accepted principles of mental health care in its emphasis on services which are accountable, multidisciplinary, comprehensive and tailored to the needs of individual users. Therefore, the costs of care programmes will have relevance for all those responsible for allocating resources or for monitoring and evaluating service delivery in mental health.

One use for costs information is to guide the budgeting of individual packages of care for people with mental health problems. Because our data relate to people with care programmes whose needs have been assessed and met as far as practicable, it can be argued that the range of costs for these packages as shown in Table 7.3 represents the costs of *adequate* care packages for people with severe and enduring mental health problems. In doing so, while not forgetting the problematic nature of the hospital costs given here, it should also be noted that none of our costs relates to London. It is estimated that in London health service costs are on average 11 per cent higher (Beecham, 1992) and local authority costs may be as much as 26 per cent higher than in the rest of the country (Bebbington with Kelly, 1993).

Information about service receipt can also help us judge services' responsiveness to need (vertical equity) under the care programme approach. For example, the unsurprising finding that more domestic assistance and monitoring were received by the older group through home care can be taken as evidence of targeting of care, while the finding that older people in our sample did not receive any psychology services and had less dental care than their younger counterparts may indicate a need for service planners to consider whether the differential is justified (by the number of elderly people with false teeth, for instance) and, if not, to address this apparent inequity. Service receipt information also helps in monitoring the process of service delivery. For example, psychiatric services for elderly people see domiciliary assessments as desirable practice (Arie and Jolley, 1982). Our finding that older people tended to receive more domiciliary visits from psychiatrists can be taken as evidence to support their achievement of this goal.

Earlier in this chapter we cited three ways in which care programming could affect costs by placing greater demands on existing resources. At the same time, the supply side of the emerging market in mental health services is changing in response to health and social services reforms. While residential accommodation is the area with the greatest diversity of providers at present, the number of providers of hospital and community health services is also increasing. Costs information is therefore essential for all participants in the mixed economy of mental health care. Commissioners need information about the costs of services to enable them to obtain value for money in the growing internal and external markets. Providers need cost information to price their services competitively. Most importantly, perhaps, all parties need to be aware of the trade-offs which occur, whereby different combinations of care, designed to meet similar needs, can have widely varying implications for agencies in a given district. Our findings concerning the different proportions of costs falling to the health service for older and younger people illustrate this problem.

Costing mental health services rarely enables us to draw definitive conclusions about such multi-faceted activities as the care programme approach, but this is not to deny the usefulness of costing. By examining the profiles of costs which emerged in this study, we have highlighted some important differences, presented a clearer picture of the relative expenditures incurred by different service providers, and suggested a framework for budgeting care packages under the care programme approach. In doing so, we hope to have illustrated how costing can be used as a tool for planning and analysis, and demonstrated its relevance to all those whose concerns include the equity and efficiency of mental health services.

The quotation at the start of this chapter claims that costing is a political activity. Of course, interpreting any research entails making value judgements about the assumptions employed along with the empirical data, as well as the choice of those data. In this chapter we have tried to detail the processes involved in costing as well as the costs produced. By giving examples of the problems which arose and hence the tentative nature of some of the results which emerged, we hope to have demonstrated something of the *craft* of costing. If cost information is demystified in this way and if costing is practised more widely, it should be possible constructively to criticise cost information using a common language and a shared repertoire of methods, rather than dismissing it out of hand as 'political'. Many skills can be turned to political ends by the unscrupulous: the danger seems to arise when those skills are in the hands of a few.

References

Arie, T. and Jolley, D. (1982) Making services work: organisation and style of psychogeriatric services, in R. Levy and F. Post (eds) *The Psychology of Later Life*, Oxford, Blackwell.

Bebbington, A.C. with Kelly, A. (1993) Area differentials in labour costs of personal social services and their relevance to Standard Spending Assessments, Discussion Paper 898, Personal Social Services Research Unit, University of Kent at Canterbury.

Beecham, J.K. (1992) Costing services: an update, Discussion Paper 844, Personal Social Services Research Unit, University of Kent at Canterbury.

Burns, T., Raftery, J., Beadsmoore, A., Mcguigan, S. and Dickson, M. (1993) A controlled trial of home-based acute psychiatric services. II: Treatment patterns and costs, *British Journal of Psychiatry*, 163, 55-61.

Challis, D.J. (1993) Case management: observations from a programme of research, *PSSRU Bulletin No. 9*, July.

Dean, C. and Gadd, E. (1990) Home treatment for acute psychiatric illness, *British Medical Journal*, 301, 1021-3.

Department of Health (1990) *Joint Health/Social Services Circular, The Care Programme Approach for People with a Mental Illness Referred to the Specialist Psychiatric Services*, HC(90)23/LASSL(90)11, Department of Health, London.

Department of Health (1993) *Health of the Nation: Mental Illness Handbook*, HMSO, London.

Dick, P., Cameron, L., Cohen, D., Barlow, M. and Ince, A. (1985) Day and full time psychiatric treatment: a controlled comparison, *British Journal of Psychiatry*, 147, 246-9.

Fenton, F., Tessier, L., Contandriopoulos, A., Nguyen, H. and Struening, E. (1982) A comparative trial of home and hospital psychiatric treatment: financial costs, *Canadian Journal of Psychiatry*, 27, 177-87.

Hoult, J., Rosen, A. and Reynolds, I. (1984) Community orientated treatment compared to psychiatric hospital orientated treatment, *Social Science and Medicine*, 18, 1005-10.

Marks, I.M., Connolly, J., Muijen, M., Audini, B., McNamee, G. and Lawrence, R.E. (1994) Home-based versus hospital-based care for people with serious mental illness, *British Journal of Psychiatry*, 165, 179-94.

Muijen, M., Marks, I.M., Connolly, J., Audini, B. and McNamee, G. (1992) The Daily Living Programme — preliminary comparisons of community versus hospital-based treatment for the seriously mentally ill facing emergency admission, *British Journal of Psychiatry*, 160, 379-84.

Netten, A. (1990) An approach to costing informal care, Discussion Paper 637, Personal Social Services Research Unit, University of Kent at Canterbury.

Netten, A. (1993) Costing informal care, in A. Netten and J. Beecham (eds) *Costing Community Care: Theory and Practice*, Ashgate, Aldershot.

Netten, A. and Smart, S. (1993) *Unit Costs of Community Care, 1992/93*, Personal Social Services Research Unit, University of Kent at Canterbury.

North, C. and Ritchie, J. (1993) *Factors Influencing the Implementation of the Care Programme Approach*, HMSO, London.

Royal College of Psychiatrists (1991) *Good Medical Practice in the Aftercare of Potentially Violent or Vulnerable Patients Discharged from Inpatient Psychiatric Treatment*, Royal College of Psychiatrists, London.

Schneider, J. (1993) Care programming in mental health services: assimilation and adaptation, *British Journal of Social Work*, 23, 383-403.

Secretaries of State (1989) *Caring for People: Community Care in the Next Decade and Beyond*, Cm 849, HMSO, London.

Secretary of State for Health (1992) *The Health of the Nation*, Cm 1523, HMSO, London.

Secretary of State for Social Services (1987) *The Mental Health Act Commission Second Biennial Report 1985-87*, HMSO, London.

Statistical Information Service (1992) *Personal Social Services Statistics 1991-92 Actuals*, Chartered Institute of Public Finance and Accountancy, London.

Stein, L.I. and Test, M.A. (1980) Alternative to mental hospital treatment, I conceptual model, treatment program, and clinical evaluation, *Archives of General Psychiatry*, 37, 392-7.

von Abendorff, R., Challis, D.J. and Netten, A. (1993) Staff activity patterns in a community mental health team for older people, Discussion Paper 981, Personal Social Services Research Unit, University of Kent at Canterbury.

World Health Organization (1991) *Evaluation of Methods for the Treatment of Mental Disorders*, WHO, Geneva.

8 Comparative Efficiency and Equity in Community-Based Care

*Jennifer Beecham, Martin Knapp and Caroline Allen**

To scatter the mentally ill in the community before we have made adequate provision for them is not a solution; in the long run not even for HM Treasury (Titmuss, 1963).

8.1 Successes and failures

Richard Titmuss reckoned the cost of premature dehospitalisation in terms of neglect and higher expenditure on police, prison and probation services, unemployment and sickness benefits, and drugs. However, the findings from studies such as that described in Chapter 5 show that hospital rundown and closure programmes can be planned and implemented in such a way as to contain the costs of community care to affordable proportions, while still maintaining — and in some important respects *improving* — the quality of life of most former inpatients. This has been the case not only with the closure of Friern Hospital, but also with the earlier Care in the Community pilot projects in England (Knapp et al., 1992). There are also encouraging results in a broadly similar initiative in Northern Ireland (Donnelly et al., 1994). But, in each case, the successful outcomes associated with community care have been achieved for former *long-stay* inpatients, and their moves from hospital have been accompanied by purposive and often quite generous funding transfers.

In this chapter we examine the experiences of a different group of people: *short-stay* hospital inpatients who move to the community without the benefit of 'dowries' or other special funding support. We describe the application of economic evaluative methods to the costing of their community care, and make comparisons with the results obtained in the Care in the Community and Friern studies of reprovision. The data on which the comparisons are based were collected in the mid- or late 1980s — prior to the introduction of the care programme approach or supervision registers — and our findings will demonstrate the need for initiatives such as these to coordinate service responses to individual needs.

The *Health of the Nation: Mental Illness Handbook* (Department of Health, 1993) suggests six criteria to use in measuring the success of treatment or care: appropriateness, equity, accessibility, effectiveness, acceptability and efficiency. These criteria are as helpful for research as they should be for practice and can stimulate or structure comparative studies of the kind described here. However, the present research was not able to follow the ideal design. The three groups were studied in three different research projects, and it therefore proved difficult to make strict like-with-like comparisons between the two long-stay groups and the short-stay group. The different instrumentation used to describe individuals' characteristics, symptoms, behaviour and quality of life causes particular problems. Nevertheless, the inter-group differences will be seen to be sufficiently stark to question the comparative efficiency and equity of community care.

8.2 Samples and methods

For each of the three samples of people with mental health problems, comprehensive service use information was collected and costed, and links between costs and individual characteristics were examined. In each study, a version of the Client Service Receipt Inventory (CSRI) was employed, and costs were attached so as to approximate long-run marginal opportunity costs (see Chapter 3). The multivariate methods used to explore the cost-characteristics links were similar to those described in Chapter 4.

The 'short-stay sample'

The first group — which we shall call the *short-stay sample* — comprised 140 people in West Lambeth discharged from psychiatric inpatient care between November 1987 and April 1988, or discharged from inpatient services or the crisis intervention team in Lewisham between November 1988 and April 1989. Each had a diagnosis of schizophrenia but no co-existing drug or alcohol problems (using the Research Diagnostic Criteria Screening Instrument; Spitzer et al., 1975). Each was to be interviewed one year after discharge, although four had died in the intervening period, one could not be traced and eleven refused to provide information. Service use data were collected for 120 people using the CSRI. Demographic and previous psychiatric service contact data were extracted from case notes, and clinical and social characteristics were assessed (Melzer et al., 1991; Conway et al., 1994). Fifty-seven per cent of the sample were men, 74 per cent had been in hospital for less than six months, and only 25 per cent had been in hospital for more than a year in their longest ever stay. Two-thirds were aged under 40 and two-thirds had never married.

The 'reprovision sample'

The first of two long-stay groups — the *reprovision sample* — was drawn from the long-running study of psychiatric reprovision initiated by the decision to begin the closure of Friern and Claybury hospitals in the mid-1980s (see Chapter 5). By August 1992, 442 former hospital residents had been interviewed one year after discharge, and service receipt and care costs calculated for 341 of them. Seventy-seven per cent of this group had a diagnosis of schizophrenia, of whom 43 per cent were women. Average age was 54 years. Sample members had spent an average of seventeen years in hospital prior to their move under this programme. In the comparisons which follow, we concentrate on those people with a diagnosis of schizophrenia.

The 'pilot projects sample'

Members of the third sample were also former long-stay psychiatric hospital residents. Each was selected to move to community residence under the Care in the Community demonstration programme funded by the Department of Health in the 1980s (Renshaw et al., 1988; Knapp et al., 1992). Eight of the 28 pilot projects provided care for people with mental health problems, and seven provided sample members: Brent, Buckinghamshire, Chichester, Greenwich, Waltham Forest, Warrington and West Berkshire. Service receipt and costs data were collected for 130 people who, during the evaluation period, had been living in the community for nine months. Most (82 per cent) had a diagnosis of schizophrenia. Average age was 51 years, and 37 per cent were women. Average length of stay in hospital had been twelve years.

8.3 Service use and costs

Each member of each sample was interviewed or assessed using a variant of the CSRI between nine and thirteen months after the hospital discharge which brought them into the study. How did the service use patterns compare?

Across the three samples, many mental health and other services were used, as would be expected given the many and various needs of people with mental health problems. Table 8.1 lists only services used by 5 per cent or more of the members of at least one sample, and another 23 services are not tabulated.

The majority of people in the short-stay sample had used hospital services in the three months prior to interview, a quarter of them having been re-admitted. People in the reprovision and pilot projects samples showed generally lower use of all hospital services, except that both these former long-stay groups made greater use of 'therapeutic' day activities provided by hospital: 14 per cent attended industrial therapy, 9 per cent hospital activity centres and 2 per cent hospital social clubs.

A high proportion in each sample had seen their GPs in the past three months, emphasising the pivotal role often played by the primary care team, although contact rates were lowest for the short-stay sample. (Indeed, 6 per cent of this sample were not even registered with a GP, none of whom received any informal care, while two-thirds had involvement with the police.) Other differences in service receipt between the short-stay and one or both of the two long-stay samples were in relation to community nurses, community-based psychiatrists, psychologists, chiropody and day care. Also of note is the comparatively high level of involvement of the short-stay sample

Table 8.1
Service use by sample

	Percentage in receipt of service		
Service	Short-stay sample %	Reprovision sample[a] %	Pilot projects sample[b] %
Hospital inpatient	27	16	11
Hospital day patient/activities	8	24	23
Hospital outpatient	57	24	30
Community psychiatry	28	63	28
Community nurse	22	31	61
Psychologist	1	16	11
Chiropodist	7	42	28
Physio/occupational therapist	3	12	11
GP	56	79	89
Dentist	18	24	25
Optician	8	17	21
Social worker	30	27	24
Local authority or voluntary sector day care	12	44	n/a
Education services	9	7	14
Criminal justice services	25	7	1
Sample size	120	262	130

a Knapp et al. (1995).
b Knapp et al. (1992).

with the police and criminal justice system. For five members of the short-stay sample, these were the *only* services used during the evaluation period.

A major component of community care is accommodation, and it should be a matter of concern that members of the short-stay sample were much less likely to be living in specialised settings with experienced, trained staff either on site or in close proximity (12 per cent of the short-stay sample; 82 per cent of the reprovision sample; 82 per cent of the pilot projects sample). Nor was this compensated by support from informal carers. Only 12 per cent of the short-stay sample lived with a partner, although one in five lived with one or both parents. Forty-two per cent lived alone and reported having no friends or relatives who spent time with them at home, leaving them socially isolated. Overall, 72 per cent received fewer than five visits per week from friends or relatives, and in 83 per cent of cases visits were from one person only. Most visits were of short duration, amounting to less than five hours per week. Visits were primarily for social reasons, and only rarely to provide personal care (11 per cent) or domestic care (6 per cent). This contrasts markedly with the long-stay samples (Knapp et al., 1992, Chap. 14; Leff et al., 1994). What the short-stay sample *did* share with the two long-stay samples was lack of paid employment (outside sheltered workshop settings) and very low levels of personal disposable income.

These different service configurations result in different costs (Table 8.2). The differences between the short-stay and each of the long-stay samples are significant ($p<0.01$). Despite the wide cost variations *within* the samples, the short-stay group *on average* received a considerably lower level of formal and informal care or support than either of the long-stay groups. On measures of *throughput* (service receipt) and *input* (costs), mental health resources would not appear to be allocated equitably.

But are these differences in service utilisation and cost between the short-stay and long-stay samples simply the result of not comparing like with like? Might it be the case that the short-stay group is less dependent: that is, less in need of health, social care and housing support?

Table 8.2
Weekly costs for the three samples (1993/94 prices)

	Weekly cost		
Service	Short-stay sample £	Reprovision sample £	Pilot projects sample £
Mean cost	357	531	423
(Standard deviation)	(303)	(234)	(145)
Sample size	120	262	130

Table 8.3
Personal characteristics, by sample

Characteristics	Short-stay sample	Reprovision sample	Pilot projects sample
Percentage male	57	63	63
Percentage single, separated, widowed or divorced	85	93	–
Percentage white ethnic group	52	88	–
Percentage under Mental Health Act section	40	0	0
Mean age at discharge from hospital (yrs)	36	54[b]	48[b]
Mean duration of stay before discharge from hospital (weeks)	28	883	834
Sample size[a]	120	341	88

a Sample size smaller on some items.
b Age at time of assessment, usually up to two years before discharge.

Table 8.4
Present State Examination (PSE) scores, by sample[a]

PSE subscore[b]	Mean (standard deviation) Short-stay	Reprovision	Test of differences (p)
Delusions and hallucinations	3.93 (5.28)	3.03 (5.69)	0.163
Specific neurotic symptoms	2.22 (2.74)	2.32 (3.49)	0.776
Non-specific neurotic symptoms	6.34 (5.73)	4.53 (5.70)	0.009
Behaviour, speech, other symptoms	3.09 (3.72)	3.55 (2.99)	0.283
Total symptom score	15.59 (12.66)	12.42[c] (12.42)	0.049
Sample size	90	308	

a The PSE was not used in the pilot projects study.
b Comparisons are possible only on these subscores. Note that higher scores indicate higher levels of mental ill health.
c n = 196.

Full comparisons between the samples are difficult because the three studies did not use the same set of research instruments to assess characteristics of individuals, but some interesting pair-wise and partial comparisons can be made. In terms of gender balance and marital status, the samples were very similar, but members of the short-stay sample were younger, more likely to be 'sectioned' under the Mental Health Act, had been hospital inpatients for shorter periods of time and were more likely to be from black or ethnic minority groups (Table 8.3). On this last point, note that King et al. (1994), in their screening for psychosis of people making contact with health services in the catchment area of a psychiatric hospital in North London, found that members of the white group were less likely than members of each of the other ethnic groups classified in the 1991 census to be given a diagnosis of non-affective psychosis or schizophrenia.

Comparisons between the short-stay and reprovision samples on the Present State Examination (PSE; Wing et al., 1974) — completed in the community a year after hospital discharge — revealed that the former scored higher on non-specific neurotic symptoms (p=0.009) and total symptom score (p=0.049). There were no significant differences between the samples in relation to: delusions and hallucinations; specific neurotic symptoms; or

Table 8.5
Disability and behaviour characteristics, short-stay sample

	Percentage at each level of dysfunction					
Disability Assessment Schedule dimension[a] or characteristic	0 %	1 %	2 %	3 %	4 %	5 %
Self-care: personal hygiene, feeding habits, keeping living space tidy	49.2	21.1	13.3	7.0	7.8	1.6
Underactivity: culturally-defined 'doing nothing', unoccupied, not conversing	36.0	20.8	15.2	18.4	6.4	3.2
Slowness: overall speed of movement and agility	54.7	18.8	12.5	9.4	3.1	1.6
Social withdrawal: active avoidance of interaction or physical proximity	31.3	19.5	10.2	21.9	13.3	3.9
Social contacts (friction): overt conflictive behaviour with staff, neighbours, others	67.7	8.9	4.8	8.1	9.7	0.8
Interests and information: interests in local and world events; efforts to obtain such information	44.5	14.8	11.7	13.3	9.4	5.5
Behaviour in emergencies: for example in relation to sickness or accident, non-routine events	72.7	3.9	10.2	8.6	3.9	0.8

a 0 = None; 1 = Minimum; 2 = Obvious; 3 = Serious; 4 = Very serious; 5 = Maximum (World Health Organization, 1988).
n=128

behaviour, speech and other symptoms (Table 8.4). Members of the short-stay sample, on average, thus displayed more symptoms of mental ill health.

A similar pattern emerges from comparisons of social skills and behaviour, although the three studies used different instruments. Table 8.5 gives the six-point scores on key items of the Disability Assessment Schedule for the short-stay sample (DAS; World Health Organization, 1988). Comparisons for some items can be made with the reprovision sample, which used a *five*-point scoring (performance rated as normal, minor, moderate or severe problems or where client does not perform at all in these areas). Information was also collected for the pilot projects sample — using a skills and behaviour checklist, rated on a three-point scale — which also allows comparisons in relation to some of the dimensions listed in Table 8.5.

Self-care. While 16 per cent of the short-stay sample were rated as having serious, very serious or maximum dysfunction, 18 per cent of the reprovision sample had severe problems or required daily supervision in relation to hygiene, toileting and tidiness. For the pilot projects sample, 3 per cent had chronically disruptive, unacceptable eating habits, and another 15 per cent needed some supervision; 1 per cent rarely washed or bathed themselves adequately without supervision or help, and another 26 per cent adequately only with help; 6 per cent rarely undertook basic housework adequately, even with supervision, and another 31 per cent only with supervision; and 4 per cent made little or no attempt to look after their own clothes and possessions, and another 32 per cent attempted to, but were untidy.

Underactivity. On the DAS scoring, maximum dysfunction is defined as doing nothing for most of the day (which described 3 per cent of the short-stay sample), very serious dysfunction is spending about eight hours a day doing nothing and needing almost continual supervision (6 per cent), and serious dysfunction refers to lack of activity for six to eight hours a day and needing occasional prompting (18 per cent). These proportions are roughly comparable with the 8 per cent of the pilot projects sample who stood or sat in one place for all or most of the time, and the 23 per cent who had some periods of extreme underactivity. Item scores are not available for the reprovision sample to allow comparison.

Slowness. Seven per cent of the pilot projects sample usually had extremely slow movement (in eating, walking, etc.), and another 15 per cent had occasional periods of extreme slowness. In the short-stay group, 2 per cent exhibited extreme slowness all or most of the time, 3 per cent exhibited marked and persistent slowness, and 9 per cent exhibited slowness most of the time. On this dimension, the long-stay group was the more dependent.

Social withdrawal. Among the short-stay sample, 17 per cent had very serious or maximum dysfunction in relation to social interaction and being in the physical presence of other people — that is, practically never mixing socially, or showing marked tendencies to self-isolation, not responding to encouragement. The comparable figure for the reprovision sample was that 16 per cent had severe problems or could not perform in this domain without supervision. Among the pilot project sample members, 6 per cent rarely or never mixed socially, and 9 per cent rarely or never initiated conversation or interaction with other people.

Social contacts — friction. A small proportion of short-stay sample members exhibited dysfunctional problems in relation to social contacts: 8 per cent had conspicuous friction with at least one person ('serious dysfunction'); 10 per cent had more generalised or more severe friction ('very serious'); and 1 per cent had serious and lasting conflict with work colleagues, neighbours, fellow students or co-residents. In contrast, 9 per cent of the pilot project sample had major rows or constant minor rows with co-residents or others.

Behaviour in emergencies. Among the short-stay sample, 9 per cent had shown incompetence, 4 per cent indifference and 1 per cent total apathy in situations which had potentially hazardous consequences. Reprovision sample members were not greatly different: 19 per cent were rated as performing badly in this domain.

We would conclude from this that the short-stay sample is no less in need of support from staff or carers than the reprovision or pilot projects samples, and in some respects would appear to have been exhibiting greater needs.

8.4 Service targeting

Horizontal equity is usually defined as the equal treatment of equals: individuals with the same health characteristics or needs should receive equivalent amounts of care or service support. It does not necessarily mean that people with the same health characteristics receive exactly the same services, for there is usually more than one way to treat a particular health problem. By contrast, vertical equity is the unequal treatment of unequals: people with different health characteristics or needs should receive different levels (and probably different types) of care or support. An equitable community mental health care system would therefore provide different packages of services in response to differences in assessed needs, where the differential allocation would be driven by social or professional value judgements and preferences, and users' views.

Although it has proved impossible to formalise the comparisons as much as one would like, the findings presented earlier suggest that the short-stay sample was *not* being supported equitably when compared with the two long-stay samples. Equivalent or sometimes higher levels of need in relation to the symptoms and consequences of mental ill health were not prompting greater levels of support. Indeed, costs were significantly lower. A natural corollary is to ask whether different people *within* a sample are receiving services which appear to reflect their different needs for support. We could view this as a 'target efficiency' question: how well are the vertical equity aims being met?

To examine these issues we estimated and compared cost prediction equations for each sample in turn. The method was exactly as described in Chapter 4 for our study of the Daily Living Programme, and in Chapter 5 for the reprovision sample itself. Ordinary least squares multiple regression techniques generated equations linking the characteristics of individuals to the comprehensive costs of their care. The 'best' equations did not emerge from a step-wise estimation procedure, but were selected so as to achieve the most satisfactory statistical results, whilst remaining both parsimonious in variable inclusion and interpretable. The best reprovision equations are given in Tables 5.5 and 5.6. These equations apply to *all* diagnoses, but tests revealed no differences between the diagnostic groups (see Knapp et al., 1995). For the pilot projects sample, two analyses are reported: one focusing on user characteristics in hospital, and the other on their characteristics in the community (Table 8.6). For the short-stay sample, the statistical exploration found fewer links with user characteristics (Table 8.7). Consider each of these three samples in turn.

The reprovision sample

As explained in Chapter 5, the cost prediction equation for the reprovision sample examined the links between users' characteristics as assessed in hospital prior to discharge and costs measured retrospectively one year after the move. Thirty-six per cent of the inter-individual variation in community care costs could be explained statistically by these characteristics (see pages 114-117). Among the influential factors are gender, marital status, age, duration of hospital residence, symptoms of mental ill health as measured by scores on the Present State Examination and the Social Behaviour Schedule (SBS), daily nursing care needs and social networks.

For a subsample of this group, other multivariate analyses had revealed links between costs and users' characteristics in the *community*, and between costs and changes in those characteristics since leaving hospital (see pages 117-119). The latter equation could explain at least 57 per cent of the inter-individual variation in community care costs. In both cases, therefore, there were significant links between users' needs-related characteristics and their care packages (as summarised by costs), with estimated coefficients interpretable as indicating reasonably good targeting. People with more symptoms of mental ill health received more support, suggesting some degree of vertical equity by the criteria usually employed.

Table 8.6
Pilot projects' cost prediction equations

	Characteristics in hospital		Characteristics in community	
Regressor variables[a]	Coeff.	Sig.	Coeff.	Sig.
Constant term (100)	145.71	.029	19.53	.106
Age at admission to hospital	-15.11	.093		
Age at onset of mental illness, squared	-0.10	.018		
Age at time of hospital assessment squared	0.19	.051		
Duration of hospital stay (years)	-26.22	.008		
Duration of hospital stay, squared	0.18	.136		
Original diagnosis: organic disorder	368.84	.007		
Behavioural problems (T1)	-377.74	.048		
Behavioural problems (T1), squared	2.58	.060		
Behavioural problems (T2)			86.53	.019
Behavioural problems (T2) squared			-0.71	.012
Schedule for Social Interaction[b] (T2)			-15.73	.034
Psychosocial Functioning Inventory[c] (T2)			4.14	.093
Cantril Morale Score[d] (T2)			-13.50	.114
Personal presentation score (T2)			-11.81	.054
Re-admission to hospital, dummy			59.04	.086
R^2	0.43[e]		0.25[e]	
F-statistic	4.25	.001	4.31	.000
Sample size	55		100	

a TI indicates hospital assessment; T2 indicates community assessment.
b Henderson et al. (1981).
c Feragne et al. (1983).
d Cantril (1965).
e Adjusted R^2=0.33 for first equation, 0.19 for second.

The pilot projects sample

Two series of analyses for the pilot projects sample are relevant to the inter-sample comparisons. The first series examined the extent to which community care costs could be explained by client characteristics in hospital. Because of missing observations on some variables, the results presented in the first

Table 8.7
Short stay sample cost prediction equation

Regressor variables	Characteristics in community Coeff.	Sig.
Constant term	14310.07	.003
Client has been subject of a 'section'[a]	9166.45	.021
No or minimum dysfunction in activity levels[b]	-12083.93	.010
Serious to maximum dysfunction in interest in local or world events[b]	11172.99	.024
No or minimum dysfunction in overall speed of movement[b]	16703.89	.001
R^2	0.21[c]	
F-statistic	7.38	.000
Sample size	114	

a Under the 1983 Mental Health Act.
b Variables taken from the Disability Assessment Schedule (World Health Organization, 1988).
c Adjusted R^2=0.18

column of Table 8.6 are based on a relatively small sample of former hospital residents (n=55). The analyses show that people with fewer behavioural problems and symptoms of mental illness in the hospital setting, relative to their peers, received relatively less costly packages of community care nine months after leaving hospital. Higher costs were also associated with organic brain disorder (as compared to other original diagnoses), shorter duration of hospitalisation, greater age at the time of the hospital assessment (in most cases this is also the age at subsequent discharge from hospital), and lower age at both the onset of mental illness and the last admission to hospital. People with more community living experience prior to their illness or hospitalisation will have taken more self-care skills into the hospital with them, reducing their dependency post-discharge.

These results suggest that — as with the reprovision sample — the widely varying costs of community care for this sample of people with long-term needs for support are not random fluctuations — the regression equation explains 43 per cent of the variation — but equally there remains quite a lot of variation to be accounted for (perhaps) by the community-assessed characteristics of users. This was the purpose of the second series of analyses, which reached the equation in the second column of Table 8.6. (A third series looked at outcomes — changes in user health and welfare between hospital and community assessments — but is not reported here because there are no comparable outcome measures available for the short-stay sample; see Knapp and Beecham, 1990.)

By the time people had settled into their new community placements, there had been some adjustment of care packages to their developing needs. Most received some form of keyworker or case (care) manager support as one of the funding conditions of the pilot programme (Renshaw et al., 1988, Chap. 8). In these circumstances we would expect to find the cost of community care responding to skills, behavioural problems, continuing symptoms of mental illness, and other felt needs as assessed *in the community*. The second equation in Table 8.6 shows that this is partly the case. Costs were higher for people displaying greater 'needs' in terms of skills, behavioural problems, symptoms, social networks and satisfaction with social contacts, life satisfaction and personal presentation. Generally, we have found the expected cost-'dependency' association (as represented, for example, by the lines in Figure 4.3 on page 94): people who are better able to lead independent lives, including maintaining high and satisfying levels of social contact, are likely to require less staff support and fewer health, social care, housing and other inputs. This finding is consistent with results from research on other client groups within carefully-designed programmes (see Conroy and Bradley, 1985, for people with learning disabilities; Davies and Challis, 1986, and Davies et al., 1990, for elderly people). One dimension of client welfare deviates from this general finding: higher scores on the morale subscale of the Psychosocial Functioning Inventory (Feragne et al., 1983) are associated with *higher* costs. We interpret this as indicating a causal connection running from service utilisation to contentment.

Examination of the links between costs and outcomes for the pilot projects sample increased the explanatory power, but missing values on some variables reduced the sample size. Significant positive associations were found between costs and hospital-community changes in relation to behaviour, life satisfaction and morale. Thus for *both* long-stay samples, higher levels of community care expenditure resulted in better user outcomes, other things being equal. (However, this was not the case for a fairly similar sample of former long-stay psychiatric hospital residents who had moved to the community in Northern Ireland: links between costs and individual characteristics were not as strong as we found for either of the two English samples; see Donnelly et al., 1994, Chap. 6.)

Short-stay sample

What happens when we use a similar approach for the short-stay sample? A series of cost prediction equations was again estimated to explore the relationship between costs, needs and other user characteristics. Symptom count variables were selected from the PSE for: delusions and hallucinations; specific and non-specific neuroses; behaviour, speech and other disorders; and total symptoms. Background characteristics were taken from the Colorado Treatment Outcome Schedule (Ellis et al., 1984) and covered: age, age at onset of schizophrenia, marital status, gender, duration of index episode, ethnicity and whether the client was currently taking medication or had ever been sectioned under the Mental Health Act. The Disability Assessment Schedule (see above) gave scores for levels of social functioning in relation to slowness, underactivity, social withdrawal, friction with social contacts, behaviour in emergencies, and interest in local and world events. Interactive terms were considered in the analyses.

The final equation has relatively low R^2 and adjusted R^2 values, giving limited evidence to suggest that resource allocation was responsive to individual characteristics (Table 8.7). Only four variables had any significant relationship with cost differences. First, if the sample member had been 'sectioned' under the 1983 Mental Health Act, their costs of community care were higher. Social functioning proved a slightly better predictor of costs, with three measures entering the equation: activity levels, interest in local or world events, and overall speed of movement. These three variables are highly inter-correlated, so interpreting their individual effects is difficult, but this does not alter our general conclusion that services appeared not to be targeted very well on need. PSE data were available for 91 members of this sample, but none of the subscores entered the equation: higher levels of clinical need were not associated with higher costs.

This tentative evidence for target inefficiency in resource allocation for the short-stay sample is supported by findings from a four-year follow-up study of those members of the sample living in West Lambeth (Conway et al., 1994). The CSRI was again used to collect service receipt data but, apart from a significant increase in the numbers of people receiving CPN support and admitted to inpatient hospital care, sample members appeared to be receiving less community support than they were three years earlier (for example, in relation to outpatient and day patient care, and GP and social work support). There was no increase in the number of people living in specialised accommodation and no apparent increase in the availability of informal care. Conway and colleagues suggest the reduction in the number of people with psychotic states may have been attributable to increased contact with psychiatric services, but there was no change over time in social functioning levels. Mean global disability scores four years after leaving hospital were associated with psychiatric inpatient admission, but provision of other services was not related to disability scores at one or four years after leaving hospital, nor to the change in global scores over time.

8.5 Towards appropriate resourcing

We can now return to the criteria of success suggested by the *Health of the Nation: Mental Illness Handbook* (Department of Health, 1993): appropriateness, equity, accessibility, effectiveness, acceptability and efficiency. Although we should again warn about the hazards of comparing across the samples because of the difficulties in making like-with-like comparisons, the evidence in this chapter offers reasons for arguing that, by these criteria, people in the short-stay sample were less well supported in the community than either of the two long-stay samples:

- Service utilisation rates were lower for the short-stay sample, with the exception of higher utilisation of hospital services (greater percentage use and higher cost).
- There were marked differences in accommodation patterns, members of the short-stay sample being less likely to live in specialised accommodation, or to receive informal support in lieu of this. Greater expenditure on accommodation for long-stay samples made more resources available for day-to-day support.
- Comprehensive costs were significantly lower for the short-stay sample.
- Inequity is shown by the generally lower service utilisation rates and costs, lower likelihood of living in specialised accommodation and lower levels of informal support despite on average *similar* or *higher* levels of need of the short-stay sample.
- The links between, on the one hand, the characteristics and needs of sample members and, on the other, their costs of care reveal reasonably strong and positive links for the two long-stay samples, but rather weaker links for the short-stay group.
- Other things being equal, better individual outcomes flowed from higher levels of support (as indicated by higher costs) within the two long-stay samples, but — although it was not possible to test this association with the same rigour — did not appear to do so within the short-stay sample.

The cumulative weight of this comparative evidence — which has been pulled together in a manner which is retrospective and opportunistic rather than purposive and planned — should be the *starting point* for a more detailed consideration of resource targeting in community mental health care. In particular, are there lessons to be learnt from the organisation, funding and delivery of community care for the two long-stay groups to guide the improvement of the quality and responsiveness of care for other people? That is, are there actions which might help to improve the efficiency and equity of the mental health care system? To conclude this chapter, we offer some suggestions for the resource environment of community care.

The accumulated findings from this exploratory study point to what we have previously called *'resource keys'* which need to be turned in order to secure good quality mental health care, particularly related to the adequacy, timeliness, distribution, coordination and flexibility of community care resources (Beecham et al., 1994; Knapp, 1995). We have also examined these resource keys elsewhere in a broader discussion of the care and treatment of people with schizophrenia (Kavanagh et al., 1995).

It hardly needs to be said that there must be enough resources for community and other mental health care, which probably means some protection or ring-fencing of funds transferred from elsewhere (such as hospital budgets) and some dedicated new funding (such as the Mental Illness Specific Grant). This is easier when the starting point for community care is hospital rundown, for the closure of inpatient places can release resources. Such resources do not get transferred automatically, but they can usually be identified (as suggested by the cost function estimates for marginal savings given in Chapter 4) and used as the basis for inter-agency negotiation. Both of the long-stay populations benefited from being part of well-resourced relocation programmes, either through special 'pump-priming' funding (in the Care in the Community programme) or through financial mechanisms or 'dowries' to transfer money from hospital to community budgets (the North London reprovision programme). For short-stay groups there is no obvious equivalent budget from which to release resources. Indeed, there is a shortage of acute inpatient provision in London, which would make any transfers difficult. For both the long-stay and short-stay groups there is a case for arguing that local authorities need to inject more resources into mental health services — *both* personal social services and housing — and that they need more central government money to enable them to do so. Capital funding is especially important.

But high-quality community care is not obtained just by throwing money at it. What, then, are the other resource keys? One other requirement is *timeliness*. The two studies of long-stay samples showed that resources and services are needed in the community *before* a hospital begins its rundown programme, as is widely recognised although not always implemented. The availability of ring-fenced funds for the long-stay groups helped to ensure that expenditure was timely. Services could be put in place *before* clients moved from hospital, comprehensive care packages could be arranged to meet individual needs, and the predictability of resources helped long-term planning. It is important, therefore, that services are planned and established early enough to ensure continuity and quality of care for those people with mental health problems who are *not* long-stay inpatients. Discharge plans and the care programme approach are steps in the right direction, but they may not be able to range over all care agencies (or at least not with real power or authority) and they do not necessarily put the necessary service or other resources in place. They may also only cover short periods of time. Another facet of the 'timeliness' requirement is thus the need to keep an eye on the *long-term* consequences of today's practice and policy decisions for users, carers, staff and budgets.

The appropriate *distribution* of responsibilities and responses is a third facet of the resource environment which needs emphasis. Inpatient hospital care funding is 96 per cent NHS, whereas only about half the cost of community care is funded from this source, and may be rather less under the post-1990 Act arrangements for funding residential and nursing home care. The obvious need in relation to people in the long-stay samples was to redistribute money between services and agencies when changing the hospital/community balance, a need which was largely achieved.

The same redistribution is required for short-stay groups: the NHS needs to recognise and help to support the important roles to be played by local authorities, and voluntary and private organisations in ensuring that care in community settings is of sufficient quality, not only to ensure a good quality of life but also to reduce the likelihood of subsequent inpatient re-admissions. There is also a need for commitment to primary health care, public health medicine based in the community and a broad-based health promotion approach which seeks to deal with socio-economic issues such as housing and employment which can prevent the exacerbation of mental health problems.

This leads in turn to the need for the *coordination* of those multi-agency resources in the pursuit of better quality community care. Coordination is needed at both strategic (macro) and tactical (micro) levels. Coordination of broad systems of care can be assisted by, for example, area-level community care plans, better information flows at the primary/ secondary care interface and by the joint commissioning of services. Coordination for individual users or 'cases' could be built around care programmes, care management or other forms of keyworking in order to assess a widely-defined range of needs, to coordinate service responses to them, to monitor progress towards goals, and to liaise with users and carers so as to elicit their preferences.

In the Care in the Community pilot programme, care management was also used as an instrument for translating broad care principles into practice, and introducing relevant financial information into planning (Knapp et al., 1992, Chap. 10). The reprovision programme had no directive to develop care management, but, as people were discharged, the administrative system attached to the financial transfer ensured that responsibility for care was accepted by the receiving district, often through a named consultant. In some areas dowry payments were contingent on care plans being drawn up.

Adequate information systems are required in order to obtain access to and make optimal use of the resources which are available. This means the employment not only of computer systems and other IT equipment but also, more importantly, staff who have or who are in a strong position to build inter-agency links and are thus in a good position to put together the information required for good coordination. It is particularly important to gather information about the work of private and voluntary sector agencies and alternative therapeutic services which can often provide complements to statutory services. Holistic approaches to mental health may be more readily found there.

Finally, there is a need for *flexibility* within the community mental health care system, both in terms of resourcing and responsiveness to individual needs and preferences. For example, certain types of specialised accommodation may become inappropriate if residents' skills and symptoms change (worsening or improving with treatment or experience). Local systems of care should be able to respond flexibly to these changes: not denying people 'homes for life' where this brings security and comfort, but equally not confining people to live in patently inappropriate accommodation.

This is *not* to say that former long-stay patients are always more favourably treated in terms of care funding. By no means every person leaving long-stay hospital is the subject of special project or dowry funding, and the coordination of their care may be cursory. The point is that people with mental health problems living in the community, whether or not they are former long-stay psychiatric inpatients, whose care is *not* covered by these resource keys often live in dire circumstances (Audit Commission, 1994; Kavanagh et al., 1995). Our findings for the short-stay sample leaving inpatient residence in the late 1980s reveal multiple deprivations and disadvantages. Despite continuing psychiatric symptoms, and sometimes high levels of social disability, these people received few care services, were unlikely to live in specialised care accommodation, and enjoyed only limited informal care support.

Legislative and other changes in the past six years have begun to address the problems which lead to inequity and inefficiency in the mental health care system and more widely, although it is not yet clear that each of these resource keys has been fully turned.

Note

* Many of the analyses and arguments in this chapter were put together when Caroline Allen was employed at the PSSRU. Data for the 'short-stay sample' were collected by David Melzer, Gary Hogman and colleagues at St Thomas's Hospital, using instrumentation and methods designed by Jennifer Beecham and Martin Knapp. Some of the data for the other samples were collected by Paul Cambridge, Angela Fitzpatrick, Angela Hallam and Corinne Thomason. The authors alone are responsible for the contents of the chapter.

References

Audit Commission (1994) *Finding a Place: A Review of Mental Health Services for Adults*, HMSO, London.

Beecham, J.K., Knapp, M.R.J., Fenyo, A.J. and Hallam, A. (1994) The costs of community care, in North East Thames Regional Health Authority, *Institution to Community: Friern Lessons Pack*, NETRHA, London.

Cantril, H. (1965) *The Pattern of Human Concerns*, Rutgers University Press, New Brunswick, New Jersey.

Conroy, J.W. and Bradley, V.J. (1985) The Pennhurst Longitudinal Study: a report of five years of research and analysis, Human Services Research Institute, Boston and Developmental Disabilities Center, Temple University, Philadelphia, Pennsylvania.

Conway, A.S., Melzer, D. and Hale, A.S. (1994) The outcome of targeting community mental health services: evidence from the West Lambeth schizophrenia cohort, *British Medical Journal*, 308, 627-30.

Davies, B.P. and Challis, D.J. (1986) *Matching Resources to Needs in Community Care*, Gower, Aldershot.

Davies, B.P., Bebbington, A.C. and Charnley, H. with Baines, B., Ferlie, E.B., Hughes, M. and Twigg, J. (1990) *Resources, Needs and Outcomes in Community-Based Care*, Avebury, Aldershot.

Department of Health (1993) *Health of the Nation: Mental Illness Handbook*, HMSO, London.

Donnelly, M., McGilloway, S., Mays, N., Perry, S., Knapp, M.R.J., Kavanagh, S., Beecham, J.K., Fenyo, A.J. and Astin, J. (1994) *Opening New Doors: An Evaluation of Community Care for People Discharged from Psychiatric and Mental Handicap Hospitals*, HMSO, London.

Ellis, R.E., Wilson, N.Z. and Foster, M.F. (1984) Statewide treatment outcome assessment in Colorado: the Colorado client assessment record, *Community Mental Health Journal*, 20, 72-89.

Feragne, M.A., Longabaugh, R. and Stevenson, J.F. (1983) The Psychosocial Functioning Inventory, *Evaluation and the Health Professions*, 6, 3, 25-48.

Henderson, S. with Byrne, D.G. and Duncan-Jones, P. (1981) *Neurosis and the Social Environment*, Academic Press, Sydney.

Kavanagh, S., Opit, L., Knapp, M.R.J. and Beecham, J. (1995) Schizophrenia: shifting the balance of care, *Social Psychiatry and Psychiatric Epidemiology*, forthcoming.

King, M., Coker, E., Leavey, G., Hoare, A. and Johnson-Sabine, E. (1994) Incidence of psychotic illness in London: comparison of ethnic groups, *British Medical Journal*, 309, 29 October, 1115-9.

Knapp, M.R.J. (1995) From psychiatric hospital to community care: reflections on the English experience, in M. Moscarelli (ed.) *The Economics of Schizophrenia*, Wiley and Sons, New York.

Knapp, M.R.J. and Beecham, J.K. (1990) The cost-effectiveness of community care for former long-stay psychiatric hospital patients, in R.M. Schleffer and L.F. Rossiter (eds) *Advances in Health Economics and Health Services Research*, JAI Press, Greenwich, Connecticut.

Knapp, M.R.J., Cambridge, P., Thomason, C., Beecham, J.K., Allen, C. and Darton, R.A. (1992) *Care in the Community: Challenge and Demonstration*, Ashgate, Aldershot.

Knapp, M.R.J., Beecham, J.K., Fenyo, A. and Hallam, A. (1995) Community mental health care for former hospital in-patients: predicting costs from needs and diagnoses, *British Journal of Psychiatry*, 166, supplement 27, 10-18.

Leff, J., Thornicroft, G., Coxhead, N. and Crawford, C. (1994) A five year follow-up of long-stay psychiatric patients discharged to the community, *British Journal of Psychiatry*, 165, supplement 25, 13-17.

Melzer, D., Hale, A.S., Malik, S.J., Hogman, G.A. and Wood, S. (1991) Community care for patients with schizophrenia one year after hospital discharge, *British Medical Journal*, 303, 1023-6.

Renshaw, J., Hampson, R., Thomason, C., Darton, R.A., Judge, K.F. and Knapp, M.R.J. (1988) *Care in the Community: The First Steps*, Gower, Aldershot.
Spitzer, R.L., Endicott, J. and Robins, E. (1975) *Research Diagnostic Criteria Instrument No 58*, New York State Psychiatric Institute, New York.
Wing, J.K., Cooper, J.E. and Sartorius, N. (1974) *The Measurement and Classification of Psychiatric Symptoms*, Cambridge University Press, Cambridge.
World Health Organization (1988) *WHO Psychiatric Disability Assessment Schedule*, World Health Organization, Geneva.

9 Reduced-List Costings

*Martin Knapp and Jennifer Beecham**

9.1 Research costs

The demands for cost information on health and social services are to be seen in the day-to-day operation of individual services, in the planning of community care services, in commissioning and contracting, in deciding on the viability of care programmes, and in performance reviews and audits. In the terminology of Chapter 1, these demands have their roots in policy, accountability, mental health practice and product development. Costs are also increasingly common and important elements of evaluative research, either as supplements to, or as integral parts of, much clinical and health services research.

However, the utilisation of cost information is rather less frequent and regular than might be expected, and certainly a lot less than is needed. There are many reasons for this, including the scarcity of economists, a shortage of good-quality data on service use patterns and their financial implications, and a common but generally indefensible hesitation to incorporate monetary magnitudes into clinical reviews, evaluations and decisions.

One very relevant reason for the rarity of costs research has been the expense of doing it. Attaching prices or costs to health care treatments is still problematic and many people also use a range of other services, especially social care, public housing and social security. It is difficult to collect this information, and difficult to attach monetary values which reflect the long-run marginal social opportunity costs of the services or other support activities (Knapp, 1993; and see Chapter 3). There are, for example, comparatively few occasions when it is sensible or acceptable to concentrate one's research attentions on just a small number of the many services which people use, or to drive a steamroller over inter-facility or inter-individual cost variations by assuming a simple average cost figure.

The problem of multiple service costing is particularly acute in relation to mental health services, where many users also need social care support and assistance with housing, and where the interactions between primary and secondary care are often numerous and sometimes complex. Support 'packages' encompassing many services and drawing on the resources of many agencies, coordinated by care managers or keyworkers appointed under the new 'care programme' arrangements (Schneider, 1993; and see Chapter 7) are increasingly the norm, not the exception. Do the multiplicity and complexity necessarily make all costs work on mental health services expensive to undertake?

The purpose of this chapter is to explore an informed short-cut to the cost evaluation of mental health services. We examine the feasibility and advisability of what we shall call *reduced-list costings* — concentrating attention on just a handful of the commonly-used and most costly services — in an effort to cut the research costs.

We should emphasise, however, that the reduced-list methodology will certainly not have universal applicability. There will be many research contexts when the approach is too crude or too limiting.

9.2 The costing methodology

As was argued in Chapter 1, and as illustrated in subsequent chapters, there are some basic principles of cost evaluation which ought to be observed. One such principle is the desirability of measuring costs comprehensively to include all components of care 'packages', unless there are good reasons for not doing so. Other principles are the need to make like-with-like comparisons, the benefits of exploring inter-user and inter-facility variations, and the importance of combining costs data with evidence on outcomes. It is primarily the first principle which is relevant for this chapter, for we are interested in *how* comprehensive costs need to be in certain practical circumstances. In fact, a more precise framing of the question addressed in this chapter is how detailed the data collection needs to be in order to calculate *sufficiently* comprehensive costs.

Of course, policy-makers and practitioners are not only interested in monetary magnitudes. They often also want to be able to examine, describe and analyse some or all of the services which people use, including some which have very little impact on the total costs of support, treatment or intervention. This is especially relevant when seeking to predict service consequences, or when commissioning support programmes. This chapter's concern with *reduced-list* costings should not therefore distract attention from these and other needs for service and costs information.

9.3 Reduced-list costs

It is inevitable in certain circumstances that one or two services will dominate the cost picture; earlier chapters offer numerous examples. For instance, hospital stays overwhelm most other service costs when looking at a long-term inpatient treatment programme, and the accommodation and living costs of a highly-staffed community facility tend to dominate total costs even where other services are used (as in the Friern and Claybury reprovision programme described in Chapter 5; and as in the other settings described in Chapter 8).

We thus re-examined some previous collections of service utilisation and cost data to reveal the proportional contributions of certain services to total package costs. These previous collections are described fully elsewhere and here we simply provide summary details. Because the research studies were conducted at different times, in different contexts, for different purposes and by different (though overlapping) groups of researchers, the classifications of services are not always identical. However, the same research instrument (the CSRI) was used throughout, and all attached costs were our best estimates of long-run marginal costs, including relevant capital elements, but excluding transfer payments (see Chapter 3).

We will detail the examination of reduced-list costs from two studies: the first is the evaluation of psychiatric reprovision for Friern and Claybury hospitals; and the second is the study of people on the caseloads of community psychiatric nurse teams in Greenwich (see Chapter 4 for more details). We then draw some conclusions as to generalisability of the reduced-list method for predicting the cost implications of care.

Psychiatric reprovision

Our study of community reprovision for the former long-stay inpatients of Friern and Claybury hospitals was described in Chapter 5. Table 9.1 reports the costs of community care for the sample of 341 former long-stay psychiatric hospital residents in the first five annual cohorts of leavers for whom we have full service use data. It gives the contributions to total cost of the ten most costly components of care packages, their cumulative contribution, and the importance of these same services for each cohort.

We can see that five services account for 94.4 per cent of the true total cost, and ten services for 98.0 per cent. In itself this is a useful finding, for it suggests that concentration on just a few services would produce cost estimates for the group as a whole which are very close to the true (full) package costs. What the reduced-list method would miss is the considerable deviation from the mean for a small number of people. The estimate based on the five most costly services was greater than 80 per cent of the true cost for 94 per cent of people, greater than 90 per cent of true cost for 87 per cent of people,

Table 9.1
Reduced-list costs: Friern/Claybury psychiatric reprovision

	Full sample contributions		Contributions by[a] annual cohort				
			85/86	86/87	87/88	88/89	89/90
Care package components	%	Cum.	%	%	%	%	%
Accommodation, living expenses	83.3	83.3	69.1	77.9	91.7	90.2	85.3
NHS day care	4.6	87.9	14.5	2.9	2.1	3.3	3.1
Hospital inpatient	2.7	90.6	5.4	5.0	0.5	1.4	5.5
Social services day care (LA)	2.2	92.8	4.5	3.7	1.1	1.7	0.4
Voluntary sector day care	1.6	94.4	0.5	1.6	1.3	0.5	2.8
Field social work	1.5	95.9	0.6	4.6	0.5	0.1	0.1
Hospital outpatient	0.7	96.5	2.3	0.5	0.2	0.5	0.2
Community nursing	0.6	97.2	1.3	0.3	0.3	0.6	0.7
Education facilities	0.5	97.6	0.3	1.7	0.2	0	0
GP	0.4	98.0	0.5	0.3	0.5	0.4	0.3
True (full) weekly cost (%)		100	100	100	100	100	100
Sample size		341	38	87	82	47	87

a By year in which patients were discharged from hospital.

and greater than 95 per cent of true cost for 74 per cent of people. The median accuracy of prediction is 97.4 per cent.

The results of reduced-list estimation for the different diagnostic groups showed some differences, although nothing particularly dramatic. For five broad diagnostic groups, the five costliest services predicted the following percentages of full cost (sample size in brackets):

- 97.7 per cent for people with organic brain disorder (12 people);
- 94.6 per cent for people with schizophrenia (262);
- 94.9 per cent for people with affective disorder (28);
- 94.9 per cent for people with neurosis or personality disorder (32); and
- 99.4 per cent for people with learning disability (3).

Of course, any fool should be able to produce encouragingly accurate reduced-list estimates with 20/20 hindsight. A better test of the accuracy of the method is whether one can predict good estimates from previous experience or evidence. The Friern and Claybury study lends itself to a simple simulation. Taking the five most costly care package components for the first annual cohort of leavers, the accuracy of predictions can be examined for the four subsequent cohorts. The five most costly services for the *second* cohort can then be taken as the basis for predicting costs for later cohorts, and so on, thus simulating a process of learning by doing. Table 9.2 shows the mean and standard deviation of the percentage of the true cost estimated from the top 5 services from earlier cohorts by these routes. Although local policies and service practices were changing over time, the sequential predictions remain quite accurate. (Of course, one can gain better predictive estimates of individual costs, given good data on individual needs and other characteristics, by using appropriate multivariate methods, as described in Chapters 4 and 8.)

The reduced-list method has therefore stood up fairly well to this first testing, but three aspects of the psychiatric reprovision programme contributed to this success. First, the transfer of finances from hospital to district health authority (community service) budgets which originally funded the reprovision of hospital services was contingent on satisfactory arrangements having been made for the community support of former inpatients. These arrangements did not usually amount to close care management of the kind recommended in *Caring for People* (Secretaries of State, 1989). It is more akin to care programming, although less likely to be a clinical than a managerial responsibility. Care programming should mean that community support is more comprehensive (which might make reduced-list costing less representative of the true cost) but also better coordinated (which should make it more predictable). As a general rule, we would expect care management or care programming to make it easier to predict the costs of community care packages.

The second and third aspects of the Friern and Claybury study which have probably contributed to the accuracy of the results generated by the reduced-

Table 9.2
Sequential prediction of costs by the reduced-list method: Friern/Claybury psychiatric reprovision

		Basis for predictions				
Estimated cost as percentage of true (full) cost		Cohort 1 'top five'	Cohort 2 'top five'	Cohort 3 'top five'	Cohort 4 'top five'	Cohort 5
Cohort 1	mean	94.9	–	–	–	–
	standard deviation	5.9	–	–	–	–
Cohort 2	mean	88.1	92.0	–	–	–
	standard deviation	14.9	10.8	–	–	–
Cohort 3	mean	95.3	95.7	96.6	–	–
	standard deviation	6.0	4.5	4.3	–	–
Cohort 4	mean	96.3	95.7	95.2	96.3	–
	standard deviation	6.4	6.8	8.0	6.6	–
Cohort 5	mean	95.0	95.1	93.2	95.5	97.0
	standard deviation	6.7	6.5	13.0	6.5	6.3

list method are the long-term ('chronic') nature of the mental health problems of each sample member and the heavy reliance on staffed accommodation in the community. The nature of the mental health characteristics of sample members means comparatively few fluctuations over time in needs (and therefore comparative few fluctuations in service responses). Reliance on staffed accommodation means that many of the service needs of individuals are met from within the accommodation facility budget (making cost prediction easier). This can be seen from Table 9.3.

Table 9.3
Reduced-list costs estimated by accommodation type: North London psychiatric reprovision

	Percentage of full cost accounted for by:			
Accommodation type	Accomm.	Top 5	Top 10	N
Residential/nursing home	91.0	97.4	98.9	164
Hostel	85.1	96.4	98.8	60
Sheltered housing	72.9	94.7	99.2	6
Staffed group home	83.3	96.6	98.7	41
Unstaffed group home	64.2	92.5	98.9	27
Adult foster placement	69.8	96.1	99.2	11
Independent living	63.2	87.7	95.9	32
All accommodation types	83.3	94.4	98.0	341

In the second examination of the reduced-list method, we therefore turn to care for people with acute mental health problems, most of whom are living in their own homes.

Community psychiatric nurse support teams

A service initiative was taken in Greenwich to re-organise part of the community psychiatric nurse (CPN) service, with individual staff acting as case managers and client advocates. The economics component of the evaluation, conducted by PSSRU, was confined to examining service utilisation and cost, and ran in parallel with the broader study of social and clinical outcomes conducted by Muijen et al. (1994).

Comprehensive service receipt data were gathered using the CSRI for a three-month pre-referral period and three consecutive treatment periods of six months. As Chapter 4 demonstrated, the evaluation found a difference in the weekly cost of all services and accommodation used by the two groups of people in the study in the first six months of the treatment period. In the longer term, the cost differences between the groups were not statistically significant (McCrone et al., 1994).

Table 9.4 summarises the contributions to (true) total cost of those services which were among the largest ten contributors during any one of the four costing periods for either of the two sample groups. The five services making the greatest contributions to total costs in the pre-referral period (accommodation, hospital inpatient and outpatient care, social services day care and CPN support) remain the most important in cost terms for the Community

Table 9.4
Reduced-list costs: Greenwich CPN teams

	Percentage contribution by group[a] and time period[b]							
	Generic group				CST group			
Care package components	T1 %	T2 %	T3 %	T4 %	T1 %	T2 %	T3 %	T4 %
Accommodation, living expenses	49.6	71.7	75.0	73.5	40.6	61.9	68.9	66.1
Hospital inpatient	41.2	16.1	12.1	17.1	49.5	14.0	16.7	18.8
Social service day care (LA)	3.5	3.3	7.8	4.5	3.7	4.8	4.6	7.0
Hospital outpatient	1.4	1.9	1.1	0.5	1.6	2.7	1.5	2.2
Health clinic	0.7							
Home help/home care	0.6	0.5		0.5				
CPN services	0.5	2.7	1.0	0.7	1.1	10.7	5.7	3.3
Education facilities	0.5						0.5	
Voluntary sector day centre	0.5	0.5		1.0		0.9	1.0	
Injection	0.4		0.3		0.4	0.7		
Community psychiatry					0.7	0.5	0.5	0.5
Police					0.5	0.5		0.3
Courts					0.3			
GP				0.4	0.3		0.6	0.6
NHS day care		1.0	0.6	0.7				
Occupational therapy		0.4						
Field social work		0.4	0.5					
Employment agency						1.7		
Free bus pass			0.3	0.3			0.4	0.3
Psychology			0.3					
Support worker								0.3
Top 5 services	96.4	95.6	97.0	96.8	96.4	94.2	95.4	94.3
Top 10	98.7	98.4	99.0	99.1	98.6	98.4	98.4	96.3
Sample size	40	35	33	30	37	36	35	32

a The generic and CST groups are defined in the text.
b Time periods are as follows: T1 = pre-referral period of 3 months; T2 = 0-6 months of treatment period; T3 = 7-12 months of treatment period; T4 = 13-18 months of treatment period.

Support Team (CST) group throughout the treatment period. A similar pattern was found for the generic group (except that CPN support replaces health clinic in the top 5 after the pre-referral period). The top 5 services account for no less than 94.3 per cent of costs.

There was also quite marked consistency over time. If we had taken the five services making the largest contributions to cost during the pre-referral period as the basis for subsequent costings, we would never have done worse than predicting 92.9 per cent of the correct figure.

If we then take the question of cost predictions one stage further, how well might we have estimated the costs of service packages for the Greenwich CST and generic team's clients if we had decided only to cost a reduced-list based on the findings from the earlier *psychiatric reprovision* study? That is, can we import findings from one study into another? Using the top 5 services from the Friern and Claybury study (the first five listed in Table 9.1), we would have been able to predict the true Greenwich CST costs with no less than 91 per cent accuracy, except in the first six months of the treatment period when the Friern and Claybury-based estimate would have been 82 per cent of the total. For the generic group, the Friern and Claybury-based predictions are better (no worse than 92.6 per cent). Thus, there is obviously some scope for taking some informed short-cuts by learning from the detail of previous research. It hardly needs to be added that such cross-fertilisation should be employed cautiously.

Other applications

We also examined the accuracy of reduced-list costings in three other contexts, again based on previous evaluations: the Daily Living Programme (see Chapter 4); the Maudsley Outreach Support and Treatment team (MOST) (Beecham et al., 1994); and our study of people with schizophrenia discharged from in-patient psychiatric services in West Lambeth and Lewisham (see Chapter 8). No-one in this last-mentioned group was covered by care programmes or care management, and generally their clinical, economic and social circumstances gave cause for concern (Melzer et al., 1991). The findings from these other reduced-list examinations will be described briefly. Added to the previous findings, they make it possible to build up a cumulative reduced list.

The services making the largest contributions to costs, and the cumulative sums of the 'top 5' and 'top 10', were all examined for each of these samples. Table 9.5 summarises the findings from each of the previous studies covered by this paper, concentrating — where there is a choice — on the longer-run costs of care packages (for example, costs in the last of the evaluation periods when we have information over time).

The five individual services separately listed in Table 9.5 (accommodation and living expenses; hospital inpatient; local authority social services day care; hospital outpatient; and NHS day care, including day patient) are those

Table 9.5
Cost contributions by reduced-list services: comparisons of studies

Service/sample and period[a]	Percentage of full cost accounted for by[b]:							N
						Top 5 sum[c]		
	Accom. %	Inpat. %	SSD day %	Outpat. %	NHS day %	Local %	Global %	
Psychiatric reprovision								
– cohorts 1 to 5	83.3	2.7	2.2	0.7	4.6	94.4	93.5	341
CPN teams (Greenwich)								
– generic group, 13-18 months	73.5	17.1	4.5	0.5	0.7	96.8	96.3	30
– CST group, 13-18 months	66.1	18.8	7.0	2.2	0.2	94.3	94.3	32
DLP evaluation								
– DLP group, 12-20 months	72.8	8.7	1.6	0.6	0.0	97.6	83.7	74
– control group, 12-20 months	70.2	18.9	2.2	1.9	3.3	96.5	96.5	68
Maudsley Outreach service								
– MOST sample	37.8	21.4	0.4	0.2	1.3	95.2	61.1	26
West Lambeth schizophrenia study								
– community sample	64.2	16.1	2.4	2.6	4.2	90.2	89.5	120

a Samples and studies are detailed in the text.
b Abbreviations are: Accom = accommodation and living expenses; Inpat = hospital inpatient care; SSD day = local authority social services department day care; Outpat = hospital outpatient; NHS day = hospital daypatient or NHS day care.
c The 'local top 5' is the sum of the contributions of the five most costly services; the 'global top 5' is the sum of the contributions of the five services separately listed in the table, these being the services which contribute most to total package costs when averaged over all of the listed studies and samples.

which, when averaged over the studies and samples listed in the table, contribute the most to full care package costs. The table also gives the cumulative sum of these five services (called the *global top 5*), as well as the cumulative sum of the five most costly services for the particular study and sample (the *local top 5*).

It can be seen that, with the exception of the MOST sample — which is made up of people who have rejected or found themselves unable to use conventional psychiatric and other support services — the five services in the *global top 5* together account for no less than 83.7 per cent of the true or full costs of care packages.

9.4 Conclusions and recommendations

This methodological investigation of detailed, comprehensive costs data for a number of samples of people with serious mental health problems has examined the possibility of concentrating research attention on just a small number of key services.

The empirical findings lead us to conclude that this short-cut approach to costing could work well in certain circumstances. It happens, however, that the five services which make up what we call the *global top 5* are rarely straightforward to cost. In particular, marked variations in accommodation types and costs between localities, and differences in the costs of inpatient treatment and local authority and NHS day services (all of them linked in part to differences in clientele) make it advisable to use local rather than national cost levels. This has obvious implications for the need for access to facility-specific accounts and for adequate researcher time.

If our aim is simply to obtain broad orders of magnitude for the costs of a programme of care or treatment for groups of users, the reduced-list method has much to commend it. Obviously its accuracy depends on the volume and quality of prior information, but we can envisage relatively few circumstances in which it would be impossible to predict the few very large contributors to total package cost. If there has been relevant previous research, or a well-worked comprehensively costed pilot sample, the ability to choose an optimum reduced-list on which to focus data collection resources will be enhanced. Moreover, the magnitude of the costing error will be known.

Conversely, of course, incomplete costs from a prior study can sometimes be rendered more comprehensive by judicious use of extraneous information from more complete service and costing accounts, as illustrated in the study by Kavanagh et al. (1993), described in Chapter 6, and in other work on the balance of provision and funding for people with schizophrenia (Kavanagh et al., 1995).

However, and to state what may by now be obvious, the reduced-list method is not recommended when:

- fully comprehensive service utilisation and cost data are needed;
- when the impact of policy or practice on seemingly peripheral services is relevant (for example, the cumulative effect on general practitioners of a hospital closure programme which concentrates replacement facilities in one locale); and
- when inter-individual differences in service use and cost are of primary importance, so that approximations based on evidence concerning group averages or assumptions concerning 'typical' service profiles could miss the considerable impact on package costs of expensive but rarely-used services for a small number of people.

Costs, however, are not just a research issue but also a pressing *practice* issue. Care managers, keyworkers and, of course, purchasers generally need to be able to predict the service and cost consequences for groups of users or whole populations, especially if they are working with devolved budgets. Reduced-list costings can provide invaluable data, but just as there are limitations to the reduced-list as a research methodology, so there are also limitations to its use in practice. It was shown, for example, that the reduced-list was not a good predictor of costs where service developments and/or care packages are some distance outside the conventional boundaries of provision, as we found when looking at the MOST services for people who were unable to use standard psychiatric services, and as would be the case with many innovations. Neither should this method be used to set inflexible individual care budgets, as greater needs may have a powerful impact on the cost implications of individual support requirements.

There is no doubt that the reduced-list methodology can provide a short-cut to estimating care costs in mental health evaluations. By reducing the time and resources required for research, the quantity of costs data should increase. As long as common sense prevails, little damage need be done to the quality of the cost information. Such an approach moves us some distance towards enabling the demands for cost information to be progressively met by good quality data built from a solid research base.

Note

* We are grateful to Eriko Kamikubo-Gould and Andrew Fenyo for statistical support, Isaac Marks for prodding us in the direction described in the paper, and to the colleagues with whom we collaborated on the studies which provide the databases for this research. A longer version of this chapter was published as 'Reduced-list costings: examination of an informed short-cut in mental health research' in *Health Economics*, **2**, 4, December 1993, pp.313-322. Reprinted by permission of John Wiley & Sons Ltd.

References

Beecham, J.K., Dansie, A. and Knapp, M.R.J. (1994) The costs of MOST, Discussion Paper 909, Personal Social Services Research Unit, University of Kent at Canterbury.

Kavanagh, S., Schneider, J., Knapp, M.R.J., Beecham, J.K. and Netten, A. (1993) Elderly people with cognitive impairment: costing possible changes in balance of care, *Health and Social Care in the Community*, 1, 69-80.

Kavanagh, S., Opit, L., Knapp, M.R.J. and Beecham, J.K. (1995) Schizophrenia: shifting the balance of care, *Social Psychiatry and Psychiatric Epidemiology*, forthcoming.

Knapp, M.R.J. (1993) Background theory, in A. Netten and J.K. Beecham (eds) *Costing Community Care: Theory and Practice*, Ashgate, Aldershot.

Knapp, M.R.J. and Beecham, J.K. (1993) Reduced-list costings: an examination of an informed short-cut in mental health research, *Health Economics*, 2, 4, 313-22.

McCrone, P., Beecham, J.K. and Knapp, M.R.J. (1994) Community psychiatric nurse teams: cost effectiveness of intensive support versus generic care, *British Journal of Psychiatry*, 165, 218-21.

Melzer, D., Hale, A.S., Malik, S.J., Hogman, G.A. and Wood, S. (1991) Community care for patients with schizophrenia one year after hospital discharge, *British Medical Journal*, 303, 1023-6.

Muijen, M., Cooney, M., Strathdee, G., Bell, R. and Hudson, A. (1994) Community psychiatric nurse teams: intensive support versus generic care, *British Journal of Psychiatry*, 165, 211-17.

Schneider, J. (1993) Care programming in mental health services: assimilation and adaptation, *British Journal of Social Work*, 23, 383-403.

Secretaries of State (1989) *Caring for People: Community Care in the Next Decade and Beyond*, Cm 849, HMSO, London.

10 Decision Analysis and Mental Health Evaluations

Alan Stewart

10.1 Introduction

Prescribing decisions are increasingly being pressured by a supply of economic information in the form of cost-effectiveness studies — or similar evaluations — of a range of pharmaceuticals. This trend has been welcomed by the government, and a set of guidelines for these economic studies has been drawn up by the Department of Health and the pharmaceutical industry (Department of Health, 1994). The content of these guidelines was discussed at greater length in Chapter 2. As that and other chapters have illustrated, the techniques of economic evaluation are also being applied to a range of other interventions, not just pharmaceuticals.

As recommended by the DH guidelines, many of these studies are using decision trees to represent clinical problems and analyse the costs and outcomes of treatment. One recent example compared alternative antidepressants for use in episodic treatment of depression among the general population (Stewart, 1994). The decision tree is given in Figure 10.1, and produced the results shown in Table 10.1. The analysis is explained below.

The figures in the table appear to be indicating a relatively narrow range of expected costs for health care providers when using drugs with extremely wide variations in acquisition cost. But what exactly do the figures in Table 10.1 mean and what benefits can this information offer to a clinician? The figures may appear to be a marketing ploy, but there is no doubt that they do have the potential to be used positively by clinicians, pharmacists and others involved in pharmaceutical prescribing or purchasing, and also by practitioners involved in evaluating alternatives in other types of care.

Figure 10.1
Treatment path for first-line use of sertraline

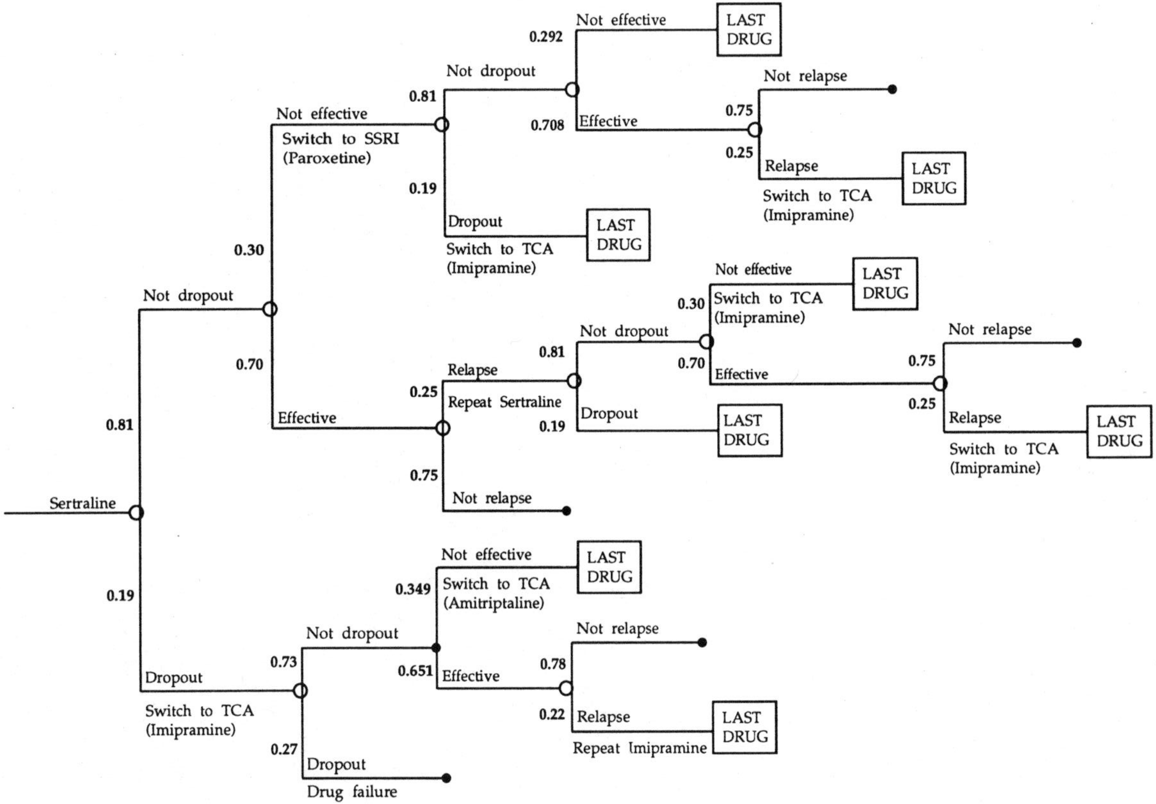

Table 10.1
Expected costs, 1992/93 prices

First-line drug	Expected costs £
Imipramine	352.38
Amitriptyline	350.79
Sertraline	401.36
Paroxetine	381.31

10.2 Decision analysis

Studies like the antidepressant evaluation described above are based on the principles of decision analysis. This mode of analysis incorporates elements of the economic theory of expected utility, and represents given clinical problems using a fairly standard diagrammatic representation and notation. In Figure 10.1 the lines represent paths through standard treatment options. The points where a clinician makes a choice between alternatives are represented by an open rectangle. Where there is uncertainty as to the outcome of an event, such as a treatment involving a possibility of success or failure, this is represented by an open circle. The endpoint of the analysis is shown by a shaded circle. The decision tree diagram lays out a defined and structured set of events that may occur in a defined sequence. This structure incorporates a number of probabilities at various points, defined as chance nodes, which generate cumulative chances of arriving at any particular endpoint in the diagram via a particular discrete path through the defined set of events. These techniques are not just used in economic analysis; they have been imported by economics as an additional means to analyse uncertainty, and have been used in many other areas and disciplines, including clinical decision-making (Thornton et al., 1992). The tree itself is just a flow diagram that visually represents decisions and outcomes in a set order.

10.3 Data sources

But where do all the data come from for this analysis? One frequent source is existing results from clinical trials, where decision analysis techniques can be used to generate retrospective economic evaluations. This has been done recently in some studies evaluating antidepressants in the context of the current debate over using selective serotonin reuptake inhibitors (SSRIs) or tricyclic antidepressants (TCAs) (Jönsson and Bebbington, 1994; Stewart, 1994), the elements of which are summarised in Box 10.1.

Box 10.1
SSRIs or TCAs? Two contrasting views

Stewart, A. (1994) Antidepressant pharmacotherapy: cost comparison of SSRIs and TCAs, *British Journal of Medical Economics*, 7, 67-79.

This model evaluated episodic antidepressant pharmacotherapy, using a tricyclic antidepressant (imipramine or amitriptyline) or a selective serotonin reuptake inhibitor (sertraline or paroxetine). Alternative drug regimens were compared in terms of expected costs per patient over a maximum of one year, as shown in Table 10.1. The study concluded that, while the cost advantage of TCAs is not as great as is usually inferred from the prescription price, there is no clear cost argument demonstrated for switching from TCAs to SSRIs.

Jönsson, B. and Bebbington, P.E. (1994) What price depression? The cost of depression and the cost-effectiveness of pharmacological treatment, *British Journal of Psychiatry*, 164, 665-673.

A model based on decision analysis principles was used to compare costs of treating depressed patients with paroxetine (an SSRI) or imipramine (a TCA). Expected costs per patient over one year were found to be similar (£430 vs £424 at 1989/90 prices), but costs per successfully treated patient (those not suffering relapse) were found to be lower for paroxetine (£785) than for imipramine (£1,024), leading the authors to argue that health service costs could be reduced by switching from TCAs to SSRIs as first-line antidepressants.

Alternatively, data are often 'synthesised' by evaluating a range of existing pieces of clinical research through a process of literature search and review that may be extended to a formal meta-analysis. This is a valuable procedure, but one that is subject to a number of possible biases: if followed it should be performed rigorously and with regard to principles laid down in the existing literature (Glass et al., 1981; Cooper and Hedges, 1994). It is important that the clinical data used are credible and rigorously constructed. If there is any doubt about this, the conclusions of economic studies may be strongly criticised, as shown in a recent exchange of views on one of the antidepressant evaluations referred to earlier (Freemantle and Maynard, 1994; Jönsson, 1994).

The critique by Freemantle and Maynard centred on the use of a specific set of pooled randomised controlled trial (RCT) results as the basis for one arm of a decision analysis report (Jönsson and Bebbington, 1994). One aspect of this clinical work, the rates for drop-outs from drug treatment, was critical to the results of the economic evaluation. This was seen as sound in terms of economic analysis, but flawed by the use of unreliable clinical data: a set of results that Freemantle and Maynard believed to exhibit many of the faults that may occur in RCTs. In his response, Jönsson defended the rigour of the underlying clinical analysis and hence the validity of the economic conclusions. This exchange emphasises the importance of using sound clinical data as a base for economic evaluations using decision analysis.

Evaluation and outputs

Moving on from this set of probabilities, the next stage in the decision tree evaluation is to carry out the cost analysis and, ultimately, the cost-effectiveness analysis. While decision analysis models calculate cumulative probabilities along their paths, they also aggregate the costs incurred at each stage of the process. Thus each endpoint has an accumulated probability of a patient arriving at that discrete point and also an aggregate expected cost for the resources utilised along the way. If one then multiplies each of these aggregate expected costs by the associated probability, the result is a weighted cost for that particular point: the sum of these weighted costs is the average expected cost of any patient being entered into the analysis at the first point in the tree.

The above process may sound complex or arithmetically tortuous, but in most studies the actual calculation of expected costs will be performed by one of a number of software packages available in the market. The analyst's role is in defining the problem and setting up the structure for analysis, then supplying the inputs of costs and clinical data.

This process therefore generates an average expected cost for all patients starting a course of treatment. For a clinician seeking to understand the economic implications of prescribing decisions, this means that for each patient entering therapy, using the selected treatment, the expected cost will equal the given figure. It should be noted, however, that this figure is based on sets of costs and probabilities that are averages, and as with all such figures there are deviations from the mean. Individual patients will vary widely in terms of their clinical progress and hence their consumption of resources and resulting costs (see Chapter 4 for more detailed discussion of cost variations). These variations are reflected *in part* in the decision tree by their completion at different endpoints, and are accounted for in the tree by the use of probabilities providing a weighting to each aggregate set of costs. There will nevertheless remain variations around the calculated costs. Ideally, the report of a decision analysis should present not just this calculated expected cost, but also the actual costs that will be incurred if patients experience specific sets of clinical outcomes. For example, the report could list costs for those who are 'cured' by the drug without any side-effects or need for repeated courses and for those at the other extreme, who do not respond and hence need other treatments. This reflects the Department of Health (1994) recommendations in their recent guidelines on presentation of disaggregated costs.

The end result — the expected cost — is therefore what we expect to happen if a specific treatment is chosen and offered as therapy to a representative sample of patients. By repeating the analysis for different drugs or therapeutic options, with differing sets of probabilities, we can evaluate the cost implications of switching from the existing option to one of a range of alternative therapies.

Testing the results

The figures from a decision tree analysis should, however, be tested and evaluated by performing thorough sensitivity analysis, as discussed in Chapter 2. During this process, the assumptions in the analysis are tested by systematically varying the values used for those key elements in the study which may be sensitive to change. The sensitivity issue area has recently been reviewed and some key aspects of its role identified (Briggs et al., 1994). For example, one can test for the uncertainty relating to variability in sample data, such as the actual packages of resources used in providing care. Not all clinicians will treat patients in the same manner. Sensitivity analysis can allow comparisons of costs where different quantities of specific items are provided. The costs of providing care within a given facility may also vary according to the intensity with which the capacity is used. The adjustments tested in sensitivity analysis allow a range of results to be generated that will cover a range of circumstances.

There may also be uncertainty as to the evidence used for efficacy: are the results obtained in the setting of a clinical trial generalisable to clinical practice? By using sensitivity analysis, one can begin to examine the impact of efficacy at levels that clinicians would expect to see in everyday practice: in other words, the likely effectiveness of a procedure or therapy rather than its efficacy as measured in the abnormal setting of a clinical trial. This is an important point: decision analysis is often used as a means to extrapolate from clinical research settings and estimate or predict what will happen in the 'real world'.

Some analyses may go beyond the calculation of costs or cost-effectiveness ratios and introduce measurement and evaluation of the quality of life, performing what is called cost-utility analysis. This particular technique of economic evaluation was discussed at greater length in Chapter 2. The general principles of criticism described here apply to cost-utility studies as well, but they also raise further issues on quality of life measurement which are dealt with in the specialist literature (Bowling, 1991; Walker and Rosser, 1993).

10.4 Summary

As was stated earlier, the basic output of economic studies using decision analysis techniques is usually an expected cost: what does that figure actually represent? It is an estimate of the average cost per patient treated that will fall on the agencies funding treatment if a very large number of patients follow the treatment pattern suggested in the study. As shown in the decision tree, various subgroups of patients will incur different figures for total costs. But over the whole range of patients, the high and low cost outcomes will balance out to give the average figure, which is the expected cost. Clinicians can compare these figures as part of the process of considering alternative types of health care intervention or modes of care. It may well be, for example, that giving in to pressures to switch to lower-price drugs will not actually help health care budgets, regardless of the impact on patient wellbeing.

So what are the key points to remember when evaluating the usefulness or veracity of decision analysis studies? At least four questions should be asked, as a check for methodological rigour.

- Does the treatment path represent a credible set of events and decisions? That is, can clinicians recognise the decision tree as representing procedures that approximate to their own practices?
- Are the data used in the study credible and valid for this particular piece of analysis?
- If data come from a clinical trial, was the trial conducted to acceptable standards and is the statistical analysis of toleration, efficacy and adverse events figures correct? Have the clinical trials results been used to justify assumptions and extrapolations that the data will not support?
- If the data are synthesised from the available literature, have rigorous meta-analysis procedures been followed? Or is the literature search and review guilty of biases, such as careful selection of papers to be used or of 'footnote chasing', where the use of references from papers known to the author shapes the final set of papers incorporated into the analysis.

All the above questions have to be considered by the reader of any economic study presenting a decision tree. If the study is accepted as having dealt with these points then it may be useful as a way for clinicians to move towards a more optimal allocation of their prescribing budgets. If the reader is unsatisfied with the rigour of the study's design, methodology and analysis, then its conclusions should be regarded with the same caution and suspicion as would be attached to a clinical trial report that did not appear to be methodologically rigorous.

But where these criteria have been met and the study is accepted as methodologically strong, then a report using decision analysis can be a valuable part of health and social policy planning. The results of intelligent sensitivity analysis can indicate areas where further research is required and also areas that have particularly significant effects on costs and outcomes. And for decision-makers faced with competing modes of care or health technologies, a well-researched and well-constructed decision analysis report can provide guidance out of the maze of alternative paths and give an indication of the best available route.

References

Bowling, A. (1991) *Measuring Health,* Open University Press, Buckingham.

Briggs, A., Sculpher, M. and Buxton, M. (1994) Uncertainty in the economic evaluation of health care technologies: the role of sensitivity analysis, *Health Economics,* 3, 95-104.

Cooper, H. and Hedges, L.V. (eds) (1994) *The Handbook of Research Synthesis,* Russell Sage Foundation, New York.

Department of Health (1994) Press release 94/251, Department of Health, London.

Freemantle, N. and Maynard, A. (1994) Something rotten in the state of clinical and economic evaluations? *Health Economics,* 3, 63-7.

Glass, G.V., McGaw, B. and Smith, M.L. (1981) *Meta-Analysis in Social Research,* Sage Publications, Beverly Hills, California.

Jönsson, B. (1994) Economic evaluation and clinical uncertainty: response to Freemantle and Maynard, *Health Economics,* 3, 305-7.

Jönsson, B. and Bebbington, P.E. (1994) What price depression? The cost of depression and the cost-effectiveness of pharmacological treatment, *British Journal of Psychiatry,* 164, 665-73.

Stewart, A. (1994) Antidepressant pharmacotherapy: cost comparison of SSRIs and TCAs, *British Journal of Medical Economics,* 7, 67-79.

Thornton, J.G., Lilford, R.J. and Johnson, N. (1992) Decision analysis in medicine, *British Medical Journal,* 304, 1099-1103.

Walker, S.R. and Rosser, R.M. (1993) *Quality of Life Assessment: Key Issues in the 1990s,* Kluwer Academic Publishers, London.

11 Have the 'Lunatics Taken Over the Asylums'? The Rising Cost of Psychiatric Services in England and Wales, 1860-1986

James Raftery

11.1 Introduction

This chapter has a different orientation from others in the book. It examines expenditure data for psychiatric provision for England and Wales in the period 1860 to 1986, and summarises analyses of these trends which were part of a recent PhD thesis (Raftery, 1993). These data show a dramatic increase in both total expenditure and unit costs over the period since 1950. The chapter considers four possible reasons for the changes observed: the so-called relative price effect; the shorter working week; equal pay for women; and the ratio of nurses to patients. The last of these is argued to be the most important factor in explaining the increase in unit costs. Finally, some implications for the costing of contemporary psychiatric services are explored.

11.2 Expenditure on psychiatric services

Two expenditure trends are reviewed in this section: total current (non-capital or revenue) costs of provision for the mentally disordered; and unit costs which indicate the cost per inpatient of the treatment and care provided. The quest must be for complete coverage — both public and private — distinguishing psychiatric illness from mental handicap. As the available time series data on expenditure on mental disorder are partial in coverage and sometimes inconsistent in their treatment of different types of expenditure, a certain amount of estimation is necessary.[1]

Current expenditure on psychiatric services

The data sources on expenditure on psychiatric services are summarised here. Three current (or non-capital) expenditure series are shown in Figure 11.1:

(a) annual public expenditure on pauper lunatics in institutions under the Lunacy Commissioners;
(b) estimated expenditure on the workhouse lunatics; and
(b) estimated private spending.[2]

Figure 11.1 shows the overall pattern of current expenditure on psychiatric services between 1870 and 1986, expressed in constant 1985 prices using the gross domestic product (GDP) deflator (Feinstein, 1972). Aggregate spending was clearly dominated by that on pauper lunatics in the institutions covered by the Lunacy Commissioners, which accounted for over 90 per cent of total spending throughout all but the earlier part of the period. Aggregate spending followed the trend in inpatient numbers up to the advent of the NHS, after which this pattern ceased to apply. Spending continued to rise as the number of inpatients fell after 1955.

Spending (in 1985 prices) ran at around £60 million per annum in 1870,

Figure 11.1
Expenditure on psychiatric services, England and Wales, 1870-1986, at 1985 prices

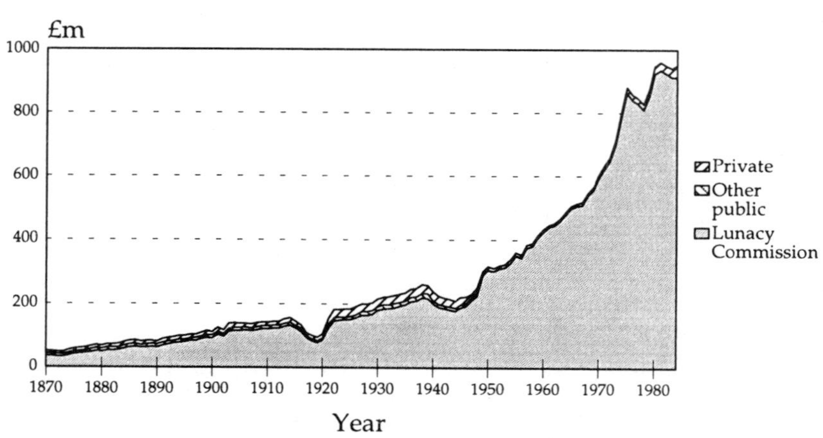

rising steadily to around £150 million by 1900. Spending continued to rise slowly to a peak of under £200 million by 1914, but then fell sharply to around £100 million during the First World War. After the war spending recovered to its pre-war level of around £200 million and resumed its steady increase to reach a peak of around £300 million by 1940. With the Second World War and a fall in the number of patients in mental hospitals, spending again fell — but less sharply than in the earlier war — to £250 million. After the Second World War, and with the coming of the NHS, spending initially continued at around the £250 million level but then began to increase rapidly, reaching £500 million by 1960 and continuing to rise despite the drop in inpatient numbers to reach some £700 million by 1970 and over £1,300 million by 1985. As shown in Figure 11.1, non-NHS spending became noticeable again by the mid-1980s so that, by 1985, such (estimated) spending accounted for some 9 per cent of the total.

Composition of spending

The data in Figure 11.1 referred only to total expenditure on the range of psychiatric facilities. With the expansion of outpatient and day patient services in recent decades, the levels of spending under these headings have become more important. The programme budget expenditure series, published through the House of Commons Social Services Select Committee (1990), provides data on spending by type of psychiatric service under the following five headings:

- inpatient costs to the NHS;
- outpatient costs to the NHS;
- day patient costs to the NHS;
- residential costs to the local authorities; and
- day care services to the local authorities.

Data under each of these headings are summarised in Figure 11.2 which indicates that, while total spending grew in real terms by around 12 per cent in the decade 1978 to 1988, the composition of that spending has shown very little change. Inpatient expenditure continued to account for around 85 per cent of total spending, or around £1,300 million, with outpatients and day patients each accounting for around £50 million, and local authority services (residential and day care combined) accounting for another £50 million. These latter services showed considerable growth in percentage terms, but from very small bases.[3]

Figure 11.2
Public expenditure on psychiatric services by programme, England, 1978-88, at 1988/89 prices

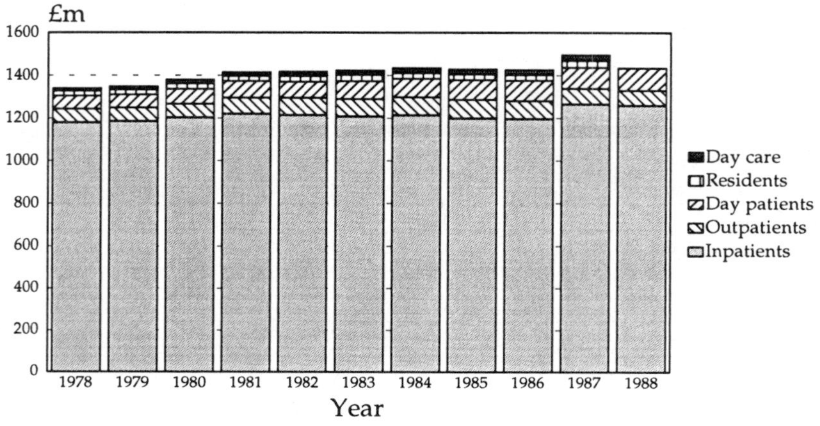

Average cost per patient

Aggregate spending is, of course, influenced by the total number of persons being financed. Unit cost data, showing the cost per patient, allow the relationship between persons and spending to be examined.

Data on average cost per place have long been available, partly because a variety of institutions provided services to both the public and private sectors, but also because the supervisory agencies (the Lunacy Commission, the Board of Control, the Ministry of Health, Department of Health) have been concerned with the quality of service as measured by the amounts spent, for example, on food. The same authorities have also used comparisons of the average cost per patient as a guide to the relative efficiency of the various institutions. Although unit costs can help assess efficiency, they omit quality entirely. Trends over time can, however, identify factors associated with changes in overall expenditures.

The average cost of maintaining a patient in county lunatic asylums,[4] as shown in Figure 11.3, remained remarkably unchanged from 1875 to 1920. Expressed in constant 1985 prices (using the GDP deflator), the cost of maintaining a pauper lunatic remained around £20 per week from 1870 through to 1920. Unit costs began to increase after the First World War, however, reaching £23 per week in 1925 and £31 in 1935. Data are not available for 1940 and 1945.

The weekly cost was £37 per week in 1950, and £38 by 1955. However, as

Figure 11.3
Cost per inpatient week, England, 1875-1986 at 1985/86 prices

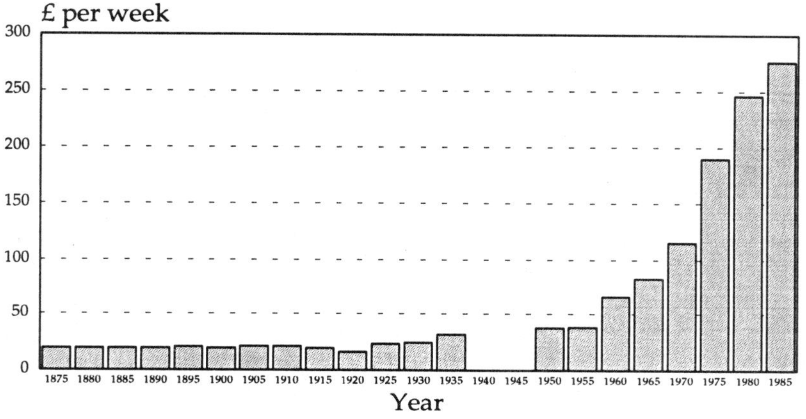

inpatient numbers began to fall, unit costs rose rapidly, doubling in each of the succeeding decades. Unit costs rose to £66 per week by 1960, £83 in 1965, £115 in 1970, and £190 by 1975. Further rises continued to take place, to around £246 in 1980, and £276 in 1985.

Taking the period 1950 to 1985, unit costs rose by a factor of seven, while inpatient numbers fell to around one-third of their 1955 level: *ceteris paribus*, such a drop in patient numbers would have pushed up unit costs by a factor of three. The seven-fold rise suggests that while the failure to adjust spending on inputs in line with patient numbers was responsible for much of the rise in unit costs, it does not explain the entire rise. This issue is explored further later in the chapter.

Components of changes in unit costs

The composition of unit costs showed considerable change, indicating a move from institutions which were provisions-intensive to ones where labour costs dominated. Provisions were the single largest component at 45 per cent of unit cost in 1875 and 48 per cent in 1880.[5] This proportion fell steadily from then onward, to 32 per cent by 1900, 29 per cent in 1910, 26 per cent in 1920 and 19 per cent in 1930. Concomitantly, the share of wages and salaries increased: from 21 per cent in 1875 to 26 per cent in 1890, 29 per cent by 1900, 31 per cent by 1910, 37 per cent in 1920 and 46 per cent in 1930.

The movements in these two components accounted for almost all the change in unit costs; no other item accounted for more than 10 per cent, with the exception of 'Necessities' which declined slightly from 11 per cent in 1875 to 10 per cent in 1930. Medical inputs, as measured by 'Surgery/dispensary', never accounted for more than a minute share of spending: 0.7 per cent of unit costs in 1875 and 1.1 per cent by 1930.

Although detailed comparison of unit costs in the period 1950 to 1986 is hindered by changes in the method whereby unit costs were compiled, with no less than four changes, the composite heading 'Patient care services' and 'Medical and paramedical support services' (which was mainly composed of labour costs) accounted for 37 per cent of the cost per inpatient in 1950/51, increasing to 49 per cent by 1970/71 and to 57 per cent by 1980/81 with a further rise to 61 per cent by 1985/6.

The overall conclusion regarding unit costs would appear to be that, while the proportion of unit costs accounted for by staff costs has been rising since 1870, it was offset by declines in other input costs so that average cost per inpatient remained largely unchanged up to 1930. Between 1950 and 1985, unit costs rose by a factor of seven or by around 10 per cent per annum in real terms. These dramatic increases appear to have been due to a continuing increase in direct patient costs, due in turn to the number and the cost of staff increasing as the number of inpatients fell.

Two points stand out. First, the current expenditure data series showed a continual rise, even though the number of inmates had fallen by 1986 to around one-third of its 1955 total. Second, the unit cost per inpatient week has risen almost exponentially in recent decades. The possible explanation of these trends is the concern of the rest of the chapter.

11.3 Analysing the increases

Four reasons may be hypothesised for the sharp cost increases described above. These are:

- the relative price effect;
- a shorter working week and unionisation;
- equal pay; and
- the ratio of nursing staff to patients.

The relative price effect

The relative price effect arises from the possibility that costs tend to rise more rapidly in certain sectors of the economy, primarily in the service sectors, than in the economy as a whole. Such an effect could result from more limited scope for productivity increases in those sectors compared to the manufacturing sector, which tends to be more capital-intensive and more subject

Figure 11.4
Mental health price index, GDP deflator and retail price index, England and Wales, 1919-1974

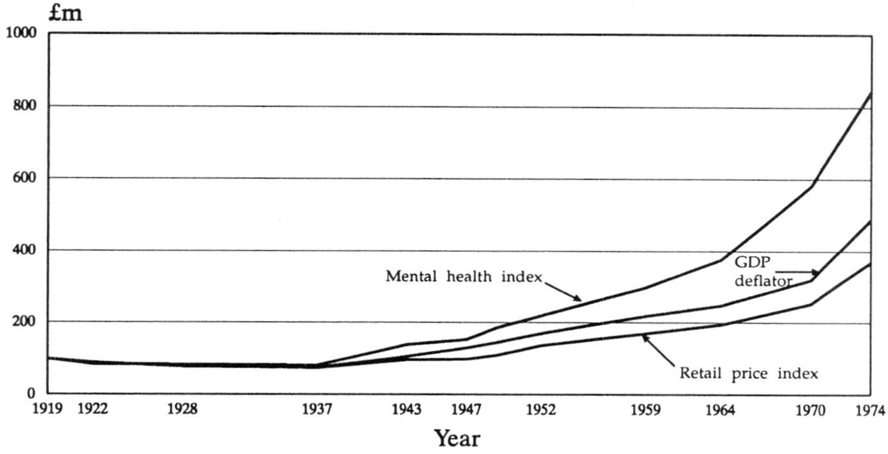

to technological change.[6] To the extent that economy-wide wage rises applied to some sectors are able to offset these by increased productivity, the unit costs in the less productive sectors would rise inexorably. O'Connor (1973) generalised this insight into the so-called 'fiscal crisis of the state' which Scull (1977) in turn invoked in explaining the rundown of the mental hospital numbers from around 1955.

The magnitude of a relative price effect is usually measured by comparing the price index for a particular product with the economy-wide price index — the GDP deflator (Heald, 1983). Unfortunately, sector-specific price indexes are seldom available, not least in the mental health services. However, a mental illness price index can be constructed for England and Wales for various years using Stanton's (1983) work on mental hospital nurses' earnings.[7] Figure 11.4 shows the resulting mental hospital price index (MHP) as well as the GDP deflator and the retail price index, all set at 100 for 1919.

Figure 11.4 provides some evidence of a relative price effect, as evidenced by the divergence between the MHP and the GDP deflator, with the former rising faster than the latter. Between 1919 and the late 1930s, the divergence was slight, but it widened during the Second World War and, after a slight post-war fall, rose steadily from the 1950s through to 1974.[8]

The percentage difference between the the MHP and the GDP deflator provides a convenient measure of the relative price effect. A continuing relative price effect would show up in a widening difference between the two indexes. A negative relative price effect applied in 1920s, but turned to a small positive effect after 1928. This gap widened in the period 1937 to 1943, fell back slightly in 1947 before widening again in 1949, with little change to 1952. Successively larger divergences were apparent in 1959, 1964 and 1970 respectively. The 1974 figure showed a narrowing of the gap from its maximum of 80 per cent in 1970.

Scull (1977) postulated that the relative price effect prompted the rundown of the lunatic asylums in the 1950s. Support for such an hypothesis would require evidence of a strong relative price effect in the decades prior to the downturn in the number of inpatients in the mid-1950s. While there is some evidence of a weak relative price effect in the 1930s and during the Second World War, the main period when a strong relative price effect operated was after 1952. Thus, the hypothesis that the relative price effect led to the decline of the psychiatric inpatient population receives little support from the data. The relative price effect was weak or absent in the pre-war period, and the major increases occurred in 1964 and 1970 (when around half of the total increase between 1919 and 1974 occurred): well after the decline in the number of inpatients had begun its course. If the policy of de-institutionalisation was prompted by the relative price effect, it was completely unsuccessful in curbing this effect.

Scull (1984), in an afterword to his earlier argument (1977), suggested in response to critics that continued increases in psychiatric expenditure might have occurred if 'decarceration' had not been developed as a policy. Applied to the relative price effect, this argument would suggest a relatively greater price effect than that observed were it not for 'decarceration'. Such an argument would, however, miss the central point that psychiatric expenditure and especially unit costs rose dramatically after 1955. Neither the empirical evidence nor the policy discussions of the time points to any concern by policy-makers with costs, let alone with the technicalities of the relative price effect.

Finally, it should be noted that the relative price effect is confined to the prices of inputs without any attention to the quantity of outputs. Given that the numbers of inpatients resident in the mental hospitals had fallen to a third of its 1955 total by 1980, unchanged relative prices would have led to a three-fold rise in unit costs, *ceteris paribus*. Unit costs rose by a factor of around four during this period (Raftery, 1993). Any relative price effect operated on top of a much stronger trend towards higher unit costs due to the decline in the number of inpatients.

Shortened working week and unionisation

These two topics can be conveniently examined together, given that trade unionisation of mental hospital nurses (known as 'attendants' until 1919) developed largely through a struggle for a reduced working week after the

Figure 11.5
Unit costs, adjusted for nurses' working hours, England and Wales, various years, at 1985 prices

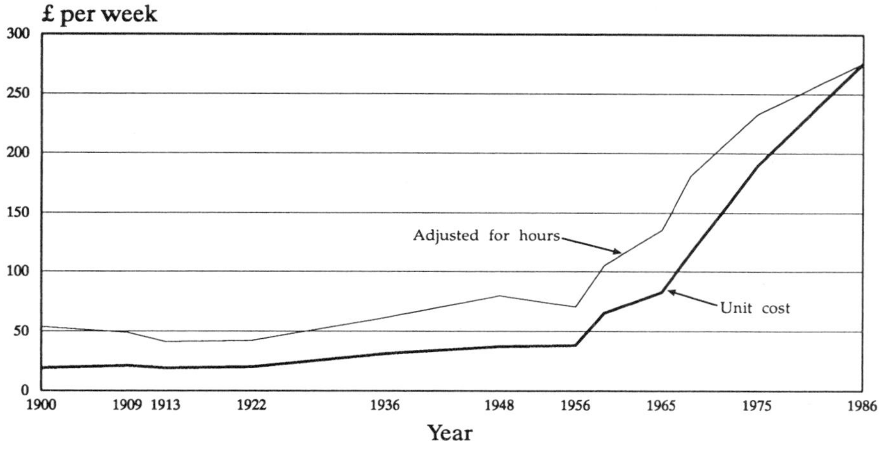

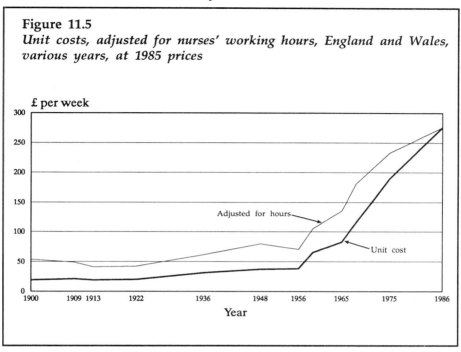

First World War (Stanton, 1983, p.90). In 1911, the average working week of mental hospital attendants was put at 84 hours, a figure which fell to a recommended 60 in 1919, but which was increased back to 66 in 1922, before falling to 54 in 1935, 48 in 1948, 42 in 1964 and 40 in 1971 (Stanton, 1983, p.98).

Figure 11.5 shows unit costs for England and Wales as in Figure 11.3, but also with an adjustment to increase costs as if the working week had been 37 hours in 1909. Although such adjustment has the effect of moderating the rate of increase by increasing the unit cost for 1909, the effect is relatively small given the magnitude of the overall increase over the period. Instead of a fourteen-fold increase in unit cost between 1909 and 1986, adjustment for hours worked yields a five-fold increase.

Equal pay

The degree to which equal pay for female nurses contributed to the increase in unit costs can be explored by assuming equal pay had applied for all years since 1909, as shown in Figure 11.6. The effect of equal pay was almost imperceptible, due to the fact that female nurses had achieved 80 per cent of the starting pay of male nurses in 1919 and 97 per cent by 1949 (Stanton,

Figure 11.6
Unit costs, adjusted for equal pay, England and Wales, 1900-1986, at 1985 prices

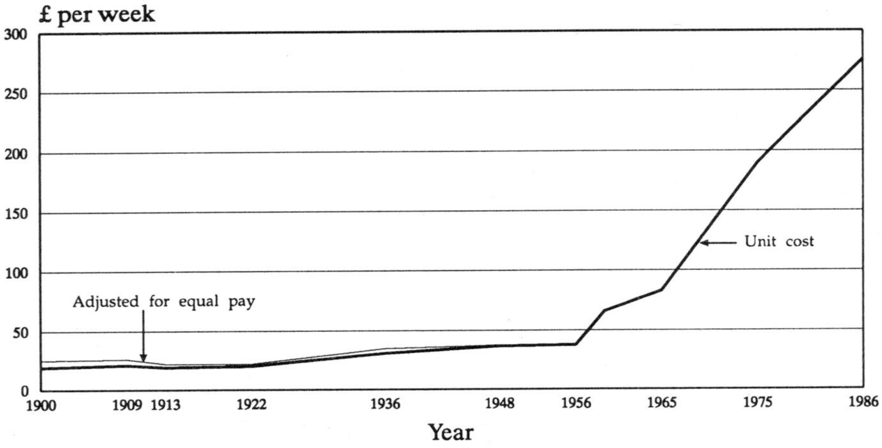

1983, p.97).

Ratio of nurses to inpatients

The central reason for the increase in unit costs was the growth in the number of nurses while the number of inpatients decreased, as shown in Figure 11.7. The number of nurses increased steadily, almost doubling from 8,300 in 1900 to 15,500 in 1922, doubling again to 31,300 by 1965, and almost doubling again to 57,800 in 1986.[9]

During the same period, the number of mental hospital inpatients fell, after peaking in 1955, with the result that the ratio of inpatients per nurse rose sharply, as shown in Figure 11.8. From just under nine inpatients per nurse in the period 1900 to 1922, the ratio fell to around six in each of the years 1923/4 to 1956. Therafter, as the number of inpatients declined and the number of nurses grew, the ratio fell sharply to 4.8 in 1959, 4.0 in 1965, 3.6 in 1968, 1.8 in 1975 and 1.0 in 1986.

While it is possible that inpatients have become more dependent and/or that the quality of nursing care has risen, neither of these factors appears to have been used prospectively to justify increased nursing inputs per patient. The level of dependency of inpatients could have changed due to the ageing of the long-stay population and perhaps due to more severe cases being

Figure 11.7
Numbers of nurses and inpatients in English psychiatric hospitals, 1948-1986 (end year data)

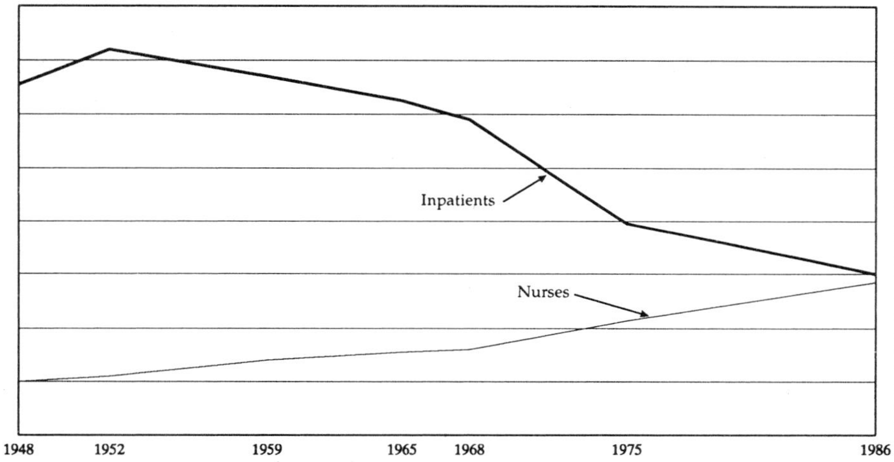

Figure 11.8
Ratio of inpatients to nurses in psychiatric hospitals, England and Wales, 1948-1986

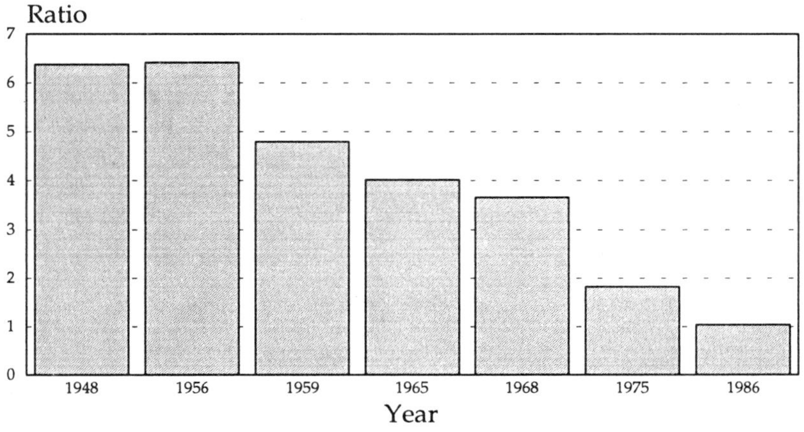

admitted. Against this, the effect of increased age on the dependency of long-stay psychiatric inpatients is unclear, and total admissions have continued to rise over the last three decades despite the reduction in overall places.

11.4 Implications

What, if any, are the implications of this for contemporary costing of mental health services? Three points seem worth exploring.

First, the rapid rise in inpatient unit costs has probably been tipping the cost balance continually in favour of non-inpatient care, as has been picked up in most studies of the relative cost-effectiveness of community-oriented psychiatric services compared to conventional inpatient services (and see Chapter 4). The development of more community-oriented psychiatric services has led to some of the costs being picked up by other agencies. Social security support for housing in the form of housing benefit in the UK in the 1970s offered scope for a shifting of the accommodation costs from the health to the social security budget, and has led to complex rule changes and legal challenges.

Second, the treatment of the costs of accommodation in economic evaluation may require revision. According to conventional economic theory, social security payments are seen as transfer payments. Since transfer payments redistribute purchasing power from the taxed to the social welfare recipient, no change in society's expenditure is involved.[10] While this approach has merits, it raises complications when applied to mental health services.

Adoption of a number of different perspectives may be helpful, and should include a public finance perspective, totalling up the costs to the public sector, whether health, social security, housing or other agencies (such as the police). Such an approach is explored in Chapter 3.

Third, moves to define standard packages of care for particular diagnoses or patients may enable the bulk of the relevant costs to be captured using relatively few cost headings. In Chapter 9, Knapp and Beecham have shown how relatively few cost headings accounted for some 90 per cent of the volume of costs captured by much more detailed measurements. To the degree that standardised packages of care can be outlined and costed, evaluations of contemporary psychiatric services may in future be able to compare like with like.

Notes

1 The earliest and most accessible expenditure series dates from 1857 but is incomplete due to being restricted to the maintenance costs of the pauper lunatics under the Lunacy Commissioners. Besides being restricted to maintenance costs (comprising direct costs such as provisions and salaries), this series excludes those paupers who were held in workhouses, and all

privately-financed patients. Expenditure on the maintenance of these 'workhouse lunatics', who accounted for around 25 per cent of all pauper lunatics from 1850 to 1880, was included in general expenditure on the workhouses, but not distinguished. Workhouse lunatics typically cost the Boards of Guardians only around 50 per cent of the cost of an asylum place.

2 While data are available on heading (a) which comprised the overwhelming majority of the places provided, the estimated expenditures under (b) and (c) have been based on the numbers of persons in each of these categories. It has been assumed that the cost per person in the workhouses was 50 per cent, and that of privately-financed lunatics 100 per cent, of the cost of pauper lunatics. Such an assumption is justified by the repeated assertions about the cost of workhouse lunatics in the literature and the fact that a growing proportion of privately-funded lunatics was cared for in the county and borough asylums. In any case, the relatively small proportions of patients in headings (b) and (c) means that little difference would be made to total expenditure if higher or lower unit costs were employed.

3 Local authority expenditure includes that on elderly people in care, some of whom suffer from mental illness. The Mental Illness Specific Grant, introduced in 1991, has increased local authority spending on mental illness.

4 Data are also available for the borough asylums which, according to the reports of the Lunacy Commissioners, kept better accounts. These have been disregarded here both because their levels were close to those of the county asylums and also because the borough asylums accounted for relatively few patients.

5 Detailed accounts were maintained of the costs of inputs purchased for the gardens and farms, as well as of the profits made by sale of their produce. Maintenance costs showed little difference between those asylums which being rural were likely to have farms, and those which were urban. Although some subsidisation may have occurred through the use of inpatient labour on the farms, it would have shown up mainly in the form of reduced provisions costs. Since the share of provisions in unit costs fell sharply over the period, no major distortion is entailed by omitting the influence of the farms.

6 The concept originates with a study by Baumol (1967) of the problems associated with funding a symphony orchestra, whose scope for productivity increases was limited by the requirement to play at a certain speed! Thus, once they had maximised their live performances and recording opportunities, they could no longer increase their productivity.

7 Since Stanton's work covered only one — albeit the largest — expenditure item, namely mental hospital nurses' pay for the years between 1919 and 1974, several assumptions have been made to compile the relevant price index. Data exist on the proportion of expenditure accounted for by the pay of mental hospital nurses and some other groups such as medical staff, professional and technical staff, cleaners and porters. The pay levels for these other groups have been assumed to have moved in line with nurses' earnings. Overall, these groups' total pay bill amounted to around 50 per cent

of that of nurses, with little differences apparent. The prices of the remainder of the inputs have been assumed to move in line with consumer prices, as measured by the retail price index.

8 The dates for which the mental hospital price index has been constructed depend on the years for which Stanton has provided data.

9 The number of mental hospital nurses rose as follows: from 8,300 in 1900, to 12,500 in 1913, 15,500 in 1922, 19,700 in 1935, 20,611 in 1949, 28,027 in 1959, 32,352 in 1969, 43,652 in 1975 and 60,000 in 1986.

10 Two main assumptions are involved: (a) that taxation does not reduce productive capacity, i.e. the disincentive effects of taxation are not large; and (b) that the pattern of spending is similar between those who are taxed and those who receive the handout. If the recipients were more likely to spend the money than those who were taxed, consumption would be boosted and vice versa.

References

Baumol, W. (1967) The macroeconomics of unbalanced growth: the anatomy of urban crisis, *American Economic Review*, 57, 415-26.

Feinstein, C.H. (1972) *National Income, Expenditure and Output of the United Kingdom, 1855-1965*, Cambridge University Press, Cambridge.

Heald, D. (1983) *Public Expenditure*, Martin Robertson, Oxford.

House of Commons Social Services Select Committee (1990) *Public Expenditure on Health Matters*, House of Commons Paper 484, HMSO, London.

O'Connor, J. (1973) *The Fiscal Crisis of the State*, St James Press, London.

Raftery, J. (1993) The economics of psychiatric services in the UK and Ireland, 1845-1985, PhD thesis, University of London.

Scull, A.T. (1977) *Decarceration. Community Treatment and the Deviant: A Radical View*, Prentice Hall, Englewood Cliffs, New Jersey.

Scull, A.T. (1984) *Decarcertation. Community Treatment and the Deviant: A Radical View*, 2nd edition with new foreword, Prentice Hall, Englewood Cliffs, New Jersey.

Stanton, K.A. (1983) The employment of nurses in public mental hospitals (England and Wales), 1909-1975, PhD thesis, University of London.

12 Mental Health Economic Evaluations: Unfinished Business

Jennifer Beecham and Martin Knapp

12.1 Introduction

For lots of good reasons — and the occasional bad one — economic evaluations are increasingly likely to be component parts of, supplements to, or even the stimulation for, clinical or other evaluations of mental health care services and systems. The need for an economics perspective — most noticeably the demand for cost-effectiveness insights — is recognised in most health care systems, and is being addressed from a number of perspectives: which drug, which location, which patient, whose funding responsibilities, when to provide treatment or support? As this book has illustrated, the search for cost-effectiveness is not confined to policy questions raised by national health care strategies or the re-organisation of local or regional systems, but has considerable currency in relation to individual programmes and individual users. Creating the right incentives and the right systems for the cost-effective delivery of care should be one of the fundamental objectives of all those concerned about the needs of people with mental health problems.

12.2 Systems, programmes and individuals

The primary aim of this book has been to introduce the principles and methods of economic evaluation as they are applied to mental health care services. Applications of these principles have been offered at three levels: for national or local systems (the macro level), for facilities, units or programmes (mezzo level) and for individual users (micro level). The book has illustrated these methods with examples from some recent evaluations (and made reference to many others) and discussed the relevance of their findings and methods for policy, practice and research.

Six tasks form the core activities of an economic evaluation. Not all of these tasks are needed or are possible in every study. Sometimes tasks are missed through oversight, because of funding or time constraints, or because the researcher does not have the technical skills to perform them. Nevertheless, each of the following should be addressed:

- collection of data on service utilisation, accommodation, medication, employment and 'informal' caregiver support in order to describe treatment or support arrangements and to calculate the costs associated with each of a number of interventions;
- description of the full and component costs, over time and by funding agency or individual, for each intervention (distinguishing total, average and marginal costs as necessary);
- examination of variations in total and component costs, analysis of their associations with the characteristics of individuals, and by reference to the nature of alternative treatments or interventions;
- collection and analysis of data on the outcomes of treatment for individuals;
- comparison, in both aggregated and disaggregated form, of the costs and outcomes of alternative treatments; and
- analysis of the links between costs, individual user characteristics (including needs) and outcomes.

Methodologically, there are few differences between macro-, mezzo- and micro-economic evaluations. It is the scale of the enterprise and the magnitude of measures that will vary, rather than the framework. At the system level, costs might be measured in tens of millions of pounds per year and outcomes as, say, a reduction in the national suicide rate or a change in the number of acute inpatient psychiatric admissions in a district. By contrast, at the programme level — for a facility or a community team — measurement might be in thousands of pounds *per month* and outcomes as the number of referrals by diagnostic group, the quality of care or changes in users' clinical symptoms or behaviour. At a finer level of detail — for an individual service user — the starting point would be their and their family's quality of life, health and general welfare. These system, programme and individual levels are not completely distinct in policy terms, nor independent methodologically. Consequently, macro, mezzo and micro evaluations will share many practical and methodological similarities, and — where possible — findings and implications should be fed back and forth between the levels.

These overlaps and links can be seen if we look at some of the earlier chapters. Chapter 6, on the care of people with dementia, discussed broad policy options with supporting cost and effectiveness evidence constructed from a number of programme evaluations. The programme-level evaluations in Chapters 5 to 9 were each built up from data for individual service users, located in the context of system re-organisations or policies. Most of these programme evaluations offered findings pertaining to individual users, so that they had relevance for the 'micro' decisions of care professionals, but some also allow generalisations to broader systems. A good system of mental health care is more than the sum of its component programmes, but the quality of the latter will fundamentally constrain the achievements of the former. Equally, the quality of a mental health care programme can be more than the sum of its achievements in improving the health and quality of life of individual users, but these improvements should nevertheless be central to the evaluation of programme effectiveness.

12.3 Unfinished business

As was argued in Chapter 1, economic evaluations are not restricted to answering questions about efficiency, although this is where most of them have been directed. Increasingly — but slowly — they have also sought to examine *distributional* implications. Generally, economic evaluations can provide answers to a wide variety of questions (Williams, 1974):

- *what* treatment or support service is more or most appropriate in given circumstances;
- *when* should treatment be provided;
- *where;*
- *to whom;* and
- *how*?

Reliable, generalisable answers to these five generic questions will assist the decision-making tasks of local mental health care purchasers and providers, central government planners, and maybe even politicians. If the term 'most appropriate' includes the criterion 'cost-effective', we can use these questions to structure a discussion of the main issues which economic evaluations can address. We will resist the temptation to use the framework of these questions to attempt a review of previous research, and instead highlight some unmet research needs and fruitful avenues for future research. We then turn to some 'why' questions, in order to address some more fundamental methodological issues.

What care service or treatment mode is more or most appropriate in given circumstances?

A number of different policy and practice questions can be subsumed under this first head. Examples of economic evaluations which address 'what' questions include those linked to clinical trials of drugs (Moore and Clip, 1994; and see Chapter 10) — including extrapolations from one country to another (Davies and Drummond, 1993) and meta-analyses (see Chapter 10). Other questions would concern new forms of home-based treatment (Burns et al., 1993), new forms of residential setting (Beecham et al., 1993) and respite care and its impacts on carers (Donaldson and Gregson, 1988).

Compared to the vast number of 'what?' questions faced daily by psychiatrists, nurses, social workers, psychologists, other care providers and policymakers, the accumulated evidence from economic evaluations is minuscule. Not surprisingly, several clinical evaluators have called for more work. For example, in relation to dementia services, recent calls have been heard for more cost-effectiveness research of home-based and institutional programmes of care (Maas and Buckwalter, 1991), alternative drugs (Grobe-Einsler, 1993), and other services and treatments (Ochs, 1991; Stoudemire et al., 1991). In relation to care or treatment for children and adolescents, people with eating disorders or those with drug misuse problems, the list of unresearched policy and practice questions would be much longer.

When should care be provided?

It is common for health economists to examine the efficacy and efficiency of preventive measures, but not — it would seem — in relation to mental health problems. Backhouse et al. (1992) listed more than 300 English language health economics studies of prevention, but only one in psychiatry. The exception was a modest evaluation of case registers published in 1980. Of course, prevention has a great many interpretations. For example, community teams, support services or pharmaceutical products could be used to prevent the development of the illness into a more serious phase, to delay relapse or admission to inpatient care, to reduce the overall probability of onset, relapse or admission, or to reduce the duration of illness or the length of time as an inpatient.

It is in the field of child psychiatry that the pressing need for more evaluation of the 'when' question is most obvious. Light and Bailey (1993) suggest that expenditure on child psychiatry services for disturbed and abused children reduces costs to education, health, social care and criminal justice services in the short term. Moreover, 'as untreated cases show a high probability of pathology in later childhood, adolescence and adulthood' (p.17), the health gain can be measured not only in terms of the child's wellbeing (reduction in pain, shame and the private horrors of abuse) but also in the prevention of poverty, criminality, injuries and self-induced illnesses. Although the cost of meeting needs for child psychiatry services may be much higher than the current resource allocation, the longer-term cost of not meeting them is arguably even higher: 'Child mental health services are a prime example of the kind of service that can provide long-term benefits in exchange for relatively cheap early intervention' (Cottrell, 1993, p.480).

Some recent research in services for elderly people with dementia examines questions relevant for all users of mental health services. O'Connor et al. (1991) found that contact from a community support team delayed admission to long-term residential care if the person with dementia lived with a carer, but speeded up admission if they lived alone. This was because people with dementia living alone do not usually come to the attention of the authorities until there is a crisis. Walsh (1991) showed that anticoagulant therapy eliminated the need for prolonged nursing home care and extended the time the person with dementia could remain at home. Brodaty and Peters (1991) found that an intensive ten-day residential carer training programme resulted in elderly people staying at home and staying alive for longer, with marked savings over the first 39 months. None of these was a full cost or cost-effectiveness study *per se*, but each illustrates the contributions which an economic evaluation can make.

In the field of (younger) adult mental health services, the timing of treatment requires further examination, but some recent programme-level studies show encouraging results to guide practice. Burns et al. (1993) and Merson et al. (1992) examined prompt or early intervention services. An evaluation of community psychiatric nursing services in Greenwich showed that the introduction of care management practices was a cost-effective alternative to standard care, but only in the first six months after referral to the service. In the longer term there were no differences (McCrone et al., 1994).

Where should care be provided?

System-level policy debates about mental health provision in many countries have been dominated for some years by the balance between inpatient and community care. In planning the *long-term* care for most people, the accumulated UK evidence should encourage further *planned and supported* moves away from hospital inpatient treatment. Chapter 5 summarised the most recent comprehensive costs evidence for people leaving hospital after many months, often years, of residence. Even though the cost and service use results presented stem from a study of only two hospitals, the data relate to many hundreds of former hospital inpatients and a number of years of community care practice. These are currently the best data available in the UK. Leff (1993) offers complementary encouragement for community-based care from an outcomes perspective.

The appropriate location of acute care is less clear and is surrounded by more controversy. This is a more complex practice issue and, therefore, a more complex research issue. Recent research tends to focus on the provision of home-based support and the provision of smaller residential units rather than hospital wards. There remain many unsolved practice problems, and a huge untouched research agenda (Kavanagh et al., 1995).

But the 'where' question should not be restricted to a comparison between hospital or community care. More information is required on where, within the range of community provision and within the developing mixed economy, cost-effective care can be provided. In North London, in the early years of psychiatric hospital reprovision, services provided by the independent sector for former hospital residents were found to be more cost-effective than those managed by the public sector after standardising for needs and outcomes. Health authority-managed services in particular were shown to be more costly than expected (Beecham et al., 1991; and see Chapter 5). Sectoral efficiency has long been a research issue in the United States. McCue and Clement (1993), for example, found that patients had longer admissions in private (for-profit) psychiatric hospitals and that public general hospitals played a more significant role than private hospitals in treating mental illness among indigent persons. Looking particularly at nursing home facilities, Weisbrod and Schlesinger (1986) found differences in quality of care and frequency of resident complaints between non-profit and for-profit providers.

A system-level examination of the location question was described in Chapter 6. A balance of care mapping was laid out for people with dementia, covering the services being used, the associated costs and some projected cost-effectiveness improvements that might be secured if the balance was altered by substituting specified new arrangements (with proven cost and effectiveness implications) for standard care. Similar work has been undertaken in relation to people with schizophrenia (Kavanagh et al., 1995). Both these studies highlight where further research is needed. There is, for example, cost-effectiveness evidence of residential care compared to different forms of domiciliary care for elderly people (Challis and Davies, 1986; Davies et al., 1990), but there is little evidence on the comparative merits of these forms of support for people with mental heath problems.

With colleagues at PSSRU and CEMH, we are currently engaged in a number of studies of alternative locations and modes of care. Some studies will later reveal the cost consequences for users' families of changing the location of service provision, a rather neglected aspect. For example, provision of outpatient rather than inpatient treatment for disturbed children may involve the family in frequent and lengthy therapy sessions at a specialist centre some distance from home. Family rather than individual therapy may have similar family cost consequences.

To whom should care be provided?

Economic evaluations of mental health care have rarely addressed this 'to whom' question, although it obviously remains fundamental to priority-setting exercises and to day-to-day practice. Surgery for epilepsy is known to be most effective for only a small proportion of people with the condition: where the patient's condition is resistant to drug therapy, where the pattern and severity of seizures is unacceptable, and where the origin of the condition is from an organic brain lesion (Rossi, 1990). Silfvenius (1988) calculated the economic costs of epilepsy and suggested that surgery will lead to functioning at a normal level for 20 per cent of patients, and that 50 per cent of those operated on will become seizure-free. The economic gain can be calculated in savings in *indirect costs* due to patients returning to or starting work, thereby reducing the costs in unemployment benefit and increasing productivity. The *direct costs* would also be reduced as there is a lower need for supervised care.

A parallel can be drawn with some of the newer drugs for schizophrenia. For example, the controversy over the efficacy of clozapine relates in part to its targeting during the US trial on particular groups of people with schizophrenia (Healy, 1993). Similarly, a study of inpatient hospital stays for risperidone treatment related only to patients with schizophrenia who completed a year of treatment and who thus tolerated the drug well (Addington et al., 1993). However, the factors which limit the generalisability of trial results might simultaneously assist in the targeting of comparatively expensive treatments.

Indications are filtering through from research evidence that this ' to whom' question might be an important consideration in the implementation of care management. Intagliata (1982) defined case management as a process 'to enhance the continuity of care and its accessibility, accountability and efficiency'. There is evidence from the US, but little from the UK, to suggest that people who are unwilling to attend hospital-based services, who show poor medication compliance and poor ability to monitor themselves, and who have frequent crises are most likely to benefit from 'assertive case-management' (Stein and Diamond, 1985, quoted in Thornicroft, 1991). Such findings lead, more generally, to the need to examine disaggregated data in order to tease out those *individual* characteristics of patients associated with different outcomes and costs.

Most studies of elderly people or their carers provide evidence of interpersonal variations, for example in relation to outcome, cost and carer stress. Torian et al. (1992) found hospital costs to be 75 per cent higher for dementing patients when compared to costs for non-dementing patients. They attributed this to the effects of the illness on mobility, nutrition and continence which led to complications of treatment and nosocomial infections. These result in using more nursing time and lengthier hospitalisations. Fries et al. (1993) reported that nursing home residents with dementia who were physically able, not undergoing rehabilitation and were without other serious medical conditions, used only slightly more staff time than residents without dementia. However, it seems that, as the dementia progressed and the physical symptoms worsened, their use of staff time increased. There are also marked differences *within* some groups of patients or users who are otherwise seen to have similar diagnoses or administrative labels. This is illustrated by the variance around the mean on virtually every cost or outcome measure in virtually every published study (and see Chapter 4).

One of the themes of this book has been to emphasise that the reasons for this cost or outcome variation need to be examined. Indeed, policy and practice decision-makers should endeavour to exploit them in the pursuit of better, more cost-effective or more appropriately distributed care, for the 'unpackaging' of aggregated data sets can reveal interesting and important inter-user differences in the effectiveness and cost of standard and innovative treatments. As was argued in Chapter 4, multivariate cost-effectiveness studies can, *inter alia*, point out *who* benefits in what circumstances, or *whose* costs are greater.

How should care be provided?

This final evaluative question is closely linked to the others, for the organisation of treatment usually cannot be separated from its location or targeting. As health and social care markets continue to develop in the UK, more information is needed about the incentives created by new financial and other mechanisms. Again, work undertaken in the US may help to point the way forward. Evidence suggests that attempts to contain costs can push up administrative overheads, resulting in fewer people being seen by mental health services, fewer illnesses treated and fewer treatment procedures covered by insurance (Bigelow and McFarland, 1989). Frank and Jackson (1989) found that pre-set budgets, rather than reimbursement after the event, were associated with a fall in admission rates and substitution of outpatient services for inpatient treatment. Capitated budgets, such as those used within the US preferred provider organisations and health maintenance organisations, as well as in the UK National Health Service, create incentives to reduce the amount of care provided. In one American study, mental health provision was found to have shifted from psychiatrists and psychologists to general physicians and social workers, resulting in lower intensity of service use by patients and lower costs (Mechanic, 1991). Systems-level information of this kind is needed to support the operation of UK markets, preferably combined with evidence on client-level outcomes (see Sederer et al., 1992) to ensure a more cost-effective service and to aid successful development of the so-called contracting culture.

This fifth evaluation question can be distinguished from the other generic questions at the programme evaluation level by its emphasis on improved *coordination* of support and treatment, whether through care programmes (North and Ritchie, 1993; and see Chapter 7), care management (Huxley, 1992) or other case-level coordinating activities which aim for better and multi-agency assessments and closer links between needs and services.

In providing care management services for elderly people in the UK, evaluations of the early experimental projects found budgetary devolution to staff with smaller caseloads and comprehensive information could produce less costly packages which were also better for elderly people and their informal carers (Challis and Davies, 1986). In the United States, an experiment which gave vouchers to clients to buy services through budget-holding case management programmes promoted choice and flexibility for clients, but also required new organisational and administrative structures to permit users to make choices (Bertsch, 1992). The results of evaluations of case management in mental health provide conflicting evidence on cost-effectiveness, although the consequences of not having such arrangements could be dire (Melzer et al., 1991; see Chapter 8). We also need to ask how coordination should be provided. Care programming is essentially a health sector process, whereas care management in the UK tends to be located in the social care sector, but the linkages and overlaps between the two need careful evaluation, and we need to isolate the factors which lead to the success of each process under given circumstances.

A host of other unanswered questions could be located within this generic 'how' question, but it should be clear from just the few examples given here that there remains an enormous amount of economic evaluation to be conducted.

12.4 Economic evaluation: a suitable case for further treatment?

While we can learn from work already undertaken, those people conducting mental health economic evaluations must not become complacent. Just as there are economic topics of interest and relevance (such as the prices of drugs, the costs of services, the valuation of capital and the remuneration of staff), so also are there economic methodologies, techniques and skills which need to be developed. We can exploit these to further our knowledge about the most appropriate way to provide mental health care and to begin to address a sixth generic question — the 'why' question. *Why* is drug, therapy or service A more cost-effective than drug, therapy or service B? *Why* do more-intensive community care programmes have better cost and outcome consequences than less-intensive programmes? *Why* do psychological therapies work better for some people than others and cost different amounts? Two of the imperatives for future evaluative work must be to 'unpack' the aggregated findings and to look carefully within the 'black box' which links inputs with outputs, costs with effectiveness. Economic and other evaluations need to pay more attention to the 'process' of mental health care. At the risk of repetition, we need to know not only *what* works, but *why*.

Another, and more obvious, imperative is to encourage more cost-effectiveness and other economic evaluations of treatment and support arrangements for people with mental health problems. These should be conducted alongside other evaluations so that the widest range of knowledge can be brought to bear on the leading practice-related and policy-inspired research questions of the next five or ten years. But we also need *better* economic evaluations. These require the development of improved or refined instrumentation and, in particular, instrumentation for service use, cost and quality of life. In our own work, we have already begun to improve and simplify the methods we use for service receipt data collection, and to standardise the concomitant calculations of unit costs for services. We need to develop better ways of evaluating the impact of services on individuals' lives, concentrating on the measurement and quantification of quality-oriented outcomes. Most importantly, we need to continue to explore the links between costs, service utilisation, needs and outcomes for people with mental health problems and their families, friends and neighbours, building on the economic theories of cost and production, other disciplines and conceptual approaches, and on work already undertaken.

Evaluators ought now to be examining some wider economic issues and economic-related outcomes. For example, to explore the long-term benefits of prevention or early intervention (as required in the study of child psychiatry) it is necessary to develop improved techniques for valuing and extrapolating costs and benefits over time. We need to put more effort into collecting and analysing data on the indirect costs of treatment and support such as lost employment, informal care and downstream personal and family consequences. There is a need to import other economic tools into the standard evaluative framework. Econometric analysis, for example, can tease out the marginal influences of socio-cultural variables (such as ethnicity, culture or gender) on psychiatric disorder, treatment and outcomes in the context of different service combinations and qualities, and they can help the research community explore more thoroughly and more appropriately the causes of cost variations. Better analyses are needed to allow the development of alternative methods of defining case mix groups, in an effort to reduce diagnostic fallibility. We need to explore the concepts of *willingness-to-pay* and *contingent valuation* in the mental health context and their use in the evaluation of programmes and services. The findings from an examination of *models of choice under uncertainty* could feed into improved decision-making for alternative interventions such as drug therapies, where side-effects are a possible but uncertain outcome.

12.5 Conclusion

This book has described, discussed and illustrated economic evaluations at the system, programme and individual levels. This final chapter has emphasised that there is a wide tract of unexplored territory. While we would argue that the discipline of economics provides a useful vehicle for the exploration, there need to be more than just economists on board. Fellow explorers should come from a range of disciplines, including psychiatry, epidemiology, psychology, sociology, social policy and statistics. Quite a number of generic questions were posed in this chapter, each of them relevant at each of the three levels. The research methods to examine such questions are, in some cases, only just beginning to be developed, but each question needs to be addressed from the basis of a theoretically sound methodology. The production of welfare model provides a framework for this task, although other approaches could equally be used. The important point is that an underpinning framework clearly defines the various research elements (for example, needs, costs and outcomes) and describes the potential relationships between them.

Unfortunately, economic analysis is probably less straightforward and less structured than it may at first appear. Indeed, some aspects of economic evaluation are perhaps more rightly described as art than science. The various modes of economic evaluation should be seen as ways of organising thought rather than as mechanistic rules for allocating resources. In consequence, results from evaluations should never replace the judgements of decision-makers, although they can usefully supplement and inform them. They can help the decision-maker formulate policy questions sensibly and logically, and then (generally) provide a *range* of answers from which the decision-maker might choose. It is not the evaluator's responsibility to determine policies; the interplay of economic appraisal and clinical and political priorities is the sensible way to proceed.

A former British Prime Minister, Alec Douglas-Home, once remarked: 'There are two problems in my life. The political ones are insoluble and the economic ones incomprehensible.' Clinicians, care workers, managers and others working in today's health and social services may share these sentiments. This book will have done little to address the first set of problems — the political ones — but we hope that economic evaluations are now considerably less incomprehensible. Better still, we hope that this book will stimulate increases in both the demand for, and the supply of, high-quality economic evaluations of mental health care.

References

Addington, D.E., Jones, B., Bloom, D., Chouinard, G., Remington, G. and Albright, P. (1993) Reduction of hospital days in chronic schizophrenia patients treated with risperidone: a retrospective study, *Clinical Therapeutics*, 15, 917-26.

Backhouse, M.E., Backhouse, R.J. and Edey, S.A. (1992) Economic evaluation bibliography, *Health Economics*, 1, Supplement.

Beecham, J.K., Knapp, M.R.J. and Fenyo, A.J. (1991) Costs, needs and outcomes, *Schizophrenia Bulletin*, 17, 3, 427-39.

Beecham, J.K., Cambridge, P., Hallam, A. and Knapp, M.R.J. (1993) The costs of Domus care, *International Journal of Geriatric Psychiatry*, 8, 10, 827-31.

Bertsch, E.F. (1992) A voucher system that enables persons with severe mental illness to purchase community support services, *Hospital and Community Psychiatry*, 43, 1109-13.

Bigelow, D.A. and McFarland, B.H. (1989) Comparative costs and impacts of Canadian and American payment systems for mental health services, *Hospital and Community Psychiatry*, 40, 805-8.

Brodaty, H. and Peters, K.E. (1991) Cost effectiveness of a training programme for dementia carers, *International Psychogeriatrics*, 3, 1, 11-22.

Burns, T., Raftery, J., Beadsmoore, A., Mcguigan, S. and Dickson, M. (1993) A controlled trial of home-based acute psychiatric services. II: Treatment patterns and costs, *British Journal of Psychiatry*, 163, 55-61.

Challis, D.J. and Davies, B.P. (1986) *Case Management in Community Care*, Gower, Aldershot.

Cottrell, D. (1993) Pound foolish: a review, *Psychiatric Bulletin*, 17, 480.

Davies, B.P., Bebbington, A.C. and Charnley, H. with Baines, B., Ferlie, E.B., Hughes, M. and Twigg, J. (1990) *Resources, Needs and Outcomes in Community-Based Care*, Avebury, Aldershot.

Davies, L.M. and Drummond, M.F. (1993) Assessment of costs and benefits of drug therapy for treatment-resistant schizophrenia in the United Kingdom, *British Journal of Psychiatry*, 162, 38-42.

Donaldson, C. and Gregson, B. (1988) Prolonging life at home: what is the cost? *Community Medicine*, 3, 200-19.

Frank, R.G. and Jackson, C.A. (1989) The impact of prospectively set hospital budgets on psychiatric admissions, *Social Science and Medicine*, 28, 8, 861-7.

Fries, B.E., Mehr, D.R., Schneider, D., Foley, W.J. and Burke, R. (1993) Mental dysfunction and resource use in nursing homes, *Medical Care*, 10, 898-920.

Grobe-Einsler, R. (1993) Clinical aspects of nimodipine, *Clinical Pharmacology*, 16, Supplement 1, S39-S45.

Healy, D. (1993) Psychopharmacology and the ethics of resource allocation, *British Journal of Psychiatry*, 162, 23-9.

Huxley, P. (1992) Social services assessment and care management: getting it right, *Journal of Mental Health*, 1, 285-94.

Intagliata, J. (1982) Improving the quality of community care for the chronically mentally disabled: the role of case management, *Schizophrenia Bulletin*, 8, 655-74.

Kavanagh, S., Opit, L., Knapp, M.R.J. and Beecham, J.K. (1995) Schizophrenia: shifting the balance of care, *Social Psychiatry and Psychiatric Epidemiology*, forthcoming.

Leff, J. (ed.) (1993) *Evaluating Community Placement of Long-Stay Psychiatric Patients, British Journal of Psychiatry*, 162, Supplement 19.

Light, D. and Bailey, V. (1993) Pound foolish, *Health Service Journal*, 11 February.

Maas, M.L. and Buckwalter, K.C. (1991) Alzheimer's disease, *Annual Review of Nursing Research*, 9, 19-55.

McCrone, P., Beecham, J.K. and Knapp, M.R.J. (1994) Community psychiatric nurse teams: cost-effectiveness of intensive support versus generic care, *British Journal of Psychiatry*, 165, 218-21.

McCue, M.J. and Clement, J.P. (1993) Relative performance of for-profit psychiatric hospitals in investor-owned systems and nonprofit psychiatric hospitals, *American Journal of Psychiatry*, 150, 77-82.

Mechanic, D. (1991) The social dimension, in S. Bloch and P. Chadoff (eds) *Psychiatric Ethics*, Open University Press, Buckingham.

Melzer, D., Hale, A.J., Malik, S.J., Hogman, G.A. and Wood, S. (1991) Community care for patients with schizophrenia one year after hospital discharge, *British Medical Journal*, 303, 1023-6.

Merson, S., Tyrer, P., Onyett, S., Lack, S., Birkett, P., Lynch, S. and Johnson, T. (1992) Early intervention in psychiatric emergencies: a controlled trial, *The Lancet*, 339, 1311-13.

Moore, M.J. and Clip, E.C. (1994) Alzheimer's disease and related dementias, *The Lancet*, 343, 239-40.

North, C. and Ritchie, J. (1993) *Factors Influencing the Implementation of the Care Programme Approach*, HMSO, London.

Ochs, M. (1991) Selecting routine outpatient tests for older patients, *Geriatrics*, 46, 39-42, 45-46, 49-50.

O'Connor, D.W., Pollitt, P.A., Brook, C.B.P., Reiss, B.B. and Roth, M. (1991) Does early intervention reduce the number of elderly people with dementia admitted to institutions? *British Medical Journal*, 302, 871-4.

Rossi, G.F. (1990) Principles of surgery for epilepsy, *Acta Neurochirurgica*, Supplement 50, 58-63.

Sederer, L., Eisen, S., Dill, D., Grob, M., Gougeon, M.L. and Mirin, S.M. (1992) Case-based re-imbursement for psychiatric hospital care, *Hospital and Community Psychiatry*, 43, 1120-26.

Silfvenius, H. (1988) Economic costs of epilepsy — treatment benefits, *Acta Neurologia Scandinavica*, 78, Supplement 117, 136-43.

Stein, L.I. and Diamond, R. (1985) A programme for difficult to treat patients, *New Directions in Mental Health Services*, 26, 29-39.

Stoudemire, A., Hill, C.D., Morris, R. and Markwalter, H. (1991) The medical-psychiatric unit as a site for outcome research in dementia/depression syndromes, *Psychiatric Medicine*, 9, 4, 535-44.

Torian, L., Davidson, E., Fulop, G., Sell, L. and Fillitt, H. (1992) The effect of dementia on acute care in a general medical unit, *International Psychogeriatrics*, 4, 2, 231-9.

Walsh, A.C. (1991) The psycho-chemical treatment of dementia: a very cost-effective therapy programme, *Medical Hypotheses*, 34, 1, 66-8.

Weisbrod, B.A. and Schlesinger, M. (1986) Public, private, nonprofit ownership and the response to asymmetric information: the case of nursing homes, in S. Rose-Ackerman (ed.) *The Economics of Nonprofit Institutions: Studies in Structure and Policy*, Oxford University Press, New York.

Williams, A. (1974) The cost benefit approach, *British Medical Bulletin*, 30, 252-6.

Name Index

Addington, D.E., 235, 239
Allen, C., 77, 80
an der Haden, W., 30, 35, 37, 56
Anderson, J., 117, 123
Arie, T., 171-172
Askham, J., 141, 152-153
Attkisson, C.C., 66, 80, 89, 100
Audini, B., 89-90, 100
Audit Commission, 6, 8, 14, 23, 192
Backhouse, M.E., 40, 54, 232, 239
Bailey, V., 12, 25, 232, 240
Baumol, W., 227-228
Bebbington, A.C., 15, 23, 34, 42, 54, 67, 69, 80, 171-172
Bebbington, P.E., 27, 57, 209-210, 214
Beecham, J.K., 15, 20, 24-25, 63, 73, 80-81, 91, 97, 100, 111, 113, 117-119, 123, 152-153, 161, 171-172, 186, 189, 192-193, 202, 206, 232, 234, 239
Bergmann, K., 131, 153
Bertsch, E.F., 237, 239
Bigelow, D.A., 236, 240
Birch, S., 48, 54
Bloor, K., 28, 58
Bond, J., 142-143, 153
Bosanquet, N., 21, 23
Bowling, A., 212, 214
Bowman, F.M., 12, 23
Bradley, V.J., 187, 192
Brayne, C., 126, 153
Brazier, J.G., 42, 54
Briggs, A., 52, 54, 212, 214
Brodaty, H., 130, 139, 153, 233, 240
Bromwich, M., 72, 80
Brugha, T., 64, 80
Buckwalter, K.C., 232, 240
Burns, T., 21, 23, 27, 31, 54, 85, 100, 159, 172, 232-233, 240
Butler, J., 77, 80
Buxton, M., 40, 54
Cairns, J., 50, 54-55
Calloway, P., 126, 153
Calnan, M., 77, 80
Cambridge, P., 62, 80
Cantril, H., 185, 192
Casmas, S.T., 97, 100
Catalan, J., 37, 55
Central Statistical Office, 134, 153
Challis, D.J., 68, 80, 134, 141, 151, 153, 159, 172, 187, 193, 234, 236, 240
Chisholm, D., 13, 23
Clark, M., 126, 153
Clement, J.P., 234, 241
Clip, E.C., 232, 241
Commonwealth of Australia, 28, 55
Conroy, J.W., 187, 192
Conway, A.S., 11, 23, 177, 188, 192
Cooper, H., 210, 214
Cottrell, D., 232, 240
Culyer, A.J., 34, 49, 55
Darton, R.A., 68, 80, 130-131, 135, 144, 147, 150, 152-154
Davidge, M., 103, 123
Davies, B.P., 15-16, 23, 34, 54, 68, 80, 134, 141, 151, 153-154, 187, 193, 234, 236, 240

Davies, L.M., 20, 24, 27, 33, 39, 55, 232, 240
Dean, C., 159, 172
Department of Employment, 144, 154
Department of Health, 5, 8, 11, 24, 27-29, 53, 55, 61, 71, 74-75, 81, 135-136, 151, 154, 157-158, 172-173, 176, 188, 193, 207, 211, 214
Department of Health and Social Security (see also Department of Health), 77, 81, 154
Derbyshire, M., 81
Diamond, R., 235, 241
Dick, P., 159, 173
Dobbs, J., 79, 81
Donabedian, A., 30, 55
Donaldson, C., 14, 24, 42, 48, 55, 139, 142-143, 153-154, 232, 240
Donker, M., 89, 101
Donnelly, M., 27, 32, 55, 62, 81, 175, 187, 193
Drummond, M.F., 8, 20, 24, 27, 30-31, 33, 39, 42-44, 53, 55, 139, 154, 232, 240
Dunn, M., 100
Dunnel, K., 79, 81
Eichelman, B., 11, 24
Elliott, R.L., 11, 25
Ellis, R.E., 187, 193
Endicott, J., 89, 100
Fadden, G.B., 41, 55
Feinstein, C.H., 216, 228
Fenn, P., 10, 24
Fenton, F., 159, 173
Feragne, M.A., 185, 187, 193
Folstein, M.F., 46, 55
Forder, J., 28, 56
Frank, E., 41, 56
Frank, R.G., 236, 240
Freemantle, N., 30, 56-57, 210, 214
Freer, C.B., 152, 154
Fries, B.E., 235, 240
Gadd, E., 159, 172
Gafni, A., 42, 48, 54, 58
Garralda, M.E., 12, 23
Gerard, K., 14, 24, 48, 56
Gilleard, C.J., 129, 154
Ginsberg, G., 47, 56
Glass, G.V., 210, 214
Glennerster, H., 27, 57
Goldacre, M., 11, 24
Goldberg, D.P., 27, 32, 56
Gorham, D.R., 37, 58, 89, 101
Grad, J., 33, 37, 56
Granzini, L., 64, 81
Gray, A., 10, 24
Greene, J.G., 130, 142, 154
Gregson, B., 139, 154, 232, 240
Gresham, M., 139, 153
Grobe-Einsler, R., 232, 240
Gurland, B., 126, 154
H.M. Treasury, 72, 81
Hadzi-Pavlovic, D., 130, 153
Häfner, H., 30, 35, 37, 56
Hallam, A., 105, 113, 123
Harrington, R., 13, 24
Hartwig, A., 11
Hatziandreu, E.J., 33, 41, 47-48, 53, 56
Haycox, A., 68, 81
Heald, D., 221, 228
Healy, D., 11, 24, 235, 240
Hedges, L.V., 210, 214
Henderson, S., 185, 193
Hofman, A., 126-127, 129, 155
Hoult, J., 89, 100, 159, 173
House of Commons Social Services Select Committee, 217, 228
Hutton, J., 27, 58
Huxley, P., 236, 240
Hyde, C., 46, 56
Intagliata, J., 235, 240
Jablensky, A., 46, 56
Jackson, C.A., 236, 240
Jackson, G., 27, 31, 56
Jenkins, R., 64, 81
Johnson, D.A.W., 28, 56
Jolley, D., 171-172
Jones, D., 105, 123
Jones, R., 32, 46-47, 56, 68, 81
Jönsson, B., 27, 30, 57, 209-210, 214
Kamlet, M.S., 41, 57
Kavanagh, S., 11, 18, 24, 33, 57, 64, 81, 150, 155, 189, 192-193, 204, 206, 233-234, 240
Kazadin, A.E., 12, 24
Kind, P., 42, 59
King, M., 181, 193
Kirk, J., 66, 81
Kitwood, T., 129, 155

Knapp, M.R.J., 1, 15-16, 19-20, 23-25, 27, 32-34, 47, 53, 57, 61-62, 68, 73, 80-81, 89-90, 92, 97, 100, 105-106, 111, 114-116, 122-124, 134-135, 142-143, 152-153, 155, 175, 177-179, 184, 186, 189, 191, 193, 195, 206
Korman, N., 27, 57
Kramer, S., 30, 58
Krawiecka, M., 46, 57
Kuipers, L., 41, 57
Laing and Buisson, 135, 141, 155
Larsen, D.H., 66, 82, 89, 101
Leff, J., 62, 82, 104, 114, 118, 121, 124, 179, 193, 233, 240
Lemmens, F., 89, 101
Levin, E., 139, 155
Light, D., 12, 25, 232, 240
Livingston, G., 126, 155
Loomes, G., 40, 57
Lukoff, D., 89, 101
Maas, M.L., 232, 240
MacDonald, A.J.D., 155
Madge, N., 13, 25
Mangen, S.P., 37-39, 58, 68, 82
Marglin, S., 49, 58
Marks, I.M., 62, 82, 89, 93, 101, 159, 173
Martin, J., 128, 145, 155
Maule, M.M., 126, 155
Mausner, J.S., 30, 58
Maynard, A., 18, 25, 27-28, 30, 56-58, 210, 214
Mayston, D., 72, 82
McCrone, P., 11, 25, 27, 38-39, 57, 62, 82, 87, 101, 201, 206, 233, 240
McCue, M.J., 234, 241
McFarland, B.H., 236, 240
McGuire, A., 14, 19, 25, 43-44, 49, 57
McGuire, T.G., 52-53, 57
McKechnie, A.A., 97, 101
McKenzie, L., 40, 57
Mechanic, D., 236, 241
Mehrez, A., 42, 58
Melzer, D., 11, 25, 62, 82, 136, 139, 150, 155, 177, 193, 202, 206, 237, 241
Mercer, A.D., 97, 101
Merson, S., 233, 241
Miller, M.L., 66, 81
Mishan, E.J., 45, 47, 49, 58
Mohide, E.A., 42, 58
Mooney, G., 34, 48, 55-56, 58
Moore, M.J., 232, 241
Morgenstern, O., 40, 59
Moriarty, J., 139, 155
Muijen, M., 38-39, 58, 86-87, 101, 159, 173, 200, 206
Murray, C., 42, 50, 58
Netten, A., 10, 19, 25, 134-135, 142, 155-156, 161-162, 173
Neuberger, H., 50, 59
Nord, E., 40, 48, 52, 58
North, C., 160, 173, 234, 236, 241
O'Connor, D.W., 141, 152, 156, 233, 241
O'Connor, J., 221, 228
O'Driscoll, C., 104, 114, 118, 124
Ochs, M., 232, 241
Office of Population Censuses and Surveys, 10, 25, 125-131, 134-136, 139, 145-147, 150-151, 155-156
Oliver, J.P.J., 43, 58
Olsen, J.A., 50, 58
Ontario Ministry of Health, 27-28, 58
Opit, L.J., 33, 58
Overall, J.E., 37, 58, 89, 101
Parsonage, M., 50, 59
Paykel, E.S., 37-38, 59-60
Pelonero, A.L., 11, 25
Pereira, J., 34, 59
Peters, K.E., 233, 240
Phanjoo, A.L., 143, 156
Pigou, A.C., 49, 59
Pitt, B., 131, 156
Pocock, S.J., 30, 59
Pudney, M., 64, 82
Raftery, J., 215, 228
Raskin, A., 37, 59
Reddy, S., 131, 156
Regier, D.A., 13, 25
Renshaw, J., 62, 82, 177, 187, 194
Revicki, D.A., 38-39, 59
Ritchie, J., 11, 25, 160, 173, 236, 241
Robertson, E., 61, 81
Robins, L.N., 12-13, 25
Rosser, R., 18-19, 25-26, 42-43, 59
Rosser, R.M., 212, 214
Rossi, G.F., 235, 241
Royal College of Psychiatrists, 173

Rutter, M., 12-13, 25
Sainsbury, P., 33, 37, 56
Sartorius, N., 42, 59
Schlesinger, M., 234, 241
Schneider, J., 150, 156, 159, 173, 196, 206
Scull, A.T., 221-222, 228
Secretaries of State, 5, 25, 26, 66, 82, 112, 124, 136, 156-159, 173
Sederer, L., 236, 241
Selai, C., 18-19, 26
Sen, A., 49, 59
Sheldon, T., 49-50, 52, 59
Shiell, A., 91, 101
Silfvenius, H., 235, 241
Smart, S., 161, 173
Spitzer, R.L., 176, 194
Stanton, K.A., 221, 223, 227-228
Stason, W.B., 36, 59
Statistical Information Service, 161-162, 173
Stein, L.I., 45, 59, 89, 101, 159, 173, 235, 241
Stern, B., 97, 101
Stern, E.S., 97, 101
Stewart, A., 207, 209, 214
Stoudemire, A., 232, 241
Sugden, R., 49, 59
Taylor, R., 130, 156
Test, M., 45, 59, 89, 101, 159, 173
Thompson, C., 28, 59, 141, 152-153
Thompson, C.M., 28, 59
Thompson, D., 64, 82
Thornton, J.G., 32, 59, 209, 214
Torian, L., 235, 241
Torrance, G.W., 40, 59
Turner, M.A., 143, 156
Twigg, J., 41, 59
van Os, J., 87-88, 101
von Abendorff, R., 162, 173
von Neumann, J., 40, 59
Wagstaff, A., 34, 55
Walker, S.R., 212, 214
Walsh, A.C., 233, 241
Weinstein, M.C., 36, 59
Weisbrod, B.A., 4, 26-27, 45-46, 52, 59-61, 82, 85, 101, 234, 241
Weissman, M.M., 37, 60, 89, 101
White, E., 38, 60
Wilkin, D., 42, 60
Wilkinson, G., 42, 60
Williams, A., 34, 49, 59-60, 231, 241
Williams, R., 12, 26
Wimo, A., 41-42, 60
Wing, J.K., 37, 60, 89, 102, 181, 194
Wistow, G., 26, 113, 124, 144, 156
Woods, J.P., 143, 156
Wooff, K., 38, 60
World Bank, 42, 60
World Health Organization, 157, 174, 181-182, 186, 194
Wright, K.G., 68, 81-82, 130-131, 152-154
Wykes, T., 46, 60
Zajdler, A., 21, 23
Zwick, R., 66, 80, 89, 100

Subject Index

accommodation, 62-65, 72, 74-75, 78-79, 86, 88-89, 103, 106-115, 117-119, 121-122, 128, 130-131, 134, 136, 138-139, 141, 143-144, 146, 160-171, 179, 188-189, 191-192, 197-198, 200-203, 204, 226, 230
accountability, 6, 9, 159, 235
accounting cost, 34, 73
acute care, 233
adaptation, 65
adolescence (psychiatric problems in), 10, 12-13, 232
adult foster placement, 107, 200
adverse event, 213
affective disorder, 13, 105, 116, 164-165, 198
after-care, 158-159
ageing, 9-11, 95, 125, 224
allocation criteria, 4, 16, 22
American Psychiatric Association, 126, 153
annuity, 72
anticoagulant therapy, 233
anxiety, 11, 19, 35, 118
appointment, 63, 65, 70, 77-79, 157, 161, 167
assessment (of need), 5, 37, 48, 54, 89, 92, 104, 117, 122, 151, 157, 160, 163, 185-186
asylum, 1-2, 99, 159, 218, 222, 227
Australia, 8, 27-28, 159
average cost, 29, 34-35, 67, 77, 91, 95, 97-98, 111, 115, 119, 161, 169, 212, 218, 220
balance of care, 8, 22, 126, 130, 134, 136, 139, 144-147, 150, 234
balance of provision, 5, 10, 95, 126, 145
behaviour, 11-14, 43, 83-84, 87, 95, 104, 106, 114, 117, 121, 129, 176, 180-183, 185-188, 230
blinding, 32
blunting of affect, 118-119
budget, 6, 8, 13, 15, 33-34, 48, 54, 63, 65, 68, 71, 74, 97-99, 107, 109, 113, 125, 142, 171-172, 190, 199-200, 205, 213, 217, 226, 236-237
budgetary devolution, 236
building, 2, 44, 52, 67-73, 75-76, 78, 151
building-block approach, 69, 75
Bulger, James, 12
burden of illness, 8
capital, 17, 29, 34, 44-45, 49, 53, 67, 71-72, 76, 103, 136, 139, 152, 161, 163, 190, 197, 215-216, 220, 237
capital charging, 72
capital cost, 46, 52, 72, 75-76, 98, 139, 151, 161
capital value, 161
capitated budget, 236
Care in the Community demonstration programme, 61, 142, 152, 177

care management, 5, 8, 11, 87-88, 109, 141, 159-160, 191, 196, 199, 202, 205, 233, 235-237
care package, 19, 21, 33, 61, 65-66, 68, 77-79, 104, 106, 109, 111-113, 115, 119-122, 136-138, 139-140, 144, 158, 160, 171-172, 183-184, 186-187, 190, 196-199, 201-203, 204-205, 211-212, 226, 236
care programme, 5, 8, 11, 45, 47, 109, 157-161, 163-164, 168, 170-172, 176, 190-191, 195-196, 199, 202, 231, 236-237
care responsibilities, 64
caregiver, 42, 230
Caregiver Quality of Life Instrument (CQLI), 42
carer, 5, 9-10, 17-18, 20, 33-34, 41-43, 46, 49, 62, 64-67, 84, 122, 125-126, 130-131, 136, 139, 141-142, 144, 158, 162, 179, 183, 190-191, 232-233, 235
carer training, 233
Caring for People, 5, 157-159, 199
case management, 62, 88, 160, 200, 235, 237
case register, 232
Chartered Institute for Public Finance and Accountancy, 73
child psychiatry, 12-13, 232, 238
childhood (psychiatric problems in), 10, 12-13, 232
Children Act, 160
chiropody, 75, 110, 121-122, 135, 167, 178
choice, 5, 10, 13, 15, 21, 28, 30, 32, 40, 62, 69-70, 72-73, 75, 202, 209, 237-238
Claybury Hospital, 105
client, 35, 53, 61-79, 84, 86-87, 92, 105-122, 136-137, 139-143, 160, 162, 169-170, 185-188, 190, 200, 202, 204, 236-237
client characteristics, 12, 17-18, 21-22, 84, 89, 91-97, 104-106, 111, 114-117, 119, 164, 170, 176, 181, 183-189, 199-200, 230, 235
Client Service Receipt Interview (CSRI), 61-64, 66, 78, 89, 92, 106, 110, 112, 122, 160, 176-177, 188, 197, 200
clothes, 163, 182
clozapine, 11, 20, 33, 38-39, 235
Clunis, Christopher, 159
cognitive therapy, 30, 52
cohort, 32, 38, 41, 110, 112, 118, 198-199, 203
commissioner, 49, 171
community care, 4-6, 9, 21-22, 28, 32, 35, 41, 61-64, 66-67, 76, 78-79, 88, 95, 97, 103-104, 107, 109, 111-115, 117, 119, 121-122, 125, 131, 136, 139, 144, 157-158, 166, 175-176, 179, 184-191, 195, 197, 199, 233-234, 237
community charge, 164-165, 170
community mental health worker, 162
community placement, 95, 105, 111, 119, 187
community psychiatric nurse, 37, 65, 86, 135, 166-167, 197, 200, 233
community support team, 86, 202, 233
comparator, 28-29, 37-38, 42, 52
comprehensive cost, 21, 43, 61, 79, 104, 111, 166, 170, 184, 189, 196, 204, 233
comprehensiveness, 20-21, 63, 104
conduct disorder, 12
confidence interval, 29, 169
consortium arrangement, 108, 113
consumption cost, 75
contract, 10, 143, 195, 236
coordination, 6, 189, 191-192
cost function, 48, 86, 91-92, 97-98, 118-119, 135, 152, 190
cost information, 4, 6, 8, 14, 20, 69, 71, 103, 111, 135, 157, 168, 171-172, 195, 205
cost minimisation, 19
cost variation, 21, 84, 88, 91-92, 97, 114, 119, 179, 184, 196, 211, 238
cost-benefit analysis, 19-20, 29, 35, 43-45, 50
cost-effectiveness, 3-6, 8, 10, 14, 19, 33, 36-39, 41, 46-47, 52, 89, 126, 136, 207, 211-212, 226, 229, 232-234, 236-237
cost-effectiveness analysis, 19, 29, 35-37, 39-40, 47, 52, 211
cost-outcome link, 20, 22, 104
cost-raising factor, 73, 106
cost-utility analysis, 19-20, 29, 35, 40-42, 47, 212

costing, 52, 61, 66-73, 75-79, 112, 134-135, 139, 144, 157, 161-163, 171-172, 175, 196, 199, 201-202, 204-205, 215, 226
council tax, 73
counselling, 30
crime, 12
criminal justice, 33, 178-179
data collection, 106, 196, 238
day care, 41, 65-67, 69-70, 73, 78, 109-110, 115, 122, 135, 143, 161, 167, 178, 198, 201-203, 217
day centre, 65, 143, 161, 166-167, 170, 201
day hospital, 143, 167
day nursery, 162
de-institutionalisation, 27, 32
decision analysis, 32, 209-213
decision tree, 207, 209, 211-213
decision-making, 84, 209, 213, 231, 236, 238-239
delphic panel, 33, 39, 41
delusion, 92-93, 116-119, 180-181, 187
demand, 4-6, 8-11, 14, 72, 122, 144, 158, 168, 171, 195, 205
dementia, 10, 13, 41-42, 104, 125-127, 129, 141, 147, 152, 164-165, 230, 232-235
demographic change, 9-10
dentist, 63, 110, 161, 167, 169, 178
Department of Health, 177
depreciation, 52-53, 67
depression, 13, 33, 37, 41, 47, 129, 207, 210
diagnosis, 37, 92, 104-105, 115-117, 126, 164-166, 176-177, 185
diagnostic fallibility, 238
diagnostic group, 13, 18, 116, 184, 198, 230
direct cost, 19, 84, 135, 226, 235
disability adjusted life year (DALY), 42
discharge from hospital, 86, 117, 163, 186
discharge practice, 105, 120
domestic accommodation, 64, 72
domiciliary assessment, 171
domiciliary care, 234
domiciliary visit, 79, 161, 167-168, 171
dose level, 28, 30
dowry, 108
drugs, 4, 9, 11, 14-15, 19, 21, 28, 30, 37-38, 63, 77, 86-87, 103, 118, 122, 129, 175-176, 188, 207, 210-211, 213, 229-230, 232, 234-235, 237-238
DSS allowance, 135
early intervention, 13, 141, 232-233, 238
econometric analysis, 238
economic analysis, 49, 209-210, 239
economic evaluation, 1, 3-4, 6, 8-10, 13-14, 16, 18-20, 22-23, 27, 29-33, 35, 37, 40, 43, 53-54, 61, 85-87, 89, 99, 104, 207, 209-210, 212, 226, 229-234, 237-239
economic theory, 66-67, 91, 111, 209, 226
economics perspective, 6, 8, 229
economy, 14, 21, 29, 33, 49, 95, 220-221
education, 14, 33, 71, 110, 115, 178, 198, 201, 232
effectiveness, 1, 6, 8, 14-15, 17, 30, 32, 36-37, 40-41, 64, 83, 126, 136, 142-144, 160, 212, 230-231, 236-237
efficacy, 8, 11, 28, 33, 83, 212-213, 232, 235
efficiency, 3-4, 6, 9, 12, 14-15, 17, 21-22, 34, 48, 84, 172, 176, 188-189, 192, 218, 231-232, 235
elderly people, 10, 16, 18, 41-42, 104, 126, 129-130, 134-136, 138-144, 146, 160, 171, 233-236
employment, 14, 35, 46-47, 64, 68, 79, 84, 89, 91, 115, 144-145, 164, 166, 201, 230, 235, 238
epilepsy, 234-235
equity, 4, 9, 14-15, 17, 21-22, 29, 33-34, 45, 143, 152, 172, 176, 183, 188-189, 192, 231
evaluation, 3-4, 17-22, 28, 30, 32, 36-38, 43-45, 47, 53, 85-92, 96, 105, 117, 139, 141, 144, 151, 168, 177, 179, 195-197, 200, 202-203, 207, 209-212, 226, 229-233, 236-239
evaluative trial, 21, 28-30, 209, 212-213, 232
expected cost, 187, 207, 209-212

expenditure account, 70-71, 73-74, 76, 106, 227
face-to-face contact, 65, 79, 162
facility-based service, 70-73, 75-78
Family Expenditure Survey, 75, 134
family health service authorities, 113, 137, 140, 169
fees, 77, 113, 161
final outcome, 17
food, 69, 71, 74, 134, 163, 218
for-profit provider, 234
foster care, 108
fuel, 125, 163
funding, 95, 113, 122, 125, 135, 137, 144, 152, 212, 227, 229-230
general hospital, 120, 167, 234
general practitioner, 21, 47, 63, 65-66, 77, 109-110, 134, 143, 161, 178, 188, 198, 201, 205
grant, 67, 113, 164, 190
group home, 62-63, 107-108, 163, 200
group worker, 162
guidelines, 27-30, 33-35, 47-49, 53, 66, 158, 207, 211
hallucination, 93, 116, 118, 180-181, 187
health authority, 6, 8, 12, 65, 67, 69, 74, 95, 97, 103, 106-108, 114, 118-119, 121-122, 136, 141-142, 150, 152, 159, 168-170, 199
health care, 1, 3-6, 9, 11-13, 15, 17-19, 21, 23, 27-28, 30-31, 34, 36, 40, 43, 45, 47-48, 53-54, 183, 189, 191-192
health gain, 8, 12, 115, 232
Health of the Nation, 5, 176, 188
health state, 40-42
healthy year equivalent, 42
hidden cost, 19, 69-70, 73
historical control, 32
home help, 65, 70, 75, 135, 167-168, 170, 201
home-based care, 88
homelessness, 159
hospital closure, 11, 205
hospital leaver, 104-105, 109
hospital-based care, 31, 86, 89, 108
hostel, 46, 63, 74, 107-108, 145, 163, 167, 200
'hotel' service, 122, 136
household, 10, 63-64, 73-75, 84, 107, 126, 128, 130-131, 134-138, 139-140, 142, 145, 150-151, 164
housing, 11, 33, 73, 84, 103, 107-108, 112-114, 134, 151, 162-163, 165, 170, 179, 187, 190, 195-196, 226
housing association, 73, 106, 113-114, 121, 163, 165, 170
Housing Association Group, 163
housing benefit, 63, 114, 170
housing subsidy, 170
income, 45, 49-50, 62, 64, 73-75, 77, 79, 89, 106, 108, 113, 122, 164-165, 179
incontinence, 119, 131, 162, 167
incremental analysis, 29, 47
independent accommodation, 107, 112
independent sector, 130-131, 234
indirect cost, 29, 69, 84, 235, 238
inflation, 68, 72, 95, 111
informal care, 10, 19, 34, 42-43, 66-67, 93, 107, 130, 134, 136, 139-141, 159, 162, 166-170, 236, 238
innovation, 5, 48, 205
inpatient, 19, 33, 35-36, 38, 46, 64, 68, 74, 88-89, 93, 95-99, 104-107, 109-112, 114-115, 117, 119-122, 135-136, 141-142, 159, 162, 166-170, 178, 197-199, 201-203, 204, 215-217, 219-220, 222, 224, 226-227, 230, 232-236
Institute of Psychiatry, 21
institution, 2, 4, 41, 103, 112, 115, 126, 130-131, 134, 139-141, 216, 218-219, 222, 232
inter-personal variation, 235
intermediate outcome, 17, 30
internal market, 5, 12, 113, 171
intervention, 8, 12-13, 17-18, 21-23, 27-28, 30-34, 36-37, 39, 41, 43-45, 47-53, 84-85, 176, 196, 207, 213, 230, 232-233, 238
keyworker, 8, 88, 157, 160, 164-165, 187, 196, 205
Lancashire Quality of Life Instrument, 43
laundry, 136, 162, 167
learning disabilities, 62, 91, 116, 129, 187-188, 198
legal aid, 162, 170

legal service, 162
like-with-like comparison, 20, 22, 86, 94, 97, 176, 188
line budget, 6
living expenses, 64, 73-74, 134, 198, 202-203
local authority, 1, 10, 13, 19, 38, 71, 73-75, 79, 103, 107-109, 113-114, 119, 125, 130-131, 135, 137-138, 140-144, 147, 152, 159, 161-163, 167-171, 178, 190-191, 202-203, 204, 217, 227
local government, 5
long-stay, 21, 32, 46, 62-64, 66, 72, 98, 107, 113-114, 117, 119, 121-122, 125, 136-138, 140-141, 143, 152, 175-179, 182-183, 187, 189-190, 192, 197, 224, 226
long-term cost, 119
longitudinal design, 63
management cost, 70
managing agency, 161
marginal analysis, 47-48
marginal cost, 18, 22, 29, 34-36, 67-69, 75, 97-98, 197, 230
marginal opportunity cost, 19, 67, 111, 134, 176
market economy, 67
markets, 5-6, 8, 14, 17, 27, 34, 43, 49, 64, 67, 72, 91, 151, 163, 171, 207, 211, 236
matched design, 22
Mental Health Act 1983, 159
Mental Illness Specific Grant, 158, 160, 190, 227
meta-analysis, 29-31, 126, 210, 213, 232
methodology, 99, 105, 111, 135, 158, 160-161, 196, 205, 213, 239
mixed economy, 5-6, 21, 109, 113, 144, 171, 234
mobility, 119, 235
monitoring, 104, 122, 157-158, 160, 171
Monte Carlo analysis, 52
multi-agency assessment, 236
multivariate analysis, 91-92, 99
National Health Service and Community Care Act 1990, 6, 113, 122, 190
National Health Service reform, 4-5, 8, 12, 54, 113, 160
needs, 5-6, 9-10, 15, 21-23, 48, 62, 83-84, 88, 92, 104-106, 109, 111-112, 115, 117, 119, 122, 142-143, 157-159, 168, 171, 176-177, 183-184, 186-187, 189-191, 199-200, 205, 229-230, 234, 236, 238-239
neuroleptic, 21, 33, 38-39
neurosis, 105, 116, 165
non-resource input, 17, 160, 168
nurse, 4, 47, 75, 79, 88, 135, 167-168, 178, 215, 221-224, 227-228, 232
nursing home, 63, 72, 75, 107, 112, 125, 128, 130-131, 135, 137-138, 140-142, 144, 147, 152, 190, 200, 233-235
occupational therapy, 65, 110, 201
Ontario, 8, 27-28
opportunity cost, 29, 34, 67-68, 72, 134, 151, 162, 195
optician, 110, 169, 178
outcome, 4, 10, 13, 15, 17-23, 28-33, 35-39, 43, 46-50, 52-54, 67, 83-85, 87-91, 111, 115, 117, 119, 121, 139, 142-143, 160, 168, 175, 186-187, 189, 200, 207, 209, 211-213, 230, 233-239
outpatient, 21, 37-38, 65, 68, 74, 78, 110, 167, 170, 178, 188, 198, 201, 203
output, 8, 17, 35, 45, 91, 151-152, 211-212, 222, 237
overhead, 76
performance review, 3, 6, 14
peripatetic service, 70, 75-77
personal aid, 65
personal expenditure, 70, 74, 139, 160, 162-165, 168, 170
personality disorder, 37, 116, 165
pharmaceutical, 8, 10-11, 27-30, 163, 207, 232
pharmacotherapy, 210
physical disability, 13, 34, 39-40, 42-43, 62, 128-129, 131, 145, 150, 165
physiotherapy, 110, 167
placebo, 28
planning, 5-6, 8, 28, 51, 76, 114, 159, 172, 190-191, 195, 213, 233
police, 46, 84, 106, 110, 169-170, 175, 178-179, 201, 226
prediction equation, 92-93, 96, 114-115, 184-187

prescribing, 28, 30, 207, 211, 213
prevention, 232, 238
price, 1, 8, 10, 17, 34, 37, 43, 61, 66-68, 91, 93, 96, 98, 111-112, 134, 136, 139, 141, 151-152, 163, 165, 171, 179, 195, 210, 213, 215-216, 218, 220-222, 228, 237
price index, 71, 151-152, 161, 163, 221, 227-228
principles for cost research, 19-20, 43, 66-68, 86, 99, 111, 159, 191, 196, 229
PRiSM, 21
private hospital, 234
private sector, 1, 72, 108, 113-114, 118, 218
privately-rented accommodation, 72, 161
process, 5, 8, 17, 20, 27, 30-32, 37, 43, 61, 69, 78-79, 89, 91, 99, 131, 144, 161, 172, 199, 210-212, 235, 237
production of welfare, 16-18, 30, 84, 91, 160, 168, 239
programme budgeting, 48
prompt card, 62
provider, 83-84, 91, 158, 168, 171-172, 207, 231-232, 234, 236
PSSRU, 85, 104, 107, 151, 161-162, 234
psychiatric hospital, 91, 95, 97, 105, 107, 115, 158, 167, 177, 187, 197, 234
psychiatric morbidity, 18, 87
psychiatric reprovision, 104, 119, 177, 197, 199, 202
psychiatry, 86, 88, 97, 104, 106, 109, 122, 157, 158, 168, 171, 176, 178, 188, 202, 205, 215-217, 226, 232, 236, 238
psychology, 4, 12, 14, 33, 110, 122, 167, 171, 178, 201, 232, 236-238
public expenditure, 9, 113, 216
public policy, 72, 77
public safety, 159
public scandal, 158
public sector, 5-6, 14, 27, 37, 47, 49, 52-53, 72-73, 107-108, 113, 145, 226, 234
purchaser, 1, 5-6, 8, 10, 12-13, 54, 76, 104-105, 205, 231
quality adjusted life year (QALY), 4, 13-14, 18, 20, 39-42, 48, 50-51, 53
quality adjustment factor, 40
quality assurance, 6
quality of life, 8, 14, 17-19, 28-29, 33, 35, 40-43, 45, 83, 141-142, 175-176, 191, 212, 230-231, 237
questionnaire, 42, 61-63, 65, 118, 145
radiography, 163
randomised controlled trial, 21-22, 30-32, 37, 41-42, 84-86, 89-90, 96-97, 210
rate of return, 72
ratings scale, 40
rationing, 15
re-admission to hospital, 19, 36-37, 64, 78, 104, 106, 109-111, 178, 191
reduced-list, 21, 196-200, 202, 204-205
regional weighting, 68, 76
reimbursement, 27, 77, 236
relatives, 9-10, 19, 35, 93, 118, 134, 142, 170, 179
rent, 2, 63, 72-73, 107-109, 113, 161-163
research instrumentation, 13-14, 18, 21, 42-43, 46, 61-62, 92, 117-118, 176, 181-182, 191, 197, 237
residential care, 5, 63, 68, 73-75, 108, 121, 125, 128, 130, 136-138, 140, 142-143, 151, 200
resource, 3-6, 8-15, 17-19, 21, 23, 29, 34-35, 37, 43, 45, 48-49, 53-54, 64, 66-68, 70-73, 77, 83-84, 91, 99, 103, 106, 110, 112, 115, 119, 126, 142-145, 152, 158, 166, 171, 205, 211-212, 232, 239
resource implication, 8, 19, 34, 67, 74, 76
resource input, 17, 30, 73, 160
respite care, 33, 135, 137-138, 139-140, 142, 167, 169, 232
retirement pension, 164
revenue, 44, 46, 67, 69, 71-76, 97-99, 103, 107, 151-152, 161, 163, 215
risperidone, 235
Rosser index, 42
salary, 67, 70-71, 75-76, 78
scarcity, 9-12, 14-15, 68, 110, 195
schizophrenia, 10-11, 13, 21, 32-33, 35, 37-38, 46, 105, 116, 129, 164-166, 176-177, 188-189, 198, 202-203, 234-235
Secretaries of State, 199, 206

Section 117, 159
sectoral efficiency, 234
selective serotonin reuptake inhibitor (SSRI), 21, 48, 209-210
self-care, 14, 18, 129, 131, 134, 182, 186
service availability, 66, 84
service component, 111
Service Entry and Numeration (SEAN), 78
service planner, 67, 114, 171
service receipt, 61, 64, 78-79, 87, 104, 106, 112, 134, 160, 162, 164-165, 167-168, 171, 176-179, 188, 200, 238
service unit, 67, 70, 74
service user, 5-6, 8, 10, 13, 15, 17-23, 32, 34, 37, 49, 77, 83-84, 87-88, 90-92, 94-95, 97, 104, 113-114, 120, 143, 158-160, 162, 164, 166-170, 183-184, 186-187, 190-191, 196, 204-205, 229-231, 233-237
service utilisation, 21, 31, 35, 37-38, 61-63, 65, 110, 126, 134, 139, 179, 187, 189, 197, 200, 205, 230, 238
sheltered housing, 108, 200
Silcock, Ben, 11, 159
social network, 18, 105, 114-115, 117-119, 121, 184, 187
social security, 62, 64, 75, 108, 113, 125, 131, 142, 163-164, 170, 195, 226
social services, 104, 108-110, 112, 136, 151, 158-160, 165, 170-171, 190, 195, 201-202, 239
social worker, 88, 109-110, 120, 161, 167, 188, 232, 236
socio-cultural variable, 238
specialist, 86, 88, 139, 142, 157, 163, 167-168, 212, 234
specialty, 136, 152
Spokes Inquiry, 158
staffing, 17-18, 30, 44, 62, 64-65, 69-71, 73, 75-79, 84, 86, 99, 106-111, 115-117, 122, 134, 144-145, 162-163, 165, 168, 179, 181, 183, 187, 190, 197, 200, 220, 227, 235-237
statistical significance, 92, 98, 119, 168
structure, 122, 159, 209, 211, 231, 237, 239
study population, 104, 108, 113
substance abuse, 164
suicide, 230
supervision register, 176
support network, 161
surgery, 163, 220, 234-235
symptom, 83-84, 89, 93, 117, 119, 121, 129, 176, 181-182, 184, 186-187, 191-192, 230, 235
target efficiency, 15, 34, 184
targeting, 171, 183-184, 189, 235-236
Team for the Assessment of Psychiatric Services (TAPS), 62, 104, 114, 119
technique, 90, 92, 184, 207, 209, 212, 237-238
transfer payment, 197, 226
tricyclic antidepressant, 47-48, 209-210
uncertainty, 29, 49, 51-52, 160, 209, 212, 238
unit cost, 19, 66-67, 71, 75, 77-78, 161, 215, 218-224, 226-227, 238
utility, 18, 40-42, 51, 68, 209, 212
value for money, 3, 6, 12, 14-15
vertical equity, 143, 171, 183-184
voluntary sector, 5, 19, 34, 64, 67, 73, 106-108, 110, 113-114, 118-119, 130-131, 135, 137-138, 141, 143-144, 147, 152, 159, 164, 167, 178, 191, 198, 201
voucher, 237
welfare economics, 43, 48
welfare shortfall, 34
wellbeing, 17-18, 32-33, 39, 49-50, 143, 160, 213, 232
willingness-to-pay, 43, 115, 238
Zito, Jonathan, 11